Integrated Critical Thinking and Clinical Reasoning in Pharmacy Practice

Integrated Critical Thinking and Clinical Reasoning in Pharmacy Practice

W. Cary Mobley, PhD, RPh
Clinical Associate Professor
Department of Pharmaceutics
College of Pharmacy
University of Florida
Gainesville, Florida

Robin Moorman Li, PharmD, BCACP, NBC-HWC
Clinical Associate Professor
Department of Pharmacotherapy and Translational Research
College of Pharmacy
University of Florida
Jacksonville, Florida

New York   Chicago   San Francisco   Athens   London   Madrid   Mexico City
Milan   New Delhi   Singapore   Sydney   Toronto

Integrated Critical Thinking and Clinical Reasoning in Pharmacy Practice

1 2 3 4 5 6 7 8 9   DSS   28 27 26 25 24 23

ISBN 978-1-264-25873-4
MHID 1-264-25873-9

This book was set in Minion Pro by MPS Limited.
The editors were Michael Weitz and Kim J. Davis.
The production supervisor was Richard Ruzycka.
Project management was provided by Poonam Bisht of MPS Limited.
The text designer was Mary McKeon; the cover designer was W2 Design.

Library of Congress Cataloging-in-Publication Data

Names: Mobley, W. Cary, editor. | Li, Robin Moorman, editor.
Title: Integrated critical thinking and clinical reasoning in pharmacy
    practice / [edited by] William Cary Mobley, Robin Moorman Li.
Description: New York : McGraw Hill, [2023] | Includes bibliographical
    references and index. | Summary: "This book explores the clinical
    reasoning of pharmacists in a variety of practices as they engage in
    clinical problem solving, and it explores the roles that critical
    thinking can play in enhancing a pharmacist's reasoning"—Provided by publisher.
Identifiers: LCCN 2022056391 (print) | LCCN 2022056392 (ebook) |
    ISBN 9781264258734 (paperback) | ISBN 9781264258741 (ebook)
Subjects: MESH: Pharmaceutical Services | Clinical Reasoning |
    Patient-Centered Care—methods | Thinking
Classification: LCC RC467.97 (print) | LCC RC467.97 (ebook) |
    NLM QV 737.1 | DDC 362.19689/082—dc23/eng/20230309
LC record available at https://lccn.loc.gov/2022056391
LC ebook record available at https://lccn.loc.gov/2022056392

Contents

Contributors

Lindsey M. Childs-Kean, PharmD, MPH, BCPS
Clinical Associate Professor
University of Florida
College of Pharmacy
Gainesville, Florida

Ericka L. Crouse, PharmD, BCPP, BCGP, FASHP, FASCP
Associate Professor
Virginia Commonwealth University
School of Pharmacy
Richmond, Virginia

Nicole Early, PharmD, BCPS, BCGP, FASCP
Associate Professor
Midwestern University
College of Pharmacy
Glendale, Arizona

Michelle Farland, PharmD, CDCES
Clinical Professor & Division Head
University of Florida
College of Pharmacy
Gainesville, Florida

Carinda Feild, PharmD, FCCM
Clinical Associate Professor
University of Florida
College of Pharmacy
St Petersburg, Florida

Robin Moorman Li, PharmD, BCACP, NBC-HWC
Clinical Associate Professor
Department of Pharmacotherapy and Translational Research
College of Pharmacy
University of Florida
Jacksonville, Florida

W. Cary Mobley, PhD, RPh
Clinical Associate Professor
Department of Pharmaceutics
College of Pharmacy
University of Florida
Gainesville, Florida

Bradley Phillips, PharmD, BCACP
Clinical Assistant Professor
University of Florida
College of Pharmacy
Gainesville, Florida

Elizabeth Pogge, PharmD, MPH, BCPS, BCGP, FASCP
Professor
Midwestern University
College of Pharmacy—Glendale Campus
Glendale, Arizona

Rebecca M. Reiss, PharmD, BCPP
Psychiatric Pharmacist Clinical Specialist
PGY1 Pharmacy Residency Program Director
Denver Health Medical Center
Denver, Colorado

Barbara A. Santevecchi, PharmD, BCPS, BCIDP
Clinical Assistant Professor
University of Florida
College of Pharmacy
Gainesville, Florida

Christine Tabulov, PharmD, BCPPS
Assistant Professor
University of South Florida Health Taneja
College of Pharmacy
Tampa, Florida

Lihui Yuan, PharmD, PhD
Instructional Assistant Professor
University of Florida
College of Pharmacy
Gainesville, Florida

Preface

As a pharmacist, critical decisions that impact patient care occur every day. Applying critical thinking and clinical reasoning skills in an efficient, objective, stepwise approach is imperative to ensure patients receive excellent medical care. Expanding knowledge and understanding of clinical reasoning and common critical thinking skills is just the beginning of growth in this area.

This book explores the clinical reasoning of pharmacists in a variety of practices as they engage in clinical problem-solving through application of the Pharmacists' Patient Care Process (PPCP) to patient cases. It also explores the roles that critical thinking can play in enhancing a pharmacist's reasoning. The general target audience for the book are second- and third-year student pharmacists, with a primary goal of helping them to discover and appreciate how critical thinking, clinical reasoning, and the PPCP can work together to optimize pharmacist-provided patient care and help them develop skills in each of these areas. A secondary goal of the book is to help third-year students prepare to successfully participate in different clinical practices during their Advanced Pharmacy Practice Experiences in their final academic year.

The book begins with an introductory chapter on the PPCP, clinical reasoning, and critical thinking, followed by eight clinical chapters split between four ambulatory care chapters, two inpatient care chapters, and two inpatient/outpatient care chapters. We purposely included a variety of practices to help the reader understand and appreciate the common and unique ways clinical reasoning, critical thinking, and the PPCP can be applied to different cases in different practice settings. The book concludes with an appendix that contains worksheets to help the reader develop critical thinking standards-based questions, apply reasoning and critical thinking in each PPCP step, and identify potential biases and approaches to avoid or mitigate them.

Topics discussed in the introductory chapter include elements of a patient-centered approach to care, the stepwise process of the PPCP, diagnostic and therapeutic (management) reasoning, common inferences and conclusions of each PPCP step, system 1 and system 2 thinking, common biases and how they can impede effective clinical reasoning, and intellectual critical thinking standards and intellectual standards-based questions that can be employed to optimize the pharmacist's reasoning in each step of the PPCP.

The clinical chapters cover ambulatory care in Chronic Pain Management, Geriatric Care Cardiology, Type 2 Diabetes Management, and Warfarin Management and inpatient care in Critical Care—Diabetic Ketoacidosis and Inpatient Psychiatry

Care—Treatment-Resistant Schizophrenia, and inpatient and outpatient care in Pediatric Care—Nephrology Service and Inpatient and Outpatient Infectious Disease Care—Transitions of Care & Outpatient Parenteral Antimicrobial Therapy (OPAT).

Knowing that our target audience would be second- and third-year student pharmacists, we set out to create a writing approach in full recognition of differences in clinical problem-solving between novice students and experienced clinicians. Experienced clinicians, through their many interactions with patients, have a great deal of experience-related knowledge stored in long-term memory. They see patterns in patient data more readily, they have automatized many clinical skills, and are better able to engage the fast and intuitive system 1 thinking described in the introduction chapter. Therefore, for the benefit of the novice students to whom this book is dedicated, we asked each clinician author to engage the reader by first describing their clinical practice and the care provided. Then, with an analytical system 2-like approach, they break down their patient care process, describing the details of their reasoning and critical thinking as they methodically worked through each step of the PPCP in problem-solving a patient case. To help the clinician authors accomplish this, we created a structure for the pain management chapter that would ultimately serve as a template for the remaining clinical chapters. We also created worksheets similar to some of those in the appendices and we worked closely with each author providing guidance, feedback, editing, and other help (eg, concept-mapping) as needed. Prior to their writing the chapters, we recommended that the authors read the introduction chapter to become thoroughly familiar with the concepts and skills we wanted them to impart to their readers.

We hope that in the writing of their chapters, the self-analysis required for these experienced clinicians to break down their patient care process and describe the details of their reasoning and critical thinking was also a process of self-discovery, where they could not only validate their reasoning, but also uncover and correct flaws in their reasoning on a pathway to self-improvement. Thus, by encouraging reasoning and critical thinking skill development in novice student pharmacists and self-analysis in experienced clinicians, it is hoped that this book can achieve its ultimate purpose for which it is dedicated: helping pharmacists provide the best care possible to their patients.

We are very grateful to all of the contributing clinician authors who tirelessly and patiently worked with us in creating their chapters, and who through their writing have allowed the reader to peer into their practice and into their excellent minds. A special thanks go to Michael Weitz, Senior Associate Global Publisher for Medical, Pharmacy & Allied Health Textbooks at McGraw Hill, and Kim Davis, Director, Medical Development at McGraw Hill, and Poonam Bisht, Senior Project Manager at MPS Limited for their enormous patience and guidance. We also thank our pharmacy students who continuously inspire us to improve our craft of teaching. Most importantly, we are each grateful to our families, whose love, support, and patience helped make the writing and editing of this textbook achievable and rewarding. Finally, we thank each other for developing and maintaining a truly synergistic and longstanding working relationship forged from community practice experience and deep interests in epistemology, reasoning, and critical thinking by Cary Mobley with the ambulatory care clinical experience and clinical reasoning acumen of Robin Moorman Li. It is a relationship that has enabled us to develop numerous exercises and programmatic training for our students and has enabled us to create this textbook, which we are grateful to be able to share with the pharmacy academic community with whom we look forward to engaging in a mutual effort to improve the clinical reasoning and critical thinking of student pharmacists.

W. Cary Mobley, PhD, RPh
Robin Moorman Li, PharmD, BCACP, NBC-HWC

Integrated Critical Thinking and Clinical Reasoning in Pharmacy Practice

Clinical Reasoning, Critical Thinking, and the PPCP—Introduction

W. Cary Mobley

CHAPTER AIMS

The aims of this chapter are to:
- Discuss how clinical reasoning, critical thinking, and the PPCP (Pharmacists' Patient Care Process) can unite to optimize pharmacist-provided patient-centered care.
- Describe elements of a patient-centered approach to care, including the roles of the biopsychosocial model of health.
- Describe each step of the PPCP.
- Describe and differentiate diagnostic reasoning and therapeutic (management) reasoning.
- List common biases and describe how they can impede effective clinical reasoning, and strategies for overcoming and combating implicit bias.
- List intellectual critical-thinking standards and intellectual standards-based questions that can be employed to optimize the pharmacist's reasoning in each step of the PPCP.

KEY WORDS

• Clinical reasoning • critical thinking • PPCP (Pharmacists' Patient Care Process) • diagnostic reasoning • therapeutic reasoning • intellectual standards • dual process theory • biopsychosocial model • patient-centered care • cognitive and implicit biases • objectivity

"Reasoning is our best guide to the truth. It is the process of systematically working toward the solution of a problem, toward the understanding of a phenomenon, toward the truth of the matter."[1]

Reasoning—the forming of conclusions, judgments, or inferences from facts or premises—is our indispensable cognitive tool that enables us to understand and explain reality; to determine truth from falsehood, what to value and why, and how to act and live; to make decisions; and to understand, explain, and solve problems. This includes solving clinical problems, for which *clinical* reasoning is employed by clinicians from a variety of healthcare disciplines to "integrate clinical information (such as histories, exam findings, and test results), preferences (eg, of the patient), medical knowledge, and contextual (situational) factors to make decisions about the care of patients."[2] The excellent clinician relies on excellent clinical reasoning to rationally investigate, understand, explain, and resolve clinical problems. Pharmacists use clinical reasoning to rationally investigate, understand, explain, and resolve *drug therapy* problems (DTPs) within the context of the patient's overall healthcare.

 KEY POINT

Pharmacists use clinical reasoning to rationally investigate, understand, explain, and resolve drug therapy problems.

To optimize the quality of our reasoning and thinking, we think critically. That is, we "skillfully take charge of the elements inherent in our thinking and impose intellectual standards on them."[3] These elements of our thinking include information and concepts, inferences and conclusions, implications and consequences, different perspectives, questions, and assumptions. The intellectual standards we apply to these elements of thinking are many, and include clarity, accuracy, and objectivity. These and others will be described later in this chapter and applied to patient problem-solving in each chapter of this book. By routinely applying critical thinking standards to our thinking, we can become more effective critical thinkers, which can improve our ability to gather, assess, and communicate relevant information, to formulate problems clearly, and to arrive at well-reasoned solutions.[4-9]

 KEY POINT

In providing patient care, pharmacists can improve their ability to gather, assess, and communicate relevant information, to formulate problems clearly, and to arrive at well-reasoned solutions by routinely applying critical thinking standards to their thinking.

This book explores the clinical reasoning of pharmacists in a variety of practices as they engage in clinical problem-solving, and it explores the roles that critical thinking can play in enhancing a pharmacist's reasoning. The clinical problem-solving model for the book will be the Pharmacists' Patient Care Process (PPCP), which is a stepwise, systematic clinical problem-solving process developed by the Joint Commission of Pharmacy Practitioners.[10,11] Through application of the PPCP to patient cases, pharmacists in different practice settings will describe their reasoning as they systematically work through each PPCP step—Collect, Assess, Plan, Implement, and Monitor. These pharmacists will also show how critical thinking can be applied to optimize the reasoning process in each PPCP step, allowing the reader to appreciate how the PPCP, clinical reasoning, and critical thinking can unite to optimize patient-centered care.

 KEY POINT

The Pharmacists' Patient Care Process (PPCP) is a stepwise, systematic clinical problem-solving process with which pharmacists, as part of an interprofessional team, can apply clinical reasoning and critical thinking to optimize patient-centered care that revolves around the patient's needs, wants, and participation.

PATIENT-CENTERED CARE

Pharmacists are part of an interprofessional team dedicated to providing patient-centered care, in which clinical problem-solving revolves around the patient's needs, wants, and participation. For a pharmacist, fully understanding patients' needs and wants requires ascertaining their thoughts and feelings about illness (their *illness experience*) and medications (their *medication experience*).[12] A patient's *illness* experience includes their ideas, understandings, and feelings about illness, including the interrelationships between their illness and various life factors such as their physical and psychological function, social relationships, and lifestyle. It also includes the patient's expectations for those who provide their care. The *medication experience* can be defined as "The sum of all of the events a patient has in his or her lifetime that involve drug therapy."[12] As with the illness experience, a patient's medication experience encompasses several factors. These include their general attitude about taking medications; their understanding, expectations, and concerns about medication therapy; and the influence of cultural, religious/spiritual, and ethical issues on their medication usage.

The patient-centered approach to care overlaps and can be combined with a biopsychosocial (BPS) model of patient care.[13] The BPS model is based on the notion that a patient's health is a function of multiple interacting factors that are present within interacting and dynamic systems.[14-28] (See **Figure 1-1.**) These systems include biological, psychological, social, and value systems. An underlying premise of the BPS model is that factors within these systems can be significant determinants of an individual's health. Biological systems include the biochemical, cellular, and physiological systems that are at the source of ill health, and include factors that

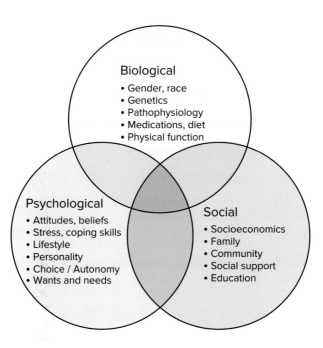

FIGURE 1-1. The biopsychosocial model of health.

can affect these systems, such as injuries, diet, physical activity, genetics, exposure to toxins or pathogens, and aging. The psychological system contains such factors as attitudes, beliefs, desire for autonomy, lifestyle, hobbies, wants, needs, stress, and coping. Social factors include interpersonal experiences and social support (eg, significant others, family, peers, friendships, loneliness), life events (eg, death of a loved one, divorce, bullying, unemployment), social policies (eg, level of freedom), socioeconomic status (eg, the standard of living), and cultural influences. An individual's value system is an important modifier of factors in psychological and social systems, because a person's values influence what kind of life to lead, goals to set, decisions to make, interactions with others, and the overall quality of life and sense of wellbeing.

In a patient-centered approach to care within a BPS framework, information acquired about factors relevant to a patient's health can be integrated into a comprehensive assessment that is unique for each patient and can serve as the foundation for one of the pharmacist's primary goals: providing the patient an individualized recommendation in accordance with the patient's "needs, goals, lifestyle, and personal and cultural values."[29] Thus, in each patient encounter, it is incumbent on the pharmacist to develop a trusting and caring rapport and be fully present as patients describe their illness experiences and medication experiences, so as to gain an understanding of potential patient-specific health determinants in the biological, psychological, and social systems. And while not all determinants for a particular patient can be readily addressed, it can still be valuable for the clinician to adopt a broad, BPS mindset in their clinical encounters and in clinical problem-solving, so as to maintain a continued alertness to potentially *significant* BPS determinants of their patient's health that should be considered in developing and implementing strategies for compassionate care.

 KEY POINT

Within a biopsychosocial framework, a comprehensive assessment that is unique for each patient can serve as the foundation for one of the pharmacist's primary goals: providing the patient an individualized recommendation in accordance with their "needs, goals, lifestyle, and personal and cultural values."

PHARMACISTS' PATIENT CARE PROCESS

The Pharmacists' Patient Care Process (PPCP) is a patient problem-solving process created by the Joint Commission of Pharmacy Practitioners, with a main purpose of promoting consistency of care across the pharmacy profession by providing a framework for clinical problem-solving that can be universally applied in a variety of pharmacy practice settings.[10,11] The PPCP has similar steps to other systematic problem-solving processes: It begins with collecting information; followed by evaluating the information to identify and define problems; followed by setting goals and generating, choosing, and implementing strategies for resolving the problems; followed by monitoring and following up to evaluate the success of the implemented strategies in achieving the goals and resolving the problems. Specifically, the PPCP is a cycle of the sequential steps of Collect, Assess, Plan, Implement, Follow-Up: Monitor and Evaluate. (See **Figure 1-2.**)

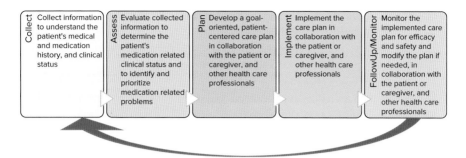

FIGURE 1-2. Steps of the pharmacists' patient care process.

 KEY POINT

The PPCP is a cycle of the sequential steps of Collect, Assess, Plan, Implement, Follow-Up: Monitor and Evaluate that can be used to guide the systematic identification, defining, and resolving of drug therapy problems as they occur within the context of the patient's overall healthcare.

A general description of each PPCP step and examples of how a pharmacist can proceed through each step are provided below. In reviewing the processes involved in each step, it is important to note that there can be variability in these processes based on the nature of the clinical practice, the specific clinical scenario, and the type of care that the pharmacist provides.

Collect—Collect information to understand the patient's medical and medication history, and clinical status.

- Collect information according to the clinical practice and setting, such as through the examination of medical records and through an interview of the patient or caregiver.
- List all existing diagnoses and any undiagnosed presenting medical conditions or patient complaints (eg, constipation, abdominal pain, rash, reason for hospital admission, etc.).
- For each listed medical condition or complaint, list all available relevant patient information that will be used to evaluate their status.
- Include in your list any information that will enable you to evaluate medication efficacy, safety, and adherence; relevant risk factors and psychosocial issues (eg, stress, family support/responsibilities, occupation, finances); and the potential need for preventative care.
- Based on data collected, the nature of the patient encounter, and the nature of the clinical practice and setting, perform assessments (eg, pain assessment) or gather further information (eg, by interview) as needed to gain a greater understanding of the patient's clinical status.
- Separately, list any other collected data that is not apparently associated with the listed conditions or complaints, which you will need to evaluate during the Assess step or which you may need to refer to another healthcare practitioner (eg, physician) for evaluation.

Assess—Evaluate collected information to determine the patient's medication-related clinical status and to identify and prioritize DTPs.

- Evaluate the information collected for each of the conditions listed in the Collect steps to determine the status of each condition and to identify any DTPs.
- Evaluate each medication for appropriate indication, effectiveness, safety, and adherence. Include reported side effects and document appropriate adherence or identified reasons for nonadherence.
- Integrate knowledge, clinical experience, and patient data to formulate and test hypotheses about actual or potential DTPs. If needed, gather further information to confirm and disconfirm any hypothesized problems or to understand more completely the status of any of the listed medical conditions.
- Include in the assessment your evaluation of relevant psychosocial issues, functional status, risks, the need for preventative care, the need for further information, and the need for referral to another healthcare practitioner for further evaluation.
- Prioritize identified problems based on their urgency and with consideration of the harm that may ensue if the problem is not addressed and how quickly the harm will manifest. Also consider the patient's priorities.
- For each problem, include problem status descriptors such as controlled or uncontrolled; acute or chronic; symptomatic or asymptomatic; mild, moderate, or severe; treated or untreated; or any combinations of these.
- For each problem, give a succinct and clear summary of your assessment of the problem, written in a manner that the reader and you can readily assess the soundness of your reasoning. Include in your summary all patient information that is critical for explaining the problem and for supporting your conclusions.
  - This includes any supporting subjective and objective data and significant contributing and moderating factors. Be certain to succinctly explain the specific relationship between the drug therapy and the associated condition (eg, is a likely cause of constipation, is dosed too low or with the wrong regimen, is inappropriate for this patient because of her age, is not indicated, etc.).
- In the assessment summary, do not include information that is irrelevant for explaining the problem and that could render your reasoning less clear.

An overarching goal for using the PPCP in patient care is to guide the systematic identification, defining, and resolving of DTPs as they occur within the context of the patient's overall healthcare. This recognizes the unique role that the pharmacist plays in an interprofessional approach to care, where clinicians and caregivers from a multitude of professions join in a collective and integrated pursuit to provide optimal patient-centered care.

There are several classification systems the pharmacists may use to identify general types of DTPs that patients may experience, including one that was developed and is continuously revised by the Pharmaceutical Care Network Europe (PCNE).[30] Another commonly used system that will be used in this book is provided in **Table 1-1**.[31]

Plan—Develop a goal-oriented, patient-centered care plan in collaboration with the patient or caregiver, and other healthcare professionals.

- List each numbered, prioritized problem with its status descriptors.
- For each problem, create a patient-centered SMART (specific, measurable, achievable, realistic, and time-bound) goal that is collaboratively determined with the patient or caregiver, and other providers when appropriate.

TABLE 1-1

Drug Therapy Problems and Their Common Causes[31]

Problem	Examples of Causes
Unnecessary drug therapy	No relevant indication for the drug, duplication of therapy, nonpharmacological therapy more appropriate, contraindication to current medication
Needs additional therapy	Need for therapy for an untreated condition, for synergistic therapy, or for preventive therapy
Ineffective drug	Drug is ineffective for the condition, more effective drug available, another dosage form or route is more appropriate, condition refractory to the drug
Dosage too low	Dose is too low for the desired response, inappropriate frequency or duration, incorrect administration, drug interaction, drug degraded
Adverse drug reaction	Undesired reaction not dose-related, unsafe medication for the patient, drug interaction, incorrect administration, allergic reaction, dosage increased or decreased too quickly
Dosage too high	Dose is too high for the indication, inappropriate frequency or duration, incorrect administration, drug interaction
Inappropriate adherence	Directions not understood by the patient, the patient forgets or prefers not to take the medication, patient cannot afford the medication, patient has difficulty administering the medication

– Structure each goal to include observable, measurable, and realistic parameters for goal achievement; the desired value or observable change for those parameters, and the expected time frame for their achievement. Objective parameters will have objective outcomes (eg, systolic blood pressure between 135 and 140 mm Hg) and subjective parameters will have subjective outcomes (eg, can work in garden without significant pain).

• In collaboration with the patient, create each goal, based on evidence-based guidelines whenever possible, with consideration of clinical outcomes of efficacy, safety, and adherence for the patient's current medications, and with consideration of significant BPS factors and the patient's overall quality of life.

• For each numbered, prioritized problem, generate a list of reasonable pharmacological and nonpharmacological strategies that could be used to achieve the SMART goals.[1]

• Eliminate options, in consideration of the goals, based on patient-centered issues such as comparative efficacy and safety, supporting evidence, the ability of the patient to adhere to the regimen, significant psychosocial factors, cost, the impact

---

[1]Note: In addition to possible new medications, strategies may also include such options as medication discontinuation, dosage or regimen adjustment, adherence or medication administration education, preventative care (eg, vaccination), and referral to another healthcare practitioner.

of the option on other patient problems (eg, comorbid conditions), and the impact of patient problems (eg, renal dysfunction) on the option.

- Indicate your specific recommendations, justified with strong rationale, for pharmacological and nonpharmacological strategies (when warranted) to achieve the patient's SMART goals.

Implement—Implement the care plan in collaboration with the patient or caregiver, and other healthcare professionals.

- For each numbered, prioritized problem and associated recommended strategy, provide:
  - The medication order in its entirety, including full drug name, dose, dosage form, route of administration, dosing interval, and duration of therapy.
  - A patient education plan for both pharmacological and nonpharmacological strategies communicated in a way that assures patient understanding. For pharmacological strategies, it may include explanations of medication action, the regimen or its proper discontinuation (where warranted), and proper medication use and storage.
  - Why and how to seek additional care, results to be expected and when to expect them, possible adverse effects to be alert to, when and how to follow-up, and other important pertinent information.
- According to the clinical practice, contribute to the coordination of care by providing documentation for other providers using an evidence-based method of communication, such as SBAR (Situation, Background, Assessment, Recommendation) or SOAP (Subjective, Objective, Assessment, Plan).

Follow-Up: Monitor and Evaluate—Monitor the implemented care plan for efficacy and safety and modify the plan if needed, in collaboration with the patient or caregiver, and other healthcare professionals.

- For each numbered, prioritized problem, write a follow-up and monitoring and evaluation plan that will include a scheduled time and method (eg, phone call, visit) of follow-up, and will consider:
  - The expected timing of goal achievement.
  - The timing of expected positive outcomes (eg, goal-related outcomes) and negative outcomes (eg, adverse effects).
  - The timing or coordination of strategies.
  - The desires and activities of the patient and other healthcare providers.
  - Parameters defined by payers (eg, insurance company).
  - The nature of the patient encounter and of the clinical practice and setting.
- Clearly describe the monitoring parameters, with the positive and negative clinical outcomes that will be used to evaluate goal attainment or potential problems associated with the strategy.

Note: The follow-up description above describes components of follow-up *plan*, which is generally created as part of the Implement step. In the actual follow-up *session* with the patient, the PPCP process begins anew with one focal point being the collection of information for assessing the outcomes of previously implemented strategies.

Some important points about the PPCP relevant to this book are the following:

1. Effective clinical reasoning is crucial in each step.
2. It is an orderly process, in that inferences and conclusions in one step lay the groundwork for reasoning in the subsequent step.
3. The application of critical thinking can improve the clinical reasoning that occurs in each step.

CLINICAL REASONING IN THE PPCP

Clinical reasoning occurs throughout the PPCP as pharmacists draw numerous inferences and conclusions as they prepare for and conduct the gathering of information in the Collect step; create explanations in the Assess step; determine goals, outcomes, and strategies in the Plan step; determine the best ways to implement strategies and educate patients in the Implement step; and evaluate achievement of outcomes and determine if changes are needed in the Monitoring and Follow-up steps.

As the clinician engages in clinical problem-solving, clinical reasoning serves two primary purposes—*diagnosis* and *therapeutic decision making*—and thus there are two main types of clinical reasoning: *diagnostic reasoning*[29,32-50] and *therapeutic reasoning* (also called *management reasoning*).[36,46,51-57] Diagnosis is defined as the "determining or analysis of the cause of or nature of a problem or situation."[58] *Diagnostic reasoning* is the reasoning involved in this process. *Therapeutic reasoning*, or *management reasoning*, is the reasoning involved in patient management. Using the PPCP framework for medication-related clinical problem-solving, diagnostic reasoning occurs mainly in the Collect and Assess steps and therapeutic reasoning occurs mainly in the Plan, Implement, and Monitoring steps. (See **Figure 1-3.**)

 KEY POINT

There are two main types of clinical reasoning: diagnostic reasoning, which occurs mainly in the Collect and Assess steps, and therapeutic reasoning, which occurs mainly in the Plan, Implement, and Monitoring steps.

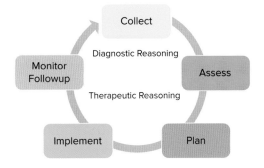

FIGURE 1-3. Diagnostic and therapeutic reasoning in the PPCP.

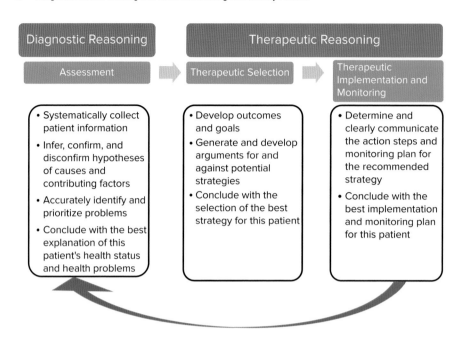

FIGURE 1-4. Diagnostic and therapeutic reasoning.

   In the Collect and Assess steps, the pharmacist engages in diagnostic reasoning about patient-related information to ultimately draw a set of conclusions that integrate to form a comprehensive explanation (assessment) of DTPs, health and functional status, risks, and needs for preventative care. With these conclusions drawn in the Assess step serving as the foundation, therapeutic reasoning is applied sequentially in the Plan, Implement, and Monitoring steps. In the Plan step, reasoning is applied to set health-related goals for addressing the patient's problems and to determine the best strategies for meeting the goals. Based on the chosen strategies, reasoning is applied to determine appropriate steps for strategy implementation and for outcome monitoring. Details of some of the cognitive activities involved in diagnostic and therapeutic reasoning are elaborated in **Figure 1-4**. Examples of common inferences and conclusions that can be drawn by the reasoning pharmacist in each PPCP step are listed in **Table 1-2**.

 KEY POINT

There are many inferences and conclusions that can be drawn by the reasoning pharmacist in each PPCP step.

ELEMENTS OF A PHARMACIST'S DIAGNOSTIC AND THERAPEUTIC REASONING

In *diagnostic reasoning*, the pharmacist infers hypotheses to explain one or more phenomena observed during the Collect step. For example, a patient on a particular medication is experiencing some physical discomfort, and the pharmacist suspects

TABLE 1-2

Common Inferences and Conclusions for Each Step of the PPCP

Collect
Collect information to understand the patient's medical and medication history, and clinical status

Clinical Reasoning—Common Inferences and Conclusions Drawn in This Step
- Type of demographic information that might be important to collect
- Possible DTPs and other hypotheses drawn from an initial review of the patient's medical record or from a patient interview
- Information needed to confirm and reject hypotheses
- The need for more detailed information
- The need for clarification
- The need for further information to obtain
- Identity of stakeholders and their roles in the patient's health and healthcare
- Specific objective information to obtain (eg, labs, physical exam, etc.)
- Assessments that should be performed (eg, risk assessment, pain assessment, etc.)
- Common psychosocial factors associated with the patient's medical conditions
- Barriers, including biases, that can impede the gathering of needed or desired information
- The point at which the Collect step, including the patient interview, can be concluded

Assess
Evaluate collected information to determine the patient's medication-related clinical status and to identify and prioritize drug therapy problems

Clinical Reasoning—Common Inferences and Conclusions Drawn in This Step
- Existing medication indication, effectiveness, safety, and adherence
- Level of achievement of previously established goals
- The need to adjust previously established goals
- The need to adjust existing medication therapy (eg, based on physiological changes)
- Potential type of data to expect, including abnormal data, based on the patient's conditions
- Patient's personal goals, values, beliefs, attitudes, expectations, abilities, commitment, and lifestyle
- Patient limitations and strengths
- Causes, precipitating factors, contributing factors, and exacerbating factors
- Risks and risk factors
- Influence and roles of different stakeholders in the patient's healthcare
- Level of severity and control of the patient's conditions
- Interrelationships between comorbid conditions
- Interrelationships between current therapeutic approaches
- Rival hypotheses: Alternative reasonable explanations for collected information
- The best explanations for collected information among the alternatives
- New drug therapy problems
- Consequences of current courses of action if unchanged
- Need for preventative care
- Need for referral or consultation
- Ranking of problems in terms of priority

Plan
Develop a goal-oriented, patient-centered care plan in collaboration with the patient or caregiver, and other healthcare professionals

Clinical Reasoning—Common Inferences and Conclusions Drawn in This Step
- Overall purpose of potential strategies (eg, cure, palliation, control, prevent complication, slow or stop progression, alleviate symptoms, etc.)
- Specific realistic outcomes to be achieved
- Measures of the outcomes that will signify goal achievement
- Achievability of the goals with known available strategies
- Relevance of the goals to the patient's attitudes, beliefs, expectations, values, and personal goals
- Reasonable time frames for achieving the goals
- Reasonable and best pharmacological strategies to meet goals
- Reasonable and best nonpharmacological strategies to meet the goals
- Evidence to support strategy selection
- Indication, effectiveness, safety, and adherence issues for proposed pharmacological strategies
- Mechanisms by which strategies can achieve the goals
- Logical interrelationship between the pathophysiology, patient assessment, goals, and potential strategies
- Benefits and risks, or strengths and weaknesses of alternative strategies
- How the proposed therapeutic strategies produce desired outcomes and potential adverse effects
- Patient's perceptions of their illness and the proposed treatment and how that may affect adherence to and outcomes of the strategy
- Complexities of treatment that should be considered
- Relationships between pharmacist-recommended strategies and strategies of other healthcare practitioners
- Capacity of patient to follow the strategy and any assistance that might be needed
- Influence of transitions of care
- The need, timeframe, method, and location for follow-up
- Appropriate monitoring parameters

Implement/Monitor/Follow-Up
In collaboration with the patient or caregiver, and other health care professionals, implement the care plan and monitor the implemented care plan for efficacy and safety and modify the plan if needed

Clinical Reasoning—Common Inferences and Conclusions Drawn in These Steps
Implement
- Steps for enacting the agreed-upon strategies
- Positive and negative consequences of implementing the strategies
- Expected duration of treatment
- Parameters to be used to evaluate treatment outcomes
- Complexities of the patient's care that may present challenges to appropriate medication use and adherence
- Potential barriers for implementation of strategies
- Likely consequences if the patient does not adhere to the prescribed regimen
- Need for patient education and training

- Communication strategy needed to achieve "proper understanding of the illness, treatment, and good adherence behavior"
- Need for assistance in implementing the strategies
- Role others might play in implementing the strategies
- Need for coordination of care
- Effective communication of the assessment and recommendations to the healthcare team

Monitoring and Follow-up

- When and how to follow-up
- What will be done at follow-up
- Clinical endpoints for monitoring
- Parameters that enable evaluation of the patient's medication experience and satisfaction with the plan
- Level of outcome achievement
- Evidence and reasons for success in meeting outcomes
- Evidence and reasons for failure to meet outcomes
- Need for revision of any elements of the assessment
- Need for revision of SMART goals
- Need for revision of strategies
- Communication strategy for providing proper feedback to the patient

(hypothesizes) that the discomfort may be due to an adverse effect of the medication the patient is taking. With a goal of creating the best explanation, the pharmacist deductively tests the hypothesis by gathering further information that can confirm the hypothesis. In pursuit of the best explanation, and to avoid premature closure on a particular hypothesis, the pharmacist must also purposefully create, test, and rule out alternate plausible explanations for the same phenomena. For example, the pharmacist can look for other potential causes of the discomfort, such as changed status of the patient's condition, the potential influence of co-occurring conditions, and the use of other medications or supplements that may elicit similar adverse effects to the medication in question. This reasoning process repeats itself for other hypotheses that the pharmacist may infer during the Collect and Assess steps, such as potential contributing factors to the patient's health problems, and strengths, barriers, and other aspects of the patient's health and healthcare.

This act of inferring hypotheses is a creative act that depends heavily on the pharmacist's domain-related knowledge and experience, which the pharmacist relies on to generate and evaluate *plausible* hypotheses. Furthermore, pharmacists rely on their knowledge for effective reasoning through all steps of the PPCP. Therefore, it is vital for each pharmacist to engage in a career-long quest of maintaining and improving their knowledge.

 KEY POINT

Since pharmacists rely on their knowledge and skills for effective reasoning through all steps of the PPCP, it is vital for pharmacists to engage in a career-long quest of maintaining and improving their knowledge and skills.

From the generation and testing of hypotheses, the pharmacist will ultimately develop a set of explanatory conclusions about causes and contributing factors for different aspects of the patient's clinical status. These conclusions will be integrated to form a comprehensive patient assessment. In applying the PPCP, this assessment will integrate explanatory conclusions about the patient's clinical condition (eg, controlled or uncontrolled), DTPs, and contributing and moderating factors. It may also include conclusions about risks, the need for preventative care, the need for more information, and about the need for consultation or referral.

In reasoning, among the criteria for good explanations is that they should be *adequate* and *true*.[59] For an explanation to be adequate, the inferred hypothesis should be *logically strong, complete,* and *informative*. A *logically strong* hypothesis is logically connected to what it is trying to explain. For example, if a drug is hypothesized to be the cause of an adverse effect, it should at a minimum make sense based on what is known about the drug. For an explanation to be *complete*, the hypothesis or set of hypotheses should account for all of the significant aspects of the information it is trying to explain. Significance is important because what is to be explained can be complex. For example, even a single condition can have multiple contributing and moderating factors and types of data to consider. So, a hypothesis or set of hypotheses may not be able to account for all of the relevant collected information, including the insignificant or trivial, but it should account for what the pharmacist considers to be significant. (Note: Significance is one of the critical thinking standards discussed later on in the text.) The final measure of adequacy of a hypothesis is *informativeness*, meaning that the hypothesis should ultimately indicate the fundamental reason or cause for what it is trying to explain. For example, it could be exposure to allergens as a cause of symptoms of allergic rhinitis, or a problem with adherence or dosing as a cause of an unmet clinical outcome.

A second criterion for a good explanation is the *truth* of the hypothesis that is used to explain the collected information.[59] Among the methods to evaluate the truth of the explanation is that in testing the hypothesis, the reasoner should find evidence for other expected consequences of the proposed hypothesis and that the hypothesis is better at explaining the totality of the evidence than all known plausible rival hypotheses.[6,60] For example, the wife of a COPD patient reports that her husband has had an increased number of emergency room visits due to COPD exacerbations after being prescribed a new inhaler. The pharmacist confirms that the inhaler is appropriate for the patient based on clinical guidelines and hypothesizes that the patient may not be using the inhaler properly. Based on that hypothesis, the pharmacist would expect the patient to be using improper technique when demonstrating its usage. If the patient demonstrates correct technique for each of the steps for inhaler usage, the pharmacist may turn to other plausible explanations for the unexpected inefficacy of the medication. Upon further investigation, the pharmacist may discover that the inhaler was not refilled on time and that the patient has experienced recent cognitive decline and depression. The pharmacist then hypothesizes a multifactorial adherence problem and refers the patient for evaluation by his physician who later confirms the pharmacist's suspicion.

In *therapeutic reasoning*, the pharmacist in the full context of the patient's overall care engages the patient, when feasible, in setting goals for therapy and helps the patient choose among the best available strategies. Based on the pharmacist's knowledge, experience, and evidence-based practice, the pharmacist generates potential strategies and develops arguments for and against them. Conclusions are drawn about the best strategies for the patient, which are those that have the best supporting argument for realistically meeting the therapeutic goals. Therapeutic reasoning continues in the implementation and monitoring steps, with conclusions drawn for optimal implementation and monitoring of the strategies.

 KEY POINT

Diagnostic reasoning and therapeutic reasoning can have some important differences worth noting, one difference being that therapeutic reasoning can be more complex than diagnostic reasoning.

Diagnostic reasoning and therapeutic reasoning can have some important differences worth noting. For diagnostic reasoning, conclusions about causes and contributing and moderating factors are reached that are objectively correct or not correct, and involve a relatively finite range of significant relationships between the factors. Although there are many potential factors (eg, BPS factors) that can contribute to the patient's problems and they can have complex interrelationships to understand for creating a comprehensive explanation, the value of this understanding may lie primarily with *therapeutic* reasoning, where the factors and complexities can be considered for optimizing the selection and implementation of therapeutic strategies. Therapeutic reasoning is inherently more complex than diagnostic reasoning mainly because there are typically multiple effective and acceptable therapeutic approaches to choose from, as opposed to the one correct conclusion or set of conclusions desired for diagnostic reasoning. Other potential sources of the greater complexity of therapeutic reasoning can include the complexities of shared decision-making between the different stakeholders in the patient's care, the potential interactions and need to coordinate therapeutic strategies of different healthcare disciplines, the need for appropriate monitoring of the plan, and the potential need for adjustments to the plan. Cook et al phrase it well: Therapeutic (management) reasoning "involves dynamic interplay among people, systems, settings, and competing priorities; involves unavoidable uncertainties; is inherently complex and situated in a dynamic biopsychosocial context."[2]

The foregoing was an overview of some of the reasoning processes pharmacists may engage in while providing care to their patients, but there is more to the field of clinical reasoning. It has been informed by decades of research in different healthcare disciplines, to which the reader is referred for deeper and broader understanding.[29,32,33,36,40,43,44,48,50,56,60–62] Among the influential theories related to clinical reasoning that may be valuable for pharmacists to become aware of is the dual-process theory of thinking that originated in the field of psychology.

TWO TYPES OF REASONING PROCESSES

 KEY POINT

An important theory of thinking for pharmacists to be aware of is the dual process theory, which describes two systems of thinking that can be engaged in reasoning and decision-making: the fast and intuitive System 1 thinking and the slower, logic-based System 2 thinking.

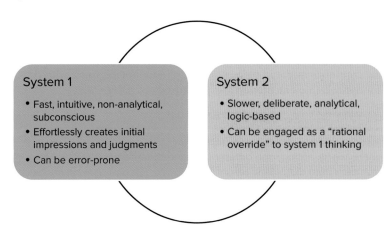

FIGURE 1-5. System 1 and System 2 thinking.

According to dual process theory, decision-making engages two systems of thinking processes: System 1 thinking and System 2 thinking.[63–66] System 1 thinking is a fast, intuitive, automatic type of thinking and System 2 thinking is a slower, deliberate, analytical, logic-based type of thinking (**Figure 1-5**). A blend of these automatic and deliberate thinking processes occurs in much of our cognitive activity.

The fast and intuitive System 1 thinking develops in individuals through repeated experiences that get stored in long-term memory. It is engaged automatically when similar experiences match the pattern of what is stored in long-term memory and can dominate much of our routine thought processes, such as the thinking that enables us to safely drive on familiar routes without the need to reason through each maneuvering position. Clinical examples include recognizing sadness or pain in patient's face or verbal communication, recognizing signs a patient may faint after receiving a vaccine injection, and recognizing signs and symptoms of a myocardial infarction. For experienced clinicians with multiple repeated experiences, it can also include the subconscious recognition of more complex patterns, or constellations of signs and symptoms that function as "illness scripts," for example, the combination of signs and symptoms that may cause a suspicion of ketoacidosis in a diabetic patient. This intuitive thinking enables the experienced clinician to subconsciously generate initial inferences or hunches that can be the basis for the next actions to take, such as beginning life-saving measures in emergency situations, or for engaging the deliberate System 2 thinking by logically analyzing the information and, if warranted, seeking further information in health records or through patient communication to verify or reject the initial hunches.

The "jumping to conclusions" that occurs in System 1 thinking saves time and mental energy, enabling quick action. It can also be very accurate, depending on the knowledge and experience of the thinker in the context of the particular situation. However, it is also prone to be mistaken, for example, when the current pattern is not a good match to what is stored in long-term memory, and the thinker does not recognize the mismatch. This may cause the clinician to "anchor" and take action on an initial impression without applying needed corrections that could lead to more accurate conclusions. System 1 thinking can also be adversely influenced by biases that exist in the subconscious, such as the biases based on a patient's physical appearance, demeanor, or behavior that can influence how clinicians subjectively feel about their patients. There are numerous other potential biases that can adversely impact the quality of one's reasoning. Some of these are discussed in the next section. Mistakes from System 1 thinking that can lead to negative consequences for the patient may also occur due to a failure to recognize and account for the complexity of the patient or of the clinical situation, or due to not having the time, cognitive energy, background knowledge, experience, or skill to effectively engage System 2 thinking to manage the complexity.

 KEY POINT

System 2 thinking can be engaged as a rational override to System 1 thinking, but it is important to be aware of fallibilities in both systems of thinking, including the role of biases.

The conscious, deliberate, analytical, logic-driven System 2 thinking can be engaged as a "rational override" to System 1 thinking, serving to monitor System 1 thinking and forcing a reassessment as needed to verify or correct the subconscious conclusions and influences of System 1. By putting themselves into the objective logical framework of System 2 thinking, clinicians can potentially rectify errors and the negative influence of bias or uncertainty in their reasoning and put themselves on a more deliberate and logical path to working through these and other challenges. To be able to recognize the need for this shift to the rational override of System 2 requires that the clinician be vigilant and mindful in their thinking so as to maintain alertness to their potential biases, uncertainties, or other potential barriers to effective reasoning.

Importantly, just as with System 1 thinking, and with reasoning in general, System 2 thinking is fallible. It is influenced by background knowledge, experience, skill, and biases of the thinker, and it can be time-intensive and cognitively demanding. Therefore, factors such as distractions, inattentiveness, sleep deprivation, fatigue, uncertainty, and the demands of the clinical practice can negatively impact the ability of the thinker to successfully engage System 2 thinking. However, the deliberate reasoning of System 2 can improve and become more efficient over time with practice employing a consistent, systematic process along with an accumulation of experience and knowledge in the domain of practice. This can be an important point for student pharmacists who as novices in their field do not have the accumulated patient-care experiences needed to develop the patterns that enable the effective System 1 thinking of experienced clinicians. Therefore, for the benefit of the students to which this book is dedicated, the clinician authors for the remaining chapters will break down their patient care process to uncover the details of their reasoning, primarily from a deliberate System 2 thinking perspective. The goal of this approach for these chapters is to help students to recognize and develop these thinking skills on their journey toward becoming excellent clinicians.

 KEY POINT

As novices in their field, student pharmacists do not have the accumulated patient-care experiences needed to develop the patterns that enable the effective System 1 thinking of experienced clinicians.

THE INFLUENCES OF BIAS

As mentioned, among the potential contributing factors to errors in reasoning are different types of bias, which can be defined as "a disposition, implicit or explicit, to reach a particular kind of conclusion or outcome, or to remain in one."[67] Potential biases include cognitive biases and implicit biases. Cognitive biases can be defined as "systematic psychological tendencies to make errors in seeking and interpreting information"[59] and implicit biases can be defined as "biases that result from the tendency to process information based on unconscious associations and feelings, even when these are contrary to one's conscious or declared beliefs." Common cognitive biases include confirmation bias, anchoring, premature closure, etc. Examples of these and other biases that can influence our reasoning are described in **Table 1-3**.

TABLE 1-3

Examples of Common Biases[64,68–79]

Bias	Description
Anchoring	Relying too heavily on the first piece of information offered. For example, creating an initial impression based on salient features in the patient's initial presentation, and failing to adjust this initial impression when warranted by later information.
Availability	Being biased toward more recent information or information that most readily comes to mind when making judgments. For example, failing to persevere and look at other information can prevent the clinician from considering plausible alternative therapeutic strategies.
Bandwagon effect	Believing and doing certain things because many others are doing so. *Groupthink* is an example that can have a detrimental impact on team decision-making and patient care.
Blind spot bias	Believing yourself to be less susceptible to bias than others. For example, this can cause the clinician to fail to adequately recognize and consider their own biases when working with patients, or fail to effectively implement de-biasing strategies.
Confirmation bias	The tendency to favor or look for information that confirms what we think, without being adequately alert to or open to refuting information, even if it is more persuasive. For example, this can cause the pharmacist to favor looking for information to confirm a hypothesis that a medication is the cause of a particular sign or symptom, at the expense of adequately considering other plausible explanations.
Diagnosis momentum	Failure to consider other plausible diagnostic conclusions when interacting with patients, due to an earlier conclusion that was accepted by others without sufficient independent scrutiny, and therefore gathered increasing momentum as the accurate diagnostic conclusion in subsequent interactions with the patient. For example, this can affect future patient workups and how handoffs are "framed" if practitioners do not properly evaluate patient information independently.

Framing effect	The tendency to allow our thinking and judgment about issues or information to be influenced by how it is presented to us (eg, how it is framed by the patient, other clinicians, or other stakeholders). As with other biases, this can cause the clinician to think without sufficient depth, breadth, or objectivity.
Fundamental attribution error	The tendency to be inappropriately judgmental and explain illnesses or behavior on internal factors of a patient, such as personality or disposition, without adequately considering external factors or circumstances. For example, there may be socioeconomic factors or certain stressors impacting a patient's health that may be significant and therefore should be considered.
Information bias	The tendency to believe that the more evidence one can accumulate to support a conclusion, the better. While gathering *sufficient* information to make a decision is important, it is also important to know the relevance and significance of that information for making the decision, and not assume that the more information the better, regardless of its significance.
Overconfidence bias	The tendency to have more confidence in our knowledge or abilities than is objectively reasonable. Overconfidence reflects a tendency to act on incomplete information, intuitions, or hunches. For example, not being self-aware of the limits of our knowledge or skills in particular situations may cause failure to adequately recognize and consider important features, complexities, or consequences in diagnostic or therapeutic decision-making.
Premature closure	The tendency to stop an inquiry or reasoning process once a decision or conclusion has been made, before it has been adequately validated.
Search satisficing	The tendency to search through the available alternatives until an acceptability threshold is met and then call off the search once something plausible is found. Although this can be valuable in formulating initial hypotheses, it can be detrimental if it stops the consideration of other plausible hypotheses.
Visceral bias	The influence of the clinician's affective response (eg, emotions or state of mind) about a patient on decision-making. This can cause a visceral arousal that may be positive or negative and can undermine objectivity and lead to poor decisions. For example, feeling friendly, humored, unsafe, untrusting, irritated, or sad about a patient can have a negative impact on a clinician's objectivity during patient interactions.

 KEY POINT

There are numerous cognitive and implicit biases that can adversely impact reasoning that pharmacists should be self-aware of and strive to mitigate.

Implicit biases comprise attitudes and stereotypes that unconsciously affect one's understanding, actions, and decisions.[80] They can be positive or negative in terms of their effect on the reasoner's perceptions, but whether positive or negative, implicit biases can adversely impact objectivity. Implicit bias can emerge from many domains, including bias towards a patient's age, weight, race or ethnicity, gender, sexual orientation, socioeconomic status, or educational background.[68] Among the strategies recommended by the Joint Commission in overcoming and combating implicit bias include the following:[80]

KEY POINT

Among the strategies for overcoming and combating implicit bias are perspective taking, emotional regulating, partnership creating, cultural understanding, bias understanding, individuating, and performing teach-back.

- Perspective-taking—Empathetically adopting the perspective of others
- Emotional regulating—Practice good emotional regulation skills
- Partnership creating—Creating a partnership with patients that together works towards common goals
- Cultural understanding—Attaining a basic understanding of the cultures in the practice's population
- Bias understanding—Understanding and respecting the potential magnitude of unconscious bias
- Individuating—Avoiding stereotypes by individuating each patient (ie, treating each patient as a distinct individual)
- Performing teach-back—Utilizing the teach-back method when educating patients

To reach the best conclusions and provide the best care for their patients, it is important that pharmacists become self-aware of implicit biases, and practice strategies for overcoming them and limiting their influence on objective, rational thought. It is also important to be aware that these biases are universal in humans and therefore exist to different degrees not only in pharmacists, but also in patients they encounter and in all other stakeholders in the patient's care, including other members of the interprofessional team. For example, biases from the patient can compromise accurate information-gathering by the pharmacist, the patient's own decision-making, and can degrade the overall quality of the clinical encounter. Regardless of their source, biases can compromise objective, rational thought. Becoming self-aware of our biases and reducing their influence on our thinking are two of the many potential benefits of engaging our critical thinking faculty, which is described next.

THE PHARMACIST AS A CRITICAL THINKER

KEY POINT

Critically thinking pharmacists "skillfully take charge of the elements of thinking and impose intellectual standards on them," and by doing so, improve their reasoning and its outcomes.

Critically thinking pharmacists "skillfully take charge of the elements of thinking and impose intellectual standards on them,"[3] and by doing so, improve their reasoning and its outcomes. There are many elements of thinking, including information we have gathered, the concepts we rely on to make sense of the information, elements of reasoning (eg, hypotheses, inferences, conclusions, premises, and assumptions), and implications, impacts, and consequences of the information and of our reasoning. Scriven and Paul offer a definition of critical thinking that further elaborates the concept: "the intellectually disciplined process of actively and skillfully conceptualizing, applying, analyzing, synthesizing, and/or evaluating information gathered from, or generated by, observation, experience, reflection, reasoning, or communication, as a guide to belief and action."[81] This definition embodies many of the thinking processes an individual will engage in (*conceptualizing, applying, analyzing, synthesizing,* and *evaluating*), what individuals think about (*information*), where the information comes from (*observation, experience, reflection, reasoning*), and the value of critical thinking (*guide to belief and action—*).

The work of Paul and Elder on critical thinking is significant and comprehensive for the field. In addition to the intellectual standards, which will be introduced below and applied throughout this book, they recognize important virtues or traits that are valuable for critical thinkers to cultivate within themselves. Among these are *intellectual empathy*—seeking to understand and reason from another's perspective; *intellectual courage and integrity*—the willingness to stay true to and stand by one's own thinking and beliefs and also to challenge them; *intellectual humility*—recognizing and considering the limits of one's knowledge and skills when reasoning; *intellectual perseverance*—a willingness to engage and maintain the pursuit of truth in the face of difficulties and obstacles; and *confidence in reason* as our best guide to truth and understanding.[5,82]

INTELLECTUAL STANDARDS OF CRITICAL THINKING

Intellectual standards are standards of critical thinking that we can use to help optimize our reasoning. These include standards for the information we gather, the knowledge we need to evaluate the information, the different perspectives to entertain, the inferences and conclusions we draw, the potential implications of our conclusions, and the logicalness of our reasoning.

The following intellectual standards will be used in this book to show how they can be applied to help pharmacists optimize their reasoning about their patients: *clarity, relevance, significance, objectivity, fairness, accuracy, precision, depth, breadth,* and *log icalness.*[7-9,83,84] One way to enable ready recall of these standards is the mnemonic: "*Clear ROAD for Logic.*"

 KEY POINT

Intellectual standards that pharmacist can employ to optimize their reasoning include *clarity, relevance, significance, objectivity, fairness, accuracy, precision, depth, breadth,* and *logicalness*, which can be recalled using the mnemonic "*Clear ROAD for Logic.*"

	Clear	R	O	A	D	Logic
Intellectual Standards	Clarity	Relevance and Significance	Objectivity[a] and Fairness	Accuracy and Precision	Depth and Breadth	Logicalness

[a]Objectivity is included here, but is not routinely presented as a separate standard in the works of Paul and Elder.

A brief description of each standard is given in **Table 1-4**. Applying these standards to problems we encounter can enable us to take command of our thinking, to keep it on track, and to help us assure that we create the best explanations and arguments and make the best decisions we are capable of.

TABLE 1-4

Critical Thinking Intellectual Standards[5–9,84,85]

Standard	Descriptions
Clarity (explicit, unambiguous, intelligible, free from confusion or doubt)	Clarity is considered a "gateway" standard, as it can be difficult or impossible to apply other standards, such as accuracy, relevance, or logicalness, if information or statements are unclear to the thinker. This also means that we need to have a clear understanding of the conceptual knowledge that we depend on when reasoning. Given that clinical reasoning involves drawing inferences and conclusions from information and premises, it is critical that information and its communication are clear, without ambiguous meanings, distortions, unclear phrasing, jargon, or faulty language usage.
Relevance (pertinent, applicable, germane)	Relevance is the standard that helps us focus on what has a close logical relationship to the problem or issue we are thinking about.
	For example, when we gather information, we will need to determine what information is relevant and how it is relevant to what we are trying to explain. When we are making an argument, we need to determine the relevance of the facts to the argument. When preparing to interview a patient, we may need to determine what further information would be relevant to obtain based on a hunch (inference) we might have. We need to determine what queries to make that will give us the information that is relevant and significant for the case. We must be able to distinguish irrelevant information from information that is relevant to the patient's health and healthcare, and we must seek to understand *how* it is relevant. Good reasoning requires that all relevant information has been considered.[86]
Significance (important, nontrivial, necessary, critical, required, impactful)	In addition to determining what is relevant, we need to determine what is most critical or significant for the explanations and arguments we are trying to make, without which our conclusions may be erroneous or weakened. Given the number of factors and their interactions that can affect a person's health, the cognitive limitations of decision makers, the limitations of resources and time to affect changes, and the consequent need to be selective in choosing which factors to address and which interventions to implement, it is important to grasp the significance of the factors in terms of their impact or potential impact on an individual's specific health problem(s) or overall health. We not only need to determine the significance of the information that we have, but we may also need to determine the information we are missing, that if not considered could degrade our ability to draw valid and complete conclusions.

Objectivity (fact-based, unbiased)	Being objective means maintaining a reality-orientation and remaining focused on seeking truth and understanding without the influence of personal beliefs, biases, emotions, fallacies, evasions, or other potential distortions of reality that can interfere with our ability to seek truth. These potential distortions, including our emotions and our biases, can creep into any step of the PPCP. For example, in the Collect step, our biases may lead to unfounded presumptions about individuals that may take us off the path of seeking accurate and relevant information, which in turn will degrade our ability to form accurate conclusions. We must strive to be objective, to become self-aware of our emotions and biases, and recognize when they are hindering any of our clinical problem-solving activities. Self-awareness can help us guard against letting those biases influence our reasoning, for example by preventing irrelevant information to factor into our thinking. Given the potential for feelings, emotions, and biases to cloud one's judgment, it is critical to be alert to their presence and remain objective and focused on the facts and reality when reasoning.
Fairness (unbiased, equitable, impartial)	Fairness entails many things, including maintaining a respect for the patient's and caregiver's humanity, with a spirit of tolerance and openness to different viewpoints, and with a goal of understanding and honoring the patient's wants and needs. There are several issues involved in patient care that require the pharmacist to be welcoming of different perspectives, including the limitations of a pharmacist's specialized knowledge in fully grasping a patient's health, the number of different healthcare strategies that may be employed, the perspectives of different stakeholders that may be involved in the patient's healthcare, and the unlikelihood that any single perspective reveals the whole truth.[59] To achieve the best explanations and arguments, the pharmacist must actively explore and be receptive to different perspectives, and when dealing with and communicating with other stakeholders, the pharmacist must maintain a sense of fairness and benevolence. That is, the pharmacist must strive to be free from bias, dishonesty, or premature judgment and must maintain a sense of civility and sensitivity, and a tolerance to diverse perspectives. Staying open to diverse perspectives and being tolerant towards perspectives that may disagree with our own can allow us to consider insights that we may not otherwise have considered.[59] It can expose us to our own flawed assumptions, rationalizations, or overconfidence, and it can expose us to ideas that can further strengthen our position or possibly take it in a different direction. And, even if the ideas and positions of others are rejected, in the process of considering them, clinicians can gain a better understanding of their own positions.[59] Applying the fairness standard to patients can also be valuable for developing trusting, caring, and open relationships that can yield more complete and accurate information, leading to better explanations about a patient's health, which can more effectively support therapeutic decision-making.
Accuracy (verifiable, valid, true, credible, undistorted)	Accuracy, or conformity with facts or truth, is indispensable to reasoning well. Given that reasoning will be based on information, propositions, and their understanding, their accuracy (trueness) is a fundamental determinant of the validity and soundness of that reasoning. The quality of our inferences and conclusions relies on the accuracy of the information and premises we are using as support. False, or insufficiently accurate information or premises, can risk false conclusions. As we are searching for truths, it is important that our information and reasoning is clear and accurate.

Precision (exact, specific, detailed)	Precision in critical thinking means exactness to the necessary level of detail for reasoning well through a particular problem or issue. For example, if a patient reports a fever or high blood sugar, it may be critical to know the precise temperature and glucose levels, respectively. Precision, or level of detail, is also important in our communications and in formulating our explanations and arguments, as they can be weakened, for example, when significant details are missing. or when there is excessive detail. Given that reasoning will be based on information, propositions, and their understanding, precision (level of detail) can be a critical determinant of the validity and soundness of that reasoning.
Depth (Roots, fundamentals, complexities, interrelationships, cause/effect, implications)	As stated previously, there are many interrelated factors that together can shape an individual's health and that should be grasped for effective clinical problem-solving, particularly when operating with a biopsychosocial mindset. Given the potential complexity of these interrelationships, it can be important to gain a deep understanding in order to determine their potential implications for the patient's health and healthcare. In reasoning about therapeutic alternatives, we must explore the potential implications and consequences of implementing various therapeutic strategies or of a failure to implement them. Thinking deeply about a patient's health can put a premium on the pharmacist to be able to associate ideas, perspectives, and insights from several disciplines and connect them to the patient's health and problems. These include the didactic disciplines of the pharmacist's education as well as the professional disciplines that comprise the interprofessional team. To achieve "interdisciplinary understanding," the clinician needs varying levels of disciplinary depth and breadth of understanding.[87]
Breadth (Comprehensive, encompassing, alternative perspectives)	Achieving breadth requires "encompassing multiple viewpoints, being comprehensive in view, and adopting a broad-minded perspective".[9] There are many potential factors that can shape an individual's health and many potential strategies from multiple professions that can be utilized in managing a patient's health. Thus, it is important to be broadminded to seek a variety of relevant information in order to gain a comprehensive understanding of an individual's health. Additionally, the clinician may need to consider a broad array of different treatment strategies towards choosing those that are best to recommend for the patient, and the clinician may need to determine how best to integrate the chosen strategies within a broad and comprehensive interprofessional plan.
Logic (Reasonable, rational, without contradiction, well-founded, sound)	Logic is the study of the methods and standards of inference.[59] It is the fundamental process that connects inferences to the information on which they are based and connects conclusions to the premises on which they are based. For an argument proposed by the pharmacist to be a good one, it must be logically *sound* in that premises are *true* and conclusions *logically follow* from them. Applying the standard of logic also involves a commitment to avoiding and uncovering logical fallacies and false assumptions when we are seeking to make logical connections.

Using Questions to Apply the Intellectual Standards of Critical Thinking

 KEY POINT

One approach that pharmacists may use to apply intellectual standards to optimize their reasoning is to ask themselves intellectual standards-based questions as they engage in clinical problem-solving using the PPCP.

One approach that pharmacists may use to apply intellectual standards to optimize their reasoning as they engage in clinical problem-solving is to ask themselves intellectual standards-based questions, such as the ones listed in **Table 1-5**. This questioning approach is commonly found throughout the works of Paul and Elder.[5-9]

TABLE 1-5	
Examples of Intellectual Standards-Based Questions	
Clear	Do I understand and express my reasoning clearly?
R (Relevance and Significance)	Am I gathering, considering, and communicating information relevant to what I am reasoning about?
	Of the relevant information I must reason about, am I considering all that is significant for basing my conclusions on, and is any significant information or are significant assumptions missing from my arguments and explanations?
	What is the significance of this particular information?
O (Objectivity and Fairness)	To what degree is my reasoning objective and free from potentially distorting influences of biases, subjective feelings, and emotions?
	Am I considering the thoughts of others with fairness, with a spirit of mutual benevolence, openness, and tolerance to opposing ideas to uncover and rectify potential errors in my reasoning?
A (Accuracy and Precision)	Am I assuring the accuracy or veracity of the information and premises I am basing my inferences and conclusions on, knowing that accuracy and truth are indispensable to sound reasoning?
	Do I have sufficient precision or detail of information or premises so that I am not basing my inferences or conclusions on information that is insufficiently exact?
D (Depth and Breadth)	Am I adequately considering the depth of interrelationships and complexities of the factors I am reasoning about, knowing that inferences and conclusions I draw depend on a grasp of how relevant factors affect each other?
	Am I gathering and considering the necessary breadth of relevant information possible to me, knowing that if anything significant is excluded, my explanations and arguments are at risk of being erroneous or incomplete, and what truths I discover may not be whole truths?
Logic (Logicalness)	Do my conclusions logically follow from my premises and are my premises true?
	Do my inferences logically follow from the information and is that information factual?
	Does my hypothesis logically explain the data? Are there better explanations for the data?
	Do I have the data, information, assumptions, premises necessary and sufficient to support my conclusions?

The questions listed in Table 1-5 are examples of general questions pharmacists can use to help assure they meet intellectual standards for a variety of cognitive activities, including clinical problem-solving. Pharmacists may also ask themselves questions more specific to PPCP-guided clinical problem-solving. Examples of these standards-based questions for each PPCP step are given in **Table 1-6**. A pharmacist can choose from these sets of questions or can create their own sets of standards-based questions according to their practice and their specific problem-solving process. The questions can be used for planning a clinical encounter, for reflection after the encounter, or metacognitively, in the midst of the clinical encounter.

TABLE 1-6

Examples of Questions Pharmacists Can Ask Themselves to Help Them Meet Intellectual Standards in Each Step of the PPCP

Collect Collect information to understand the patient's medical and medication history, and clinical status.	
Clear	In written or oral communication, did I communicate in a way that I was clearly understood by the patient or other stakeholders?
	In written and oral communication, did I clearly understand the patient or other stakeholders?
	Am I communicating with vocabulary that the patient understands and is free of jargon that the patient may not understand?
	Am I verifying that the patient understands me?
	Am I asking questions as needed to clarify what the patient is communicating to me?
	Are there any potential barriers to clear communication with the patient or other stakeholders?
	Am I clear on the meaning of the data that I have collected and am analyzing?
Relevance and Significance	Based on initial information that I have gathered, what relevant and potentially significant additional information do I need to gather to effectively evaluate this patient's clinical status and healthcare needs?
	Prior to collecting information, did I determine what was the most significant aspect of a problem or issue that needed to be addressed?
	Have I gathered sufficient information to form a strong conclusion?
	Am I missing important relevant information, such as the patient's age, social status, family support, financial capability, and other potentially significant psychosocial information?
	Am I missing information that could be significant for accurately evaluating this patient?
Objectivity and Fairness	Have I gathered information objectively, to the best of my ability, in the pursuit of truth and understanding, without the influence of bias or emotions?
	Am I maintaining a presence throughout my interactions in a way that respects patient autonomy, encourages open communication, encourages patient participation in care, suspends premature judgment, and enables me to clearly and comprehensively understand the patient's wants and needs?

	Were there any biases that potentially influenced my gathering of information, such as visceral bias, framing effect from a handover, bandwagon effect, confirmation bias, or anchoring?
	Are there limitations or barriers that prevent me from collecting sufficient information?
Accuracy and Precision	What level of detail do I need for specific information I am gathering?
	Have I considered and assured the accuracy of the subjective and objective information?
	Have I collected information with sufficient accuracy and precision that will enable me to draw sound conclusions on medication effectiveness, safety, and adherence?
	Have I collected information with sufficient accuracy and precision that will enable me to draw sound conclusions on any factors negatively impacting the patient's medication use experience?
Depth and Breadth	In my practice, what are the common biopsychosocial patient factors to inquire about because of their potential significance for assessment and therapeutic planning?
	Am I able to evaluate the depth or level of complexity needed to fully assess this patient?
	Have I gathered information from a sufficiently broad array of categories to enable me to fully assess this patient and to determine potential complexities?
	Have I gathered enough information for a complete assessment?
	Have I acquired enough information about the patient's strengths that can be possibly leveraged for optimal patient care, including physical, psychological, social, cultural, and spiritual strengths?
Logic	As I inferred hypotheses during this step, did I seek information that could confirm or strengthen them as well as information that could reject or weaken them?
	Am I able to combine information from multiple sources needed to form an integrated understanding?
Assess Evaluate collected information to determine the patient's medication related clinical status and to identify and prioritize drug therapy problems.	
Clear	Were there any problems with clarity that could hinder my reasoning, such as ambiguous meanings, distortions, unclear wording and phrasing, faulty language usage, or other problems with communication?
	Were there any deficiencies in the clarity of my understanding of the relevant knowledge needed to develop sound inferences, conclusions, explanations, and arguments?
	Is my assessment expressed with sufficient clarity, accuracy, and precision to properly support the planning and implementation of therapeutic strategies and to be understood and evaluated by other stakeholders?

Relevance and Significance	Have I evaluated all subjective and objective information for its relevance and significance to the patient's health?
	Is there significant information that I am missing or was unable to obtain through appropriate sources?
	Is there significant existing information that I am not adequately considering?
	Have I distinguished relevant from irrelevant information?
	Does my assessment explain all the significant aspects of the information I have collected?
	Have I evaluated the significance of the contributing factors to this patient's health problems?
	In assessing the patient's medical problems, drug therapy problems, risk, and need for preventative care, were the most significant contributing factors identified and considered when developing and evaluating therapeutic alternatives?
Objectivity and Fairness	To what extent do I uncritically accept what I am told by my supervisors, consultants, peers, patients, and others?
	Was I willing to change my position when the evidence led to a more rational conclusion?
	In service to my patient, to what extent:
	• Have I analyzed my beliefs that may impede my ability to think critically?
	• Am I willing to yield my positions when sufficient evidence is presented against them?
	• Am I willing to stand my ground against the majority or in the face of criticism?
	• Do I strive to recognize and eliminate self-deception or self-interest when reasoning through clinical issues?
	• Do I seek to understand others reasoning and objectively use insights from others, when warranted, to strengthen or correct my own reasoning?
	Have I objectively evaluated this information and formed conclusions without influence of my emotions or biases, such as visceral bias, framing effect from a handover, bandwagon effect, confirmation bias and anchoring?
Accuracy and Precision	Is there any information for which I have inadequate details or insufficient accuracy to effectively draw conclusions?
	Are my conclusions expressed with sufficient clarity, accuracy, and details to enable other stakeholders to readily understand and evaluate my reasoning?
Depth and Breadth	Have I been thorough in summarizing all known factors significant to the patient's medical problems?
	Do I have strategies for grasping complex clinical issues, such as interrelationships between the patient's different clinical problems and their causes and contributing factors?
	Have I identified the root causes of the patient's problems and the most significant contributing and moderating factors?
	Do I grasp and am I able to articulate the complexity of this case and the factors that are contributing to this complexity?
	Is the complexity or difficulty of this case exceeding my capacity to create a logically sound and clear assessment?

	In my assessment, did I think deeply enough to consider the potential consequences and implications of changes being made in this patient's healthcare as well as the potential consequences and implications of no changes being made?
Logic	Have I identified and considered the assumptions I am making when drawing conclusions?
	Did I consider other explanations for this patient's signs and symptoms?
	To what extent are there contradictions or inconsistencies in the way I deal with clinical issues?
	Have I considered information that rejects or does not support my conclusions?
	Does my assessment adequately express the complexity of this patient's health and DTPs?
	Have I considered the implications of my conclusions being incorrect?
	Are the inferences and conclusions I have made in my assessment logically sound, with full consideration of all available factors, without contradictions or unsupported assumptions?
Plan Develop a goal-oriented, patient-centered care plan in collaboration with the patient or caregiver, and other health care professionals.	
Clear	Were the SMART goals and strategies for achieving them developed with a clear understanding by the patient of what is achievable for meeting their healthcare wants and needs?
	Have the SMART goals set for this patient been clearly stated, including their timeframe and expected outcomes?
	In reasoning about the best therapeutic options for this patient, was there knowledge or information where I needed a greater clarity or accuracy?
	In my written and oral communications, was I clear and consistent with my use of language, terminology, and concepts?
	In presenting the plausible therapeutic strategies, did I assure that the patient and other stakeholders clearly understood the benefits and risks of each option, and were not overwhelmed with the information I presented to them?
Relevance and Significance	Were the SMART goals and strategies for achieving them developed in consideration of the most significant factors affecting this patient's health and the most significant expected outcomes?
	Were the SMART goals and strategies for achieving them developed with a consideration of the relevance of the evidence for the potential therapeutic strategies for this patient?
	Were the SMART goals and strategies for achieving them developed with a consideration of relevance and significance of the patient's prognosis, physiological variables, and other conditions?
	Are the SMART goals and strategies for achieving them clearly aligned with my assessments in the Assess step?

Objectivity and Fairness	In helping the patient develop SMART goals, did I clearly understand the patient's wants, needs, and values, and did the patient clearly understand the rationale for the desired goals?
	Were the SMART goals and strategies for achieving them developed without the undue influence of emotions or biases?
	Were the SMART goals and strategies for achieving them developed with a fair consideration and participation of the patient and relevant stakeholders?
	Did I detect any bias, narrowness, or contradictions in other stakeholder's perspectives?
	Have I sought the opinions of others for identifying and considering alternative strategies?
	In formulating my opinion, was I able to reason well with different points of view, particularly those that I disagreed with?
	Was I able to critically examine and evaluate my interests, beliefs, and assumptions?
	Did I adhere to sound principles and evidence when persuading others of my position?
	Did I distort matters to support my position?
	Was the plan mutually developed with the patient in a manner that empowers the patient to self-manage their health and health behaviors?
	In fairness to the patient and other stakeholders, do I adequately understand the roles of other providers in this patient's care and recognize when it is best to refer the patient to other providers when I am at the limit of my knowledge or scope of practice?
Accuracy and Precision	Did I identify details about the different options that are important for conveying to the patient?
	Were any of my communications possibly too detailed so as to hinder understanding?
	In reasoning about the best therapeutic options for this patient, was there knowledge or information where I needed a greater accuracy?
	Were there any sources of information where there were concerns of credibility, accuracy, or reliability?
	Though medications are my expertise, in reasoning about the best non-pharmacological options for this patient, do I have sufficiently accurate and clear knowledge needed to make these recommendations?
Depth and Breadth	Were the SMART goals and strategies for achieving them developed in consideration of their relevance to this patient's personal goals, values, beliefs, attitudes, expectations, abilities, commitment, and lifestyle?
	Were the SMART goals and strategies for achieving them developed with consideration of the complexities that could be involved in this patient's care?
	Was the plan developed with sufficiently broad and deep consideration of all of the significant contributing factors and the complexity of this patient's health?
	In developing my recommendations, have I thought broadly about different, complimentary strategies that may be integrated into a comprehensive plan for this patient's care?

Logic	Were the SMART goals and strategies for achieving them developed in consideration of what was realistically achievable for this patient?
	Do the SMART goals and strategies for achieving them make logical sense based on disease pathophysiology, a full assessment of the patient, clinical guidelines, and potential therapeutic strategies?
	Do the recommended therapeutic strategies for achieving the SMART goals represent those that had the best arguments for goal achievement based on the patient assessment, the SMART goals, available options?
	Am I able to articulate the relevant evidence and rationale to support my conclusions?
	Do my arguments for my recommended strategies rest in any way on false, biased, or doubtful assumptions?
	Were the strategies that I have chosen to recommend supported by current evidence or guidelines?

Implement/Monitor/Follow-Up
In collaboration with the patient or caregiver, and other health care professionals, implement the care plan and monitor the implemented care plan for efficacy and safety, and modify the plan if needed.

Clear	Are the steps for implementing the strategies clearly understood and outlined and provided with enough clarity, accuracy, and details to facilitate their implementation by the patient and others involved in the patient's care?
	In developing and providing clear education to the patient, have I carefully considered potential ambiguities, jargon, poor grammar, or other potential causes of unclear understanding by the patient?
	Is my oral and written communication to fellow professionals clearly conveyed and understood? This includes SBAR, SOAP notes, and other forms of professional communication.
Relevance and Significance	Have my written and oral communications with all stakeholders focused on what is relevant and avoided what is irrelevant?
	To facilitate successful implementation of strategies that may be complicated to the patient, have the most significant actions for strategy implementation been determined, outlined, and conveyed?
	Have the most significant elements of monitoring been determined, outlined, and conveyed?
Objectivity and Fairness	Has the implementation plan been developed fairly, taking into full consideration that the patient can become overwhelmed with the actions needed for successful implementation, particularly when faced with multifaceted or complex strategies presented to the patient in a single short encounter?
	Have the implementation and follow-up plans been developed in fair consideration of the patient's wants, needs, and abilities?
	Have the implementation and follow-up plans been developed in fair consideration of the roles and responsibilities of caregivers, family members, and other stakeholders?
	In fairness to the patient, has the implementation plan been developed and communicated with an empathetic understanding of their perspectives and in a manner that assures the patient is empowered to self-manage their health and health behaviors?

Accuracy and Precision	Have the monitoring and evaluation parameters been listed with appropriate accuracy and precision in accordance with evidence and guidelines?
	Does the patient understand the importance of implementing the strategies accurately and the potential consequences of deviating from instructions?
Depth and Breadth	Does the patient understand any significant complexities of the strategies and how to manage them?
	In thinking broadly about this patient's care, have I identified all of the stakeholders involved in this patient's care, including providers, family members, caregivers, and payers, and have I considered their integral contributions to achieving the identified health outcomes?
	Are there any difficulties or complexities associated with the strategies that the patient will need help in managing?
	Have I outlined what is needed for coordinating care between different providers?
Logic	Is there a strong logical connection and alignment between the details of the implementation, monitoring, and follow-up plans—with the assessment, the goals, and the chosen strategies—so as to optimize the chances for successful outcomes and minimize the risks of untoward consequences?
	Are the steps for implementation logically outlined?
	Is the timing for follow-up logically supported by evidence for the time needed for the outcomes to manifest?

CONCLUSION

The provision of excellent patient care requires excellent clinical reasoning by healthcare providers, including pharmacists who use clinical reasoning to rationally investigate, understand, explain, and resolve drug therapy problems within the context of the patient's overall healthcare. Among the ways that pharmacists can optimize their reasoning in the care they provide to their patients is to apply intellectual standards of critical thinking as they engage in a systematic patient problem-solving process such as the Pharmacists' Patient Care Process (PPCP). These intellectual standards include clarity, relevance, significance, objectivity, fairness, accuracy, precision, depth, breadth, and logicalness. Together they can be applied in each step of the PPCP to help the pharmacist develop the highest quality explanations and arguments required to provide the highest quality of compassionate, patient-centered care.

Summary Points

- Pharmacists are part of an interprofessional team dedicated to providing patient-centered care, in which clinical problem-solving revolves around the patient's needs, wants, and participation. This approach to care includes developing an understanding of the patient's illness and medication experiences and can be combined with a biopsychosocial model of patient care that recognizes multiple interacting factors involved in a patient's health that can inform the development of individualized recommendations, unique for each patient.
- The PPCP is a cycle of the sequential steps of Collect, Assess, Plan, Implement, Follow-Up: Monitor and Evaluate that can be used to guide the systematic

identification, defining, and resolving of drug therapy problems. There are two general types of reasoning that occur in the PPCP: diagnostic reasoning, which occurs mainly in the Collect and Assess steps, and therapeutic reasoning, which occurs mainly in the Plan, Implement, and Monitoring steps.

- In their thinking about a patient case, pharmacists can engage a combination of fast and intuitive System 1 thinking and slower, logic-based System 2 thinking. Fallibility exists in both systems of thinking, including those due to biases. Among the common biases that can impede effective clinical reasoning are cognitive biases, such as confirmation bias and overconfidence bias, and implicit biases, such as those related to a patient's age, weight, gender, race, or ethnicity. Among the strategies to combat these biases are perspective taking, cultural understanding, and individuation.

- In providing patient care, pharmacists can improve their ability to gather, assess, and communicate relevant information, to formulate problems clearly, and to arrive at well-reasoned solutions by routinely applying critical thinking standards to their thinking. This can be accomplished by pharmacists asking themselves intellectual standards-based questions as they engage in clinical problem-solving using the PPCP.

References

1. Scriven M. *Reasoning*. New York, NY: McGraw-Hill; 1976.

2. Cook DA, Durning SJ, Sherbino J, Gruppen LD. Management reasoning: implications for health professions educators and a research agenda. *Acad Med*. 2019;94(9):1310-1316.

3. Paul R, Elder L. *Critical Thinking: Tools for Taking Charge of Your Learning and Your Life*. Upper Saddle River, NJ: Prentice Hall; 2001.

4. Paul R. Critical thinking: what, why, and how. *New Dir Community Coll*. 1992;1992(77):3-24.

5. Paul R, Elder L. *The Miniature Guide to Critical Thinking Concepts and Tools*. 8th ed. Lanham, MD: Rowman & Littlefield Publishers; 2019.

6. Elder L, Paul R. Critical thinking: a stage theory of critical thinking. part I. *J Dev Educ*. 1996;20(1):34-35.

7. Elder L, Paul R. Critical thinking: intellectual standards essential to reasoning well within every domain of human thought, part 3. *J Dev Educ*. 2013;37(2):32-33.

8. Elder L, Paul R. Critical thinking: intellectual standards essential to reasoning well within every domain of thought. *J Dev Educ*. 2013;36(3):34-35.

9. Paul R, Elder L. Critical thinking: intellectual standards essential to reasoning well within every domain of human thought, part two. *J Dev Educ*. 2013;37(1):32-33.

10. Bennett M, Kliethermes MA, American Pharmacists Association. *How to Implement the Pharmacists' Patient Care Process?* Washington, DC: American Pharmacists Association; 2015.

11. Boyce EG. The pharmacists' patient care process and more. *Am J Pharm Educ*. 2017;81(4):62.

12. Cipolle RJ, Strand LM, Morley PC. Chapter 4. Patient-centeredness in pharmaceutical care. In: Cipolle RJ, Strand LM, Morley PC, eds. *Pharmaceutical Care Practice: The Patient-Centered Approach to Medication Management Services*. 3rd ed. New York, NY: The McGraw-Hill Companies; 2012.

13. Turabian JL. Patient-centered care and biopsychosocial model. *Trends Gen Pract*. 2018;1(3):1-2.

14. Borrell-Carrió F, Suchman AL, Epstein RM. The biopsychosocial model 25 years later: principles, practice, and scientific inquiry. *Ann Fam Med*. 2004;2(6):576-582.

15. Gatchel RJ, Peng YB, Peters ML, Fuchs PN, Turk DC. The biopsychosocial approach to chronic pain: scientific advances and future directions. *Psychol Bull*. 2007;133(4):581-624.

16. Karunamuni N, Imayama I, Goonetilleke D. Pathways to well-being: untangling the causal relationships among biopsychosocial variables. *Soc Sci Med*. 2021;272:112846.

17. Smith RC, Fortin AH, Dwamena F, Frankel RM. An evidence-based patient-centered method makes the biopsychosocial model scientific. *Patient Educ Couns.* 2013;91(3):265-270.

18. Smith RC. Making the biopsychosocial model more scientific-its general and specific models. *Soc Sci Med.* 2021;272:113568.

19. Engel GL. The clinical application of the biopsychosocial model. *Am J Psychiatry.* 1980;137(5):535-544.

20. Sadler JZ, Hulgus YF. Clinical problem solving and the biopsychosocial model. *Am J Psychiatry.* 1992;149(10):1315-1323.

21. Wade DT, Halligan PW. The biopsychosocial model of illness: a model whose time has come. *Clin Rehabil.* 2017;31(8):995-1004.

22. Schneiderman N, Ironson G, Siegel SD. Stress and health: psychological, behavioral, and biological determinants. *Annu Rev Clin Psychol.* 2005;1:607-628.

23. Slavich GM. Life stress and health: a review of conceptual issues and recent findings. *Teach Psychol.* 2016;43(4):346-355.

24. Booth FW, Roberts CK, Laye MJ. Lack of exercise is a major cause of chronic diseases. *Compr Physiol.* 2012;2(2):1143-1211.

25. Fava GA, Sonino N. From the lesson of George Engel to current knowledge: the biopsychosocial model 40 years later. *Psychother Psychosom.* 2017;86(5):257-259.

26. Kusnanto H, Agustian D, Hilmanto D. Biopsychosocial model of illnesses in primary care: a hermeneutic literature review. *J Family Med Prim Care.* 2018;7(3):497-500.

27. Saxena A, Paredes-Echeverri S, Michaelis R, Popkirov S, Perez DL. Using the biopsychosocial model to guide patient-centered neurological treatments. *Semin Neurol.* 2022;42(2):80-87.

28. Young-Hyman D, de Groot M, Hill-Briggs F, Gonzalez JS, Hood K, Peyrot M. Psychosocial care for people with diabetes: a position statement of the American Diabetes Association [published correction appears in diabetes care. 2017;40(2):287] [published correction appears in Diabetes Care. 2017;40(5):726]. *Diabetes Care.* 2016;39(12):2126-2140.

29. Rogers JC. Eleanor Clarke Slagle Lectureship—1983; clinical reasoning: the ethics, science, and art. *Am J Occup Ther.* 1983;37(9):601-616.

30. *PCNE Classification for Drug-Related Problems. V9.1* Pharmaceutical Care Network Europe Association 2020. Available at https://www.pcne.org/upload/files/417_PCNE_classification_V9-1_final.pdf.

31. Cipolle RJ, Strand LM, Morley PC. Chapter 5. Drug therapy problems. In: Cipolle RJ, Strand LM, Morley PC, eds. *Pharmaceutical Care Practice: The Patient-Centered Approach to Medication Management Services.* 3rd ed. New York, NY: The McGraw-Hill Companies; 2012.

32. Arocha JF, Wang D, Patel VL. Identifying reasoning strategies in medical decision making: a methodological guide. *J Biomed Inform.* 2005;38(2):154-171.

33. Bolton JW. Varieties of clinical reasoning. *J Eval Clin Pract.* 2015;21(3):486-489.

34. Cappelletti A, Engel JK, Prentice D. Systematic review of clinical judgment and reasoning in nursing. *J Nurs Educ.* 2014;53(8):453-458.

35. Chernushkin K, Loewen P, de Lemos J, Aulakh A, Jung J, Dahri K. Diagnostic reasoning by hospital pharmacists: assessment of attitudes, knowledge, and skills. *Can J Hosp Pharm.* 2012;65(4):258-264.

36. Cockcroft PD. Clinical reasoning and decision analysis. *Vet Clin North Am Small Anim Pract.* 2007;37(3):499-520.

37. Croskerry P. A universal model of diagnostic reasoning. *Acad Med.* 2009;84(8):1022-1028.

38. Edwards I, Jones M, Carr J, Braunack-Mayer A, Jensen GM. Clinical reasoning strategies in physical therapy. *Phys Ther.* 2004;84(4):312-335.

39. Furze J, Nelson K, O'Hare M, Ortner A, Threlkeld AJ, Jensen GM. Describing the clinical reasoning process: application of a model of enablement to a pediatric case. *Physiother Theory Pract.* 2013;29(3):222-231.

40. Haig BD. Scientific method, abduction, and clinical reasoning. *J Clin Psychol.* 2008;64(9):1013-1018.

41. Hawkins DR, Paul R, Elder L. *The Thinker's Guide to Clinical Reasoning.* Dillon, CA: Foundation for Critical Thinking; 2010.

42. Johnsen HM, Slettebø Å, Fossum M. Registered nurses' clinical reasoning in home healthcare clinical practice: A think-aloud study with protocol analysis. *Nurse Educ Today.* 2016;40:95-100.

43. Kassirer JP, Wong JB, Kopelman RI. *Learning Clinical Reasoning*. 2nd ed. Philadelphia, PA: Wolters Kluwer Health/Lippincott Williams & Wilkins Health; 2010.

44. Norman G. Building on experience: the development of clinical reasoning. *N Engl J Med*. 2006;355(21):2251-2252.

45. Nusair MB, Cor MK, Roduta Roberts M, Guirguis LM. Community pharmacists' clinical reasoning: a protocol analysis. *Int J Clin Pharm*. 2019;41(6):1471-1482.

46. Purvis J. Clinical reasoning: the analysis of medical decision making. *Ulster Med J*. 2016;85(3):151-152.

47. Rutter PM, Harrison T. Differential diagnosis in pharmacy practice: time to adopt clinical reasoning and decision making. *Res Social Adm Pharm*. 2020;16(10):1483-1486.

48. Simmons B. Clinical reasoning: concept analysis. *J Adv Nurs*. 2010;66(5):1151-1158.

49. Vertue FM, Haig BD. An abductive perspective on clinical reasoning and case formulation. *J Clin Psychol*. 2008;64(9):1046-1068.

50. Young ME, Thomas A, Lubarsky S, et al. Mapping clinical reasoning literature across the health professions: a scoping review. *BMC Med Educ*. 2020;20(1):107.

51. Abdoler EA, O'Brien BC, Schwartz BS. Following the script: an exploratory study of the therapeutic reasoning underlying physicians' choice of antimicrobial therapy. *Acad Med*. 2020;95(8):1238-1247.

52. Anakin MG, Duffull SB, Wright DFB. Therapeutic decision-making in primary care pharmacy practice. *Res Social Adm Pharm*. 2021;17(2):326-331.

53. Cook DA, Sherbino J, Durning SJ. Diagnostic vs management reasoning-reply. *JAMA*. 2018;320(17):1818-1819.

54. Kumar VD, Basheer A. Does management reasoning constitute the backbone of the clinical learning environment? Conceptual analysis of the existing notions. *J Adv Med Educ Prof*. 2021;9(1):54-58.

55. Parsons AS, Wijesekera TP, Rencic JJ. The management script: a practical tool for teaching management reasoning. *Acad Med*. 2020;95(8):1179-1185.

56. Patel JJ, Bergl PA. Diagnostic vs management reasoning. *JAMA*. 2018;320(17):1818.

57. Wright DFB, Anakin MG, Duffull SB. Clinical decision-making: an essential skill for 21st century pharmacy practice. *Res Social Adm Pharm*. 2019;15(5):600-606.

58. Diagnosis. In: *Dictionary.com*. Available at https://www.dictionary.com/browse/diagnosis. Accessed July 23, 2021.

59. Kelley D, Hutchins D. *The Art of Reasoning: An Introduction to Logic*. 5th ed. New York, NY: W.W. Norton & Company; 2021.

60. Facione NC, Facione PA. *Critical Thinking and Clinical Reasoning in the Health Sciences: An International Multidisciplinary Teaching Anthology*. Millbrae, CA: California Academic Press; 2008.

61. Higgs J, Jensen GM, Loftus S, Christensen N. *Clinical Reasoning in the Health Professions*. 4th ed. Edinburgh; New York, NY: Elsevier; 2019.

62. Norman G. Methods for the analysis of clinical reasoning. *Annu Conf Res Med Educ*. 1977;16:352-353.

63. Marcum JA. An integrated model of clinical reasoning: Dual-process theory of cognition and metacognition. *J Eval Clin Pract*. 2012;18(5):954-961.

64. Norman GR, Monteiro SD, Sherbino J, Ilgen JS, Schmidt HG, Mamede S. The causes of errors in clinical reasoning: cognitive biases, knowledge deficits, and dual process thinking. *Acad Med*. 2017;92(1):23-30.

65. Pelaccia T, Tardif J, Triby E, Charlin B. An analysis of clinical reasoning through a recent and comprehensive approach: the dual-process theory. *Med Educ Online*. 2011;16:10.3402/meo.v16i0.5890.

66. Kahneman D. A perspective on judgment and choice: mapping bounded rationality. *Am Psychol*. 2003;58(9):697-720.

67. Beaulac G, Kenyon T. Critical thinking education and debiasing. *Informal Logic*. 2014;34(4):341-363.

68. Balakrishnan K, Arjmand EM. The impact of cognitive and implicit bias on patient safety and quality. *Otolaryngol Clin North Am*. 2019;52(1):35-46.

69. Croskerry P, Singhal G, Mamede S. Cognitive debiasing 1: origins of bias and theory of debiasing. *BMJ Qual Saf*. 2013;22(Suppl 2):ii58-ii64.

70. Croskerry P. From mindless to mindful practice: cognitive bias and clinical decision making. *N Engl J Med*. 2013;368(26):2445-2448.

71. Elston DM. Cognitive bias and medical errors. *J Am Acad Dermatol.* 2019;81(6):1249.

72. Mailoo V. Common sense or cognitive bias and groupthink: does it belong in our clinical reasoning? *Br J Gen Pract.* 2015;65(630):27.

73. Miles RW. Cognitive bias and planning error: nullification of evidence-based medicine in the nursing home. *J Am Med Dir Assoc.* 2010;11(3):194-203.

74. Molony DA. Cognitive bias and the creation and translation of evidence into clinical practice. *Adv Chronic Kidney Dis.* 2016;23(6):346-350.

75. O'Hagan T, Fennell J, Tan K, Ding D, Thomas-Jones I. Cognitive bias in the clinical decision making of doctors. *Future Healthc J.* 2019;6(Suppl 1):113.

76. O'Sullivan ED, Schofield SJ. Cognitive bias in clinical medicine. *J R Coll Physicians Edinb.* 2018;48(3):225-232.

77. Smith JR. Cognitive bias: a potential threat to clinical decision-making in the neonatal intensive care unit. *J Perinat Neonatal Nurs.* 2017;31(4):294-296.

78. Cognitive Bias Codex—180+ biases, designed by John Manoogian III (jm3).jpg. 2016. Available at https://commons.wikimedia.org/w/index.php?title=File:Cognitive_Bias_Codex_-_180%2B_biases,_designed_by_John_Manoogian_III_(jm3).jpg&oldid=503397534. Accessed July 23, 2021.

79. Yuen T, Derenge D, Kalman N. Cognitive bias: Its influence on clinical diagnosis. *J Fam Pract.* Jun 2018;67(6):366-372.

80. Implicit bias in health care. *Quick Safety.* 2016;23. Available at https://www.jointcommission.org/resources/news-and-multimedia/newsletters/newsletters/quick-safety/quick-safety-issue-23-implicit-bias-in-health-care/implicit-bias-in-health-care/#.ZAqSIhXMKUk.

81. Scriven M, Paul R. Defining critical thinking: a draft statement for the National Council for Excellence in Critical Thinking. Published 1996. Available at http://www.criticalthinking.org/pages/defining-critical-thinking/766. Accessed July 26, 2021.

82. Elder L, Paul R. Critical thinking: developing intellectual traits. *J Develop Educ.* 1998;21(3):34-35.

83. Paul R, Elder L. Critical thinking: nine strategies for everyday life, part I. *J Develop Educ.* 2000; 24(1):40.

84. Paul R, Elder L. Critical thinking: intellectual standards essential to reasoning well within every domain of human thought, part 4. *J Develop Educ.* 2014;37(3):34-35.

85. Paul R, Elder L. *Critical Thinking: Tools for Taking Charge of Your Professional and Personal Life.* 2nd ed. Indianapolis, IN: FT Press; 2014.

86. Moore DT, Joint Military Intelligence College (U.S.). *Critical Thinking and Intelligence Analysis.* Washington, DC: Center for Strategic Intelligence Research, Joint Military Intelligence College; 2006.

87. Repko AF, Szostak R. *Interdisciplinary Research: Process and Theory.* 3rd ed. Los Angeles, CA: Sage; 2017.

2

Ambulatory Care— Chronic Pain Management Clinic

Robin Moorman Li

CHAPTER AIMS

The aims of this chapter are to:
- Discuss the roles of a systematic patient care process and clinical reasoning in assessing and resolving medication-related problems as part of a collaborative effort to provide patient-centered care in chronic pain management.

- Illustrate common medication-related problems encountered in an example chronic pain management case using clinical reasoning and critical thinking techniques through utilization of the Pharmacists' Patient Care Process.

KEY WORDS
- Chronic Pain • Osteoarthritis • Clinical reasoning • Clinical problem-solving •
Medication-related problems • Pharmacists' Patient Care Process • Critical thinking •
Cognitive biases

INTRODUCTION

Pharmacy practice in ambulatory care provides many opportunities for managing a variety of chronic disease states. Chronic pain management is one type of ambulatory care practice in which pharmacists can play a very impactful role in patient assessment, patient safety, treatment plan development, and in-depth patient education.

Pain is defined by the International Association for the Study of Pain (IASP) as "an unpleasant sensory and emotional experience associated with, or resembling that associated with, actual or potential damage." Chronic pain is pain that occurs for greater than 3 months or beyond the common healing time.[1] At least 50 million Americans suffer from chronic pain and 19.6 million of these patients are classified as suffering from high-impact chronic pain, which is considered chronic pain that frequently limits life or work activities.[2] In the United States alone, the yearly direct medical costs, costs of lost productivity, and cost of disability programs associated with chronic pain are estimated at a combined 560 billion dollars.[2] Primary care providers have increased the utilization of ambulatory pharmacists for a variety of multidisciplinary chronic disease state management programs including chronic pain management.[3] The Pain Management Best Practices Inter-Agency Task Force published recommendations focusing on acute and chronic pain management. These recommendations emphasized care should be individualized, multimodal, and multidisciplinary. It has been demonstrated that including pharmacists in multidisciplinary teams improves efficiency and overall patient care.[4]

 KEY POINT

When treating acute or chronic pain, care should be individualized and include multimodal and multidisciplinary treatment approaches.

OUR PRACTICE—AN OUTPATIENT PHARMACIST-RUN PAIN CLINIC

Our practice is an outpatient pharmacist-run clinic working under a collaborative agreement with primary care providers (PCPs), where pharmacists participate in the medical management of patients who struggle with chronic pain. Pharmacists receive referrals from the PCPs to perform risk assessment, medication therapy management, and extensive patient education. The patient population in this clinic ranges in age from 20 to 64 years old who present with a chronic painful condition, such as fibromyalgia, neuropathic pain-related disorders, cancer-related pain, pain due to a previous injury, and a variety of joint pains due to osteoarthritis (OA) and injuries. Some patients are managed on nonpharmacological and nonopioid therapies, while others are also managed with opioid therapy. Additionally, some PCPs refer patients for the evaluation of the appropriateness of an opioid trial.

UTILIZING CRITICAL THINKING SKILLS IN OUR PRACTICE

In this practice, critical thinking must be utilized continually throughout the entire patient care process. For example, the pharmacist will need to constantly question and reflect on all information gathered to determine if it is factual and reliable.[5] As a treatment plan is considered, pharmacists must reflect to verify the decisions are evidence-based and cognitive biases have been identified and addressed.[5] **Table 2-1** provides a list of sample standards-based questions that can be applied to assure that intellectuals standards for thinking are met as the pharmacist provides pain medication therapy management (MTM). Proper application of these standards will also help develop and foster an effective collaborative relationship with the patient. This will enable the pharmacist to gain a clear comprehensive understanding of the patient's clinical status and healthcare needs to develop the best strategy for optimal analgesia while limiting potential side effects.

TABLE 2-1

Sample Standards-Based Questions That Can Be Applied to Assure That Intellectual Standards for Thinking Are Met as the Pharmacist Provides Pain Medication Therapy Management

Clarity (explicit, unambiguous, intelligible, free from confusion or doubt)	• Has all information been collected from the patient to ensure clarity regarding pain levels, activity, sleep quality, medication use, and side effects? • Have I documented the information I have obtained in a clear format so others may clearly understand? • Have I utilized validated tools to aid in proper collection of information, pain assessment, and risk mitigation?
Relevance (pertinent, applicable, germane)	• What collected information during the interview/pain assessment is relevant? • As I work through the process, is it clear I am following proper standards of care and clinical pain management guidelines?
Significance (important, nontrivial, necessary, critical, required, impactful)	• What significant information have I gathered from the patient, caregivers, and other providers' clinic notes? • Have I evaluated all information to determine what is clinically relevant and significant, and then can I use that information to develop an effective treatment plan?
Objectivity (fact-based, unbiased)	• Are there biases that could affect my judgment (eg, race, gender, religious and political beliefs)? • Have I worked to identify any biases and worked to verify my objectivity? • Have I identified when emotion could possibly impact my objectivity? When this occurs, do I identify this is occurring and work to focus on the objective facts rather than the emotions? • Am I able to establish proper patient-provider boundaries and recognize when I am being taken advantage of as a provider?
Fairness (unbiased, equitable, impartial)	• What perspectives do I need to consider: the patient, the caregivers, the providers? • How do I ensure I am empathically and impartially considering the perspectives of others? • Can I use my professional judgment to fairly evaluate patients with a past history of substance abuse without penalizing them in the future when they adhere to clinic policies?
Accuracy (verifiable, valid, true, credible, undistorted)	• Through the collection step, including the patient pain assessment, what information gathered should I spend some extra time evaluating for clarity and accuracy? • What other deeper questions can I ask the patient to verify the information accuracy? • What other steps can I take to verify information provided or documented that could be considered inaccurate?
Precision (exact, specific, detailed)	• What are some proper questions that can be asked during the patient interview to obtain specific details regarding the pain experience, impact associated with the pain, use of medication, and potential side effects of medications? • While educating the patient, what level of detail should be provided to the patient? What format of education is appropriate for this particular patient (eg, handout, teach-back method)?

Depth (roots, fundamentals, complexities, interrelationships, cause/effect, implications)	• When assessing the patient's pain: what are the pain generators and what impact are they having on the patient's overall pain reports? • When considering treatment recommendations, what medical complexities must be considered when choosing proper therapy and dosing, and when considering potential side effects? • How are psychological and social factors impacting the overall pain experience?
Breadth (comprehensive, encompassing, alternative perspectives)	• What are the proper questions to ask to identify psychological impacts associated with the perception of pain? • Who are the stakeholders aside from the patient? Family members, caregivers? What providers are involved in this patient's care who can be impacted with changes to medication therapy?
Logic (reasonable, rational, without contradiction, well-founded, sound)	• How do I evaluate the logicalness of my hypotheses? • Have I worked to identify assumptions and address these accordingly? • What are the steps I need to take to evaluate my alternative explanations associated with the problems I am focusing on?

 KEY POINT

Utilizing critical thinking skills when managing patients who suffer from chronic pain is necessary to identify all important factors impacting the patient that can negatively or positively impact the perception of pain.

APPLICATION OF THE PHARMACISTS' PATIENT CARE PROCESS IN OUR PRACTICE

In the application of the Pharmacists' Patient Care Process (PPCP) for providing care to chronic pain patients referred to our clinic, the pharmacist begins by collecting information about the patient—first by chart review, then by patient interview. The patient interview will include a pain assessment and other assessments, such as a biopsychosocial assessment. From this collected information, a comprehensive patient assessment is completed in the Assess step. This comprehensive assessment serves as the basis for developing SMART goals with the patient, followed by the generation of viable treatment strategies from which the best multimodal treatment plan for the patient is created. In the ensuing implementation step, the treatment plan is effectively communicated to the patient and to other healthcare providers, and a proper monitoring and follow-up plan is developed and communicated.[6]

As mentioned, the process of patient care provided by pharmacists in our practice begins with the gathering of information about the patient. For deeper understanding of this Collect step, details are provided in the next section. This will be followed by a patient case review in which all PPCP steps will be elaborated with the clinical reasoning and critical thinking that can be employed by a pharmacist care-provider who engages in a systematic and deliberate clinical problem-solving process.

THE COLLECTION OF PATIENT INFORMATION IN OUR PRACTICE

The Collect process begins with a chart review that will serve as the basis for an effective patient interview. A complete chart review is vital to understand the complexities associated with chronic pain. This thorough review can include the following:

- Evaluation of recent history or physical examinations from PCPs and specialists
- Diagnostic information that can provide further insight on the pain generators that can be targets for nonpharmacological and pharmacological treatment recommendations
- Prior evaluations of the pain complaint(s) by providers
- Past treatment regimens used in an attempt to control pain-related issues
- Other related concerns associated with the treatment approach

 KEY POINT

Many patients have a very long history of chronic pain issues. Completing a very detailed history as part of the Collect process will help gain a better understanding of how chronic pain is impacting the patient physically, emotionally, and socially.

Table 2-2 provides a more complete listing of data that can be collected in preparation for a pain management MTM session along with the rationale for collecting the specified data.

TABLE 2-2

Examples of Data That Can Be Collected During Chart Review in Preparation for a Pain Management MTM Session[51]

Data to Collect During Chart Review	Rationale for Collecting Specific Data
Patient characteristics: age, weight, comorbidities, current lab results (eg, renal/hepatic function, basic metabolic panel, complete blood cell count)	Understanding dosing of medications and sensitivity to side effects can depend on several patient characteristics and lab results. The relevance of various lab results will vary based on the patient's comorbidities.
Etiology of pain; diagnosis associated with pain	Determining the type of pain the patient is experiencing (nociceptive/inflammatory, neuropathic, nociplastic) can help drive the treatment recommendations.
Imaging results, if available	Understanding of possible contributing factors associated with the pain reports can be improved with knowledge of imaging results.
Current and past medications used to treat pain (including all adjuvants)	A pharmacist must have a complete understanding of all medications the patient is currently taking, how the patient is taking them, adherence, and the possible side effects associated with the medications. Additionally, it is important to have a complete list of all medications that have been previously prescribed, the efficacy, any side effects, and reasons for discontinuation to identify if a possible re-challenge could be considered or if that treatment option is not a possibility due to the past effects.
Current and past nonpharmacological interventions used in managing pain	All nonpharmacological options currently in use or previously tried should be explored to identify the efficacy, side effects, and reasons for discontinuation. This can provide ideas for possible treatment options and also can rule out treatments that have previously been attempted.

Last date of referring-MD visit	If the patient is prescribed opioids for chronic pain, certain states require re-evaluation and confirmation of the treatment plan every 3 months. Documenting the last date of this visit will help ensure this requirement is met.
MD plans for treatment and goals of therapy	The pharmacist should verify the MD's plans for the treatment and goals of therapy if mentioned in the previous notes or in the referral to ensure the team is in alignment.
PDMP (Prescription Drug Monitoring Plan) fill history (if applicable)	The PDMP is a valuable resource to track the fill history of controlled substances. Checking the PDMP site is important with all patients even if controlled substances are not currently prescribed by the patient's particular office.
Urine drug screens: past results; review pattern of results, identify any concerns (if applicable)	Any past urine drug screens should be evaluated to identify any unexpected results. If there are unexpected results, further review should be completed to determine what steps were taken to verify the results. Identifying patterns can be helpful when completing risk mitigation.
Past pill count results, if available	Pill counts are utilized more commonly with controlled substances to help in monitoring adherence. Reviewing results of pill counts can help identify if there is a pattern that needs to be considered when developing a treatment plan.
ER visits: reason/frequency, was visit due to uncontrolled pain?	Reviewing the frequency and reasons for emergency room visits should be completed during a chart review. If the ER visits are related to chronic pain conditions, this could lead to important educational topics that can be covered with the patient to ensure proper utilization of the ER system and review possible self-management techniques that can be attempted if possible during a flare of a chronic pain condition.
Past medical history which could be a contributing factor to pain-related issues	Reviewing all past medical history will aid in identifying possible contributors to pain. Many diseases can be pain generators such as cancer, stroke, PVD, etc. It is important for the pharmacist to review the patient's current and past medical history and consider what could be contributing to the overall pain experience. Additionally, depression and anxiety are commonly seen in patients who suffer from chronic pain[2,4] and should be considered when reviewing this information as well.
If the patient is prescribed >50 mg oral morphine equivalents or taking an opioid with concomitant CNS depressants (eg, gabapentinoids, muscle relaxants, benzodiazepines, hypnotics): Naloxone history: • Active prescription written • Confirmation patient picked naloxone up from the pharmacy • Date of last naloxone prescription (within 1 to 2 years or time of product expiration)	It is important to consider naloxone if a patient is exposed to opioid therapy.[4] Screening the patient for risk of opioid-induced respiratory depression (OIRD) can help determine if the patient is a candidate of naloxone. If a prescription for naloxone has been provided to the patient, it is important to follow-up with the patient and verify the device has been obtained. Follow-up education on the proper use of the device and ensuring the device is within date are also important steps associated with the naloxone process.[4]

Insurance coverage	The pharmacist should be aware of the type of insurance coverage the patient has due to formulary concerns and overall prices of drugs. Copays for higher-tier drugs could be a barrier for patients and should be explored with the patient when discussing treatment plans.
Pharmacogenomic testing if available	Pharmacogenomic testing can prove beneficial when developing a treatment plan. Many of the medications utilized in the treatment of chronic pain are affected by metabolizing enzymes impacted by genetic variations.

With a thorough review of the patient chart completed, the pharmacist enters the MTM session well-equipped for an effective patient-centered interview that continues the Collect step. Part of this interview may include questions to strengthen or weaken the initial working hypotheses developed during the chart review. These can include hypotheses about potential causes for increased pain experiences, related contributing factors, and medication-related problems. In the process of testing these hypotheses through questioning, the pharmacist can gain a better perspective on the patient's perception of specific issues in question and can identify other hypotheses that need to be ruled out. Additionally, this is a time when the pharmacist may identify educational opportunities that can occur during the course of the interview.

 KEY POINT

There are many patient education opportunities that can arise during the PPCP. It is important pharmacists identify and use these opportunities effectively to improve the patient's understanding of important aspects of chronic pain and treatment options.

In addition to testing hypotheses made during the chart review, there are numerous other types of data to gather and common assessments to perform during the pain management MTM session with the patient. Many of these areas of inquiry are listed in **Table 2-3** and the interview will include inquiries about coexisting comorbidities, history of substance abuse, past or current treatment strategies, including medications, (prescription and over-the-counter), interventional treatments, complementary and integrative health strategies, psychological treatment, and nonpharmacological strategies. This comprehensive review of treatment strategies will allow the pharmacist to assess these areas in greater detail with the patient, thus gaining a better understanding of the treatment history, including efficacy, possible side effects, and reasons for discontinuation if applicable.

There is significant subjectivity of the pain experience and there are limits to the ability of objective data, such as laboratory values, in attaining a comprehensive assessment of the patient's pain experience.[20] Therefore, an important goal for interviews in chronic pain management is the collection of subjective information from the patient. To effectively acquire this information, it is important to develop a professional rapport with the patient at the onset of the interview, since topics covered during these assessments can become sensitive and uncomfortable.

TABLE 2-3

Patient Interview: Examples of Data That Can Be Collected During the Patient Interview

Patient's description of the following topics:
- Past injuries that could be contributing to the overall pain experience
- Current pain description
  - Duration
  - Intensity
  - Location
  - Description of pain sensations: nociceptive (eg, sharp, stabbing, dull, aching) vs neuropathic (eg, burning electrical) in nature
  - Pattern of pain
  - Cognitive impact from pain sensations

Assessment tools (not all-inclusive)
- Brief Pain Inventory (BPI) (available in long and short forms)[7,8]
- McGill Pain Questionnaire (MPQ)[9]

Pain assessment–related questions—pain ratings:
- At rest
- "good day" pain rating
- "bad day" pain rating
- "average" pain rating
- First thing in the morning
- One hour after taking pain medication

Assessment tool (not all-inclusive)
- Numerical rating scale (NRS)[10]
- Defense and Veterans Pain Rating Scale (DVPRS)[11]

Activity levels
- Typical day's activities
- Activities patient desires to increase if pain was not a limiting factor

Sleep quality
- Contributing factors to sleep interruption (eg, stress, nocturia, pain)
- Nap frequency during the day

Functional abilities
- Current abilities
- Goals to increase abilities (specific examples)

Assessment tool
- DoD/VA Pain Supplemental Questions[11]

Contributing factors to pain levels:
- Specific activities which increase pain experience
- Specific activities which improve overall pain experience
- Timing of pain-related experiences
- Current stress levels and approach to managing stress

Patient's perception of pain impact on current life
- Overall life satisfaction

Biopsychosocial assessment tools available to aid in assessment (not all-inclusive)
- Pain Self-Efficacy Scale (PSEQ)[12]
- Patient Health Questionnaire (PHQ-9)[13]
- Patient Health Questionnaire (PHQ-15)[14]
- Pain Catastrophizing Scale (PCS)[15]
- Adverse Childhood Events (ACE)[16]
- Generalized Anxiety Disorder (GHD-7)[17]
- STOP-BANG questionnaire for obstructive sleep apnea.[18]

Patient's goal for pain treatment
- Goal pain ratings
- Current functional abilities
- Functional improvement goals

Past and current nonpharmacological treatment approaches
- Effective nonpharmacological treatment strategies
- Ineffective nonpharmacological treatment strategies
  – Length of time treatment attempts were made

Risk mitigation
- Completion of the opioid risk assessment tool (ORT)[19]
- Further questions on substance use (current and past)
- If patient is currently using medical cannabis or cannabidiol (CBD)
  – Indication for use: medical or recreational?
  – Strength of cannabis or CBD currently used
    – %THC/CBD, how many mg
    – Strain(s) of THC
  – Route of cannabis (eg, oral, vaporized, smoked)
  – Route of CBD (eg, oral mucosal, vaporization, topical/transdermal, sublingual, ingestion)
  – Frequency of use
  – Perceived effectiveness for pain

Complete medication review:
- Current medications: indication, use pattern, missed doses, identified side effects, perceived efficacy
- Past medications used for pain (including adjuvants): indication, length of trial, dosing, reasons for discontinuation
- Insurance coverage, access issues, copayment costs
- Pharmacogenomic information if available

Naloxone (if applicable)
- Confirm patient has the devices
- Confirm where patient stores the devices
- Review patient's understanding of the purpose of naloxone, proper use of naloxone, and family member/caregiver training on proper use of the naloxone device
- Expiration date of current naloxone devices

 KEY POINT

In pain management, much of the information collected is very subjective. Therefore, it is important for the pharmacist to build an effective professional rapport with the patient to help assure the information collected is complete and accurate.

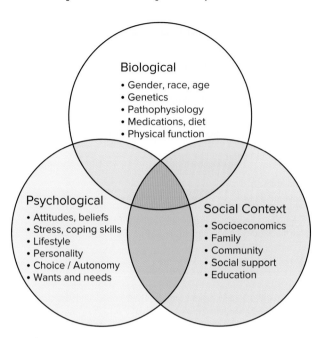

FIGURE 2-1. The biopsychosocial model of health.

There will be various assessments also performed during the Collect step. One of the assessments will be a comprehensive pain assessment, where it is suggested to complete this assessment using a biopsychosocial approach. (See **Figure 2-1.**) Due to the complexity of chronic pain, the biopsychosocial model has proven effective in developing a multipronged approach to improving overall function and quality of life (QOL). This model focuses on all aspects of the patient, recognizing the biological, psychological, and social factors associated with the chronic pain experience.[21] This is emphasized in the Pain Management Best Practices Inter-Agency Task Force Report: "a critical part of providing comprehensive care is a thorough initial evaluation, including assessment of both the medical and the probable biopsychosocial factors causing or contributing to a pain condition."[4]

 KEY POINT

The experience of chronic pain can impact all aspects of a patient's life. Utilizing the biopsychosocial approach while assessing a patient can help the pharmacist better understand how the patient is impacted by chronic pain.

This background knowledge of chronic pain management MTM and our practice is applied below with an in-depth analysis of a fictitious case of a patient presenting with osteoarthritic knee pain and current conditions. This analysis will illustrate the reasoning that occurs during each PPCP step and will demonstrate how critical thinking can be applied to optimize the reasoning process in each step. The primary goal of this analysis is to enable the reader to grasp how the PPCP, clinical reasoning, and critical thinking can combine to optimize patient-centered care.

The Case of Catherine T.: Overview

Catherine T. is a 76-year-old female who presents to the primary care clinic with a chief complaint of bilateral knee pain. She reports she has had knee pain over the last 2 years, but the pain seems to have worsened over the last 6 months. The only treatment she has tried to control her knee pain includes over-the-counter (OTC) naproxen, which resulted in stomach pain after taking one tablet twice daily for 2 weeks. After experiencing this side effect, she has been hesitant to take any medications before obtaining approval from her doctor. She mentions that she has tried some ice therapy on both knees when the pain was high. Her PCP evaluated her today and confirmed her pain is due to OA of both knees and has completed the comprehensive patient assessment. Medical management is indicated. She has been referred to the clinical pharmacy services for evaluation of her current medications and development of a new treatment regimen to manage her bilateral knee pain secondary to OA.

Current pain rating (DoD pain assessment scale): 7/10 Low: 5/10 High: 10/10 three to four times a week. Goal: 2/10

Activity: The patient reports her activity continues to decrease as her pain increases. She explains she was working part-time at a library 3 times a week, but this has decreased to no more than once per week since pain levels prevent her from leaving the house. Current Activities of Daily Living (ADLs): doing dishes, general housework. She visits family when possible but since her pain has worsened, she has found she has decreased her social interactions, including family visits. The patient admits her lifestyle has become progressively more sedentary over the last 2 years as her pain has worsened.

Sleep quality: Insomnia has been a problem since she was young but worsened when her husband passed away 3 years ago. She cannot adjust to sleeping in the bed alone and the feelings of loneliness and sadness are heightened at night. She discussed this with her PCP, and he had her complete a screening tool for depression that indicated she had mild depression. Her doctor told her he will continue to monitor her depression, but no medications have been initiated. She has noticed her mood and insomnia have also worsened as her activities have decreased over the last few years due to her limitations associated with her severe knee pain. Her knee pain has worsened her insomnia causing her to awaken several times a night, as she finds it difficult to find a comfortable position and turning in her sleep leads to sharp stabbing pain in both of her knees.

Diet: She admits her diet is poor, consisting of mainly carbohydrates and fast food with limited fruit and vegetables.

Past Medical History:

Hypertension × 30 years (controlled) based on recent blood pressure readings in flowchart in EMR

Mild Depression (not treated)

Chronic Insomnia (not treated)

GERD (controlled)

Allergic Rhinitis (controlled)

Bilateral knee pain (OA) (not controlled)

Type 2 DM (controlled)

Obesity

Last emergency room visit due to pain conditions: No ER visits recently
Insurance Coverage: Medicare

CLINICAL REASONING, CRITICAL THINKING, AND THE PPCP FOR THE CARE OF CATHERINE T.

The following series of tables delineates the PPCP as it is applied for the provision of pharmacy care to Catherine T. (CT). For each step, from Collect to Monitor, there is a description of the pharmacist's clinical reasoning along with examples of how the critical thinking standards can be applied to optimize the pharmacist's clinical reasoning. Clinical reasoning is described in terms of the conclusions drawn along with case information or premises on which the conclusions are based. Critical thinking intellectual standards are expressed in the form of past-tense statements, instead of the question format introduced in Chapter 1. This is because the case analysis was performed in *reflection* upon the clinical encounter. An exception to this past-tense format of critical thinking statements is with the Collect step, where the future tense is used to illustrate how the standards can be applied in *preparation* for the clinical encounter. As a reminder, the critical thinking standards are embodied in the mnemonic Clear ROAD for Logic. They are clarity, relevance, significance, objectivity, fairness, accuracy, precision, depth, breadth, and logic.

Collect

In this step, the pharmacist collects the subjective and objective information about the patient in order to understand the relevant medical and medication history and clinical status of the patient. This will include information from the chart review conducted by the pharmacist in preparation for the MTM session and verified with the patient during the session. It will also include assessments, such as a pain assessment, performed by the pharmacist during the session.

COLLECT: Current Medications and Immunizations	
Conclusions	Rationale: Information or Premise to Support the Conclusion
Perform a full and complete medication review with the patient during the pain management consult. *(Collected during the chart review and the interview)* Match each medication with its indication. Evaluate efficacy and any current side effects and drug interactions. Verify adherence to each medication.	• Though the focus will be on the pain regimen during this visit, it is vital the pharmacist has a good understanding of the complete medication regimen • Confirming the indication with each medication can help identify any medications that might not be indicated any longer or can identify possible duplications of therapy. • Identifying possible drug–drug interactions or possible side effects is a fundamental role of pharmacists, as are the determination of adherence patterns and any barrier to adherence. • A thorough medication review can also help uncover any other drug therapy problems.
During the medication review for each medication, reinforce with the patient the indication and purpose, proper dosing and use, and possible side effects that can occur.	• Reinforcing medication purpose and use with the patient can be a great help to improve overall adherence and the patient's understanding of the entire treatment regimen.

Determine if immunizations are up-to-date. *(Collected during the chart review)*	• It is important to assure that the patient's immunization status is up-to-date to ensure she is protected. This is especially true for elderly patients who may be at greater risk for complications and morbidity associated with preventable infections.

Critical Thinking Checks for the Collect Plan for This Patient's Current Immunizations and Medications

In the medication review for this patient, it will be important to collect information with sufficient **accuracy** and **precision** that will enable me to draw sound conclusions on medication effectiveness, safety, and adherence, and any barriers negatively impacting the patient's medication use experience.

As optimizing medication use is an essential part of my practice, it will be critical in our discussion of medications that I **clearly** understand the patient and that she clearly understands me.

Given that the patient has several medical conditions and takes several medications, it will be important for me to think **deeply** as we discuss her medication usage, so that I can gather the information needed for me to grasp the complexity of her medication experience.

 KEY POINT

It is vital the pharmacist reviews and explores all aspects of the entire medication profile, not just the medications associated with chronic pain.

Collected Current Medication and Immunization Information Entered into Health Record

Current medication regimen:
- Loratadine 10 mg po daily; Indication: seasonal allergies; The patient takes daily; no ADRs
- Lisinopril 10 mg po daily; Indication: hypertension (controlled); The patient takes daily; no ADRs
- Omeprazole 20 mg po daily; Indication: GERD (controlled); The patient takes daily; no ADRs
- Metformin 500 mg po bid; Indication: Diabetes (controlled); The patient takes bid; minor GI ADRs (gas) but patient takes as prescribed

Current immunizations:
Influenza vaccine: up-to-date
Pneumococcal vaccine: up-to-date
Zoster vaccine: completed

COLLECT: Allergies, Vitals, Labs

Conclusions	Rationale: Information or Premise to Support the Conclusion
Verify the patient's allergy status. When entering any allergies into the system, report specific effects that the patient experienced. *(Collected during the chart review and the interview)*	Verifying all allergies on a regular basis is an important step for patient safety. Additionally, providing specific information regarding the allergic reaction will help in assessing if this is a true allergy or a drug intolerance.

Collect the patient's current vital signs, height, weight, and pertinent labs. *(Collected during the chart review and the interview)*	• Reviewing the vital signs during the visit can identify if further follow-up with the patient's PCP is needed for concerns such as elevated blood pressure. Some patients experiencing high levels of pain could exhibit elevated heart rate, respiratory rate, and possibly blood pressure. However, many patients who have chronic pain will not demonstrate changes in vital signs caused by higher pain levels.[22] • Monitoring the weight of patients with OA can be vital for the progress and care of their condition. For example, even a 5% weight loss can help improve overall pain associated with OA.[23] Also, certain medications used in chronic pain management have been associated with weight gain, which would be an additional reason for weight monitoring. • Reviewing pertinent labs based on comorbidities and current medications is important to identify any dosing concerns or other problems that can occur with certain medications such as elevated liver enzymes or reduced kidney function.
If a patient is diabetic, it is important to focus on the diabetes control by evaluating the current A1C. *(Collected during the chart review)*	• Patients who have diabetes are at risk of developing painful diabetic peripheral neuropathy, which can contribute to the overall pain presentation.[24] • This is also an excellent opportunity to reinforce the importance of proper blood sugar control through exercise, diet, and adherence to her diabetes medication to reduce risks of micro- and macrovascular complications.[24]

 KEY POINT

Clearly documenting all information regarding allergies, including specific reactions is needed to help healthcare providers determine if the reported allergy is a true allergy or an adverse drug reaction.

Critical Thinking Checks for the Collect Plan for This Patient's Allergies, Vitals, and Labs

When gathering information on allergies, it will be important for me to obtain **precise** descriptions in order to accurately determine the true nature of the patient's response to the medications.

The **relevant** information I should collect includes the patient's weight, due to its potential impact on OA and its care, and its relationship to comorbid conditions. Relevant labs include those related to liver and kidney function due to their potential impact on medication disposition.

Collected Allergies, Vitals, and Labs Information Entered into Health Record

Allergies: PCN: Hives

Adhesive Tape: Hives

Vitals: BP: 132/83 P: 74 R: 18 Temp: 98.6°F

Labs: Comprehensive Metabolic Profile (CMP): WNL

CrCl: 64 mL/min

A1C: 6.8%

Weight: 196 lbs

Height: 64 in

COLLECT: Social History

Conclusions	Rationale: Information or Premise to Support the Conclusion
Complete a full social history of the patient. *(Collected during the interview)*	When considering the biopsychosocial model, we need to collect psychosocial information from the patient, which includes personal living situations, health behaviors, and personal choices. Low socioeconomic status can be a contributing factor for chronic pain conditions such as chronic low back pain.[4] Examples of social factors that can be collected include: • Marital status • Current employment status/history • Living environment • Financial stability/concerns • Well-being of self, family • Education history • Hobbies • Dietary habits • Exercise habits • Usual ADLs
Collect information about patient's occupation. *(Collected during the chart review and the interview)*	Factors associated with the patient's current or past occupation can be possible contributing factors to painful conditions. For example, development of OA can be attributed to repetitive movements through various occupations and activities.[25]
Collect information on who lives with the patient. *(Collected during the interview)*	Evaluating a patient's perception of social interactions can help evaluate the patient's loneliness and social isolation. Both of these factors have been demonstrated to have a relationship with musculoskeletal pain.[26] Additionally, initiation of certain medications that are commonly known to cause CNS side effects could increase fall risk, which needs to be considered at all times but especially if a patient lives alone.
Collect information on substance use. *(Collected during the chart review and the interview)* This includes past and present use of tobacco, alcohol, and illicit substances. If currently used, determine frequency and quantity of use. *(Collected during the chart review and the interview)*	Substance use can have a negative impact on overall health. Additionally, if opioids are part of the treatment plan or are being considered, it is important to screen the patient for current or past substance use as part of the risk mitigation strategy.[27]

Critical Thinking Checks for the Collect Plan for This Patient's Social History

Information to gather that may be **significant** for evaluating this patient includes potential catastrophizing information, psychosocial contributing factors to her pain experience and effects of her pain on psychosocial factors, information about her other conditions and medications (indications, safety, efficacy, and adherence), and substance use.

To gather the most **accurate** information needed to optimize my reasoning, **clear** communication with the patient will be critical. This includes communicating with vocabulary that the patient understands, verifying understanding, and asking questions as needed to clarify what the patient is communicating.

Given the potential sensitivity of information obtained for social history, it will be important for me to maintain a presence that will **fairly** respect her autonomy, encourage open communication, encourage her participation in her care, and will enable the gathering of information needed to help me clearly and comprehensively understand her wants and needs.

To maintain **fairness** in our interaction, I must remain alert to any biases that might potentially influence my gathering of information.

Collected Social History Information Entered into Health Record

Social History:

+Tobacco 1 ppd × 60 years; the patient voices no interest in smoking cessation treatment or reducing her smoking at this time

Denies current ETOH or history of abuse

Denies current or past illicit substance use

Widowed ×3 years; CT lives alone, 1 son lives nearby, visits infrequently.

Retired

Dietary habits: skips breakfast, admits to limited fruits/vegetables, commonly eats TV dinners since it is difficult to cook for one person

Limited exercise; walking limited distances as tolerated

COLLECT: Pain Assessment

Conclusions	Rationale: Information or Premise to Support the Conclusion
Perform a thorough pain assessment Examples areas to inquire about pain ratings when the pain is high, when pain is at its lowest level, pain ratings before taking pain medications and 1 h after taking medications, pain levels before and after a typical activity. *(Collected during interview)*	Assessing the patient's pain is critical for pain evaluation and all aspects of management. Asking the patient to rate her current pain level is a start but inquiring more deeply into the pain level ratings is important for understanding the full pain experience.
Collect information on what provokes the patient's pain and how the patient treats her pain when the pain ratings are high, and also evaluate the effectiveness of these approaches. *(Collected during interview)*	Identifying what provokes the pain and what the patient finds is effective in relieving pain can also be critical for pain evaluation and all aspects of management.

Critical Thinking Checks for the Collect Plan for This Patient's Pain Assessment

For fully assessing the patient's pain experience, it is important to ascertain with good **accuracy** and **precision** the patient's reported pain experience under a **broad** array of conditions.

Collected Pain Assessment Information Entered into Health Record

Pain Assessment Information:

(Completing a full pain assessment during this visit will occur during the Collect step of the PPCP. There are many aspects of the pain assessment the pharmacist should focus on)

- Current pain rating (DoD pain assessment scale): 7/10 Low: 5/10 High: 10/10 three to four times a week. Goal: 2/10
- DoD pain supplemental questions
  - Activity: 8/10
  - Sleep: 10/10
  - Mood: 7/10
  - Stress: 9/10
- Pain is described as a stabbing sensation especially when walking or moving after periods of rest. Aching sensation occurs during rest, especially at night.

COLLECT: Biopsychosocial Assessment

Conclusions	Rationale: Information or Premise to Support the Conclusion
Evaluate the social and economic impacts the patient has experienced with her limitations from her chronic pain. *(Collected during interview)*	Inability to fully participate in social activities and work because of pain can have significant negative impacts on a patient's QOL and pain experience. The result can be social isolation and reduced financial independence.
Collect information on the negative effects of her pain on her functioning and QOL and also on her coping strategies for managing pain-related issues. *(Collected during interview)*	Chronic pain can have devastating negative impacts on a patient's QOL, sleep patterns, and overall activity.[28] Developing proper coping mechanisms can improve a patient's overall perception of pain.
Identify any catastrophizing statements voiced during the interview. *(Collected during interview)*	Catastrophizing has been shown to amplify the pain experience and increase the sense of suffering and translates into a higher perception of pain.[22]
Collect information about the patient's depression. *(Collected during the chart review and the interview)*	Depression and pain can be mutually impactful to each other. Furthermore, there are adjuvant medications that treat pain and depression. Thus, it is important to characterize the patient's depression, its control, and the PCP's therapy plan.

Critical Thinking Checks for the Collect Plan for This Patient's Biopsychosocial Assessment

In conducting this patient's biopsychosocial assessment, I must communicate in a way that she **clearly** understands me and I clearly understand her. I must communicate with vocabulary that she understands, verify her understanding, and ask her questions as needed to clarify what she is communicating.

Information for which **accuracy** and **precision** is critical includes the patient's pain reports, pain impact on ADLs, and current treatment approach (in order to understand its impact on the patient and to make an inference that her reported pain is not well controlled on current regimen).

In conducting a biopsychosocial assessment, in **fairness** to this patient, it will be important for me to maintain a presence in a way that respects her autonomy, encourages open communication, encourages her participation in care, suspends premature judgment, and enables me to clearly and comprehensively understand her wants and needs.

Collected Biopsychosocial Assessment Information Entered into Health Record

Biopsychosocial Assessment:

A common assessment suggested to identify the global personal effects of chronic pain is the biopsychosocial aspect. The biopsychosocial assessment focuses not only on the biological aspects of pain, but focuses on the psychological and social impacts.

Information obtained from our patient CT during the initial interview:

Biological:

Bilateral knee pain is not well controlled on her current regimen (ice therapy prn) as evidenced by current pain rating 7/10 (range 5/10 on good days, 10/10 on bad days, which occur three to four times a week). Pain is negatively impacting her QOL, ADLs, and social interactions. Sedentary lifestyle and poor diet have contributed to her obesity, which can also contribute to her elevated pain levels and progression of OA.

Treatment regimen:

She is not currently taking any medications for her pain. However, she did report a trial of naproxen resulted in increased GERD symptoms.

Ice therapy: Applies ice therapy to both knees when pain is elevated and limiting ADLs.

Psychological:

Catherine T. shares during the visit that she continues to struggle with the loss of her husband. She has discussed this with her PCP resulting in a screening for depression. A diagnosis of mild depression has been listed in chart and the treatment plan indicates the PCP is currently monitoring her symptoms and no pharmacological treatment has been initiated. Depression can negatively impact her perception of pain and a worsening pain experience could contribute to worsening depression symptoms.[4]

Social:

Activities are decreasing secondary to bilateral knee pain. Part-time work at the library has decreased from three times a week to once weekly. Her son lives close by but her frequency of visiting her son and his family have decreased over the last few years. She attributes this to her difficulty in ambulating secondary to bilateral knee pain. It is clear her social activities have been negatively impacted by her bilateral knee pain.

COLLECT: Pain Treatment History	
Conclusions	Rationale: Information or Premise to Support the Conclusion
Collect information related to the patient's experience with physical therapy (PT). Inquire how long she attended the PT sessions and if she continues to do the exercises. *(Collected during interview)*	There are many times a patient will report attending one or two PT sessions and then stop due to increasing pain from the therapy or perceived lack of progress. Increased soreness following these sessions is common as the exercises include utilizing muscles that might have been sedentary for an extended period. However, the benefits associated with the therapy can be substantial since it can improve overall conditioning over time. This presents an excellent counseling opportunity, since a better general description of what can be gained from PT can improve the chances of the patient completing the PT regimen and help the patient meet treatment goals.
Collect information that may help identify potential barriers to optimal medical care. *(Collected during the interview)*	There are many potential barriers to optimal medical care, including financial difficulties that can decrease adherence to appointments and purchasing medications, limited transportation options leading to missed appointments and inability to pick up medications, and limited mobility due to pain-related issues that again can result in missed appointments and medication adherence issues. Pharmacists must screen for barriers and develop solutions to overcome them.
Complete a full assessment of previous pharmacological pain management regimens. *(Collected during interview)*	There may be past medications used for pain by the patient that may have worked or failed. Characterizing this medication experience can be valuable for therapeutic planning. For example, inquiring on why a patient stopped a previous medication can provide insight into drug intolerances. Additionally, identifying the starting and ending doses of the medication can help identify possible root causes of drug intolerances (eg, starting dose too high, rapid titration of dose) or it can be used to determine if improper proper target dosing was the source of a drug's ineffectiveness.
Complete an assessment of current and past nonpharmacological approaches to pain management, including interventional and complementary approaches. *(Collected during interview)*	Complementary and interventional approaches to pain management may have been utilized by patients. These will have varying levels of effectiveness and impact on the overall pain management strategy. It is important to collect information about these approaches, including duration of treatment, immediate effects, and extended effects, to help determine if options should be discarded and what other options can be considered.

Critical Thinking Checks for the Collect Plan for This Patient's Pain Treatment History

Obtaining a pain treatment history will be critical for me to ascertain the patient's medication experience and for optimal therapeutic decision-making. Therefore, it will be essential for me to communicate **clearly,** communicating with vocabulary that the patient understands, verifying understanding, and asking questions as needed to clarify what the patient is communicating.

To obtain the most **accurate** information during the interview, it will also be important for me to act in **fairness** in a way that respects her autonomy, encourages her open communication, and encourages her participation in care.

Pain management is multidimensional. Therefore, it will be important to gain a **broad** understanding of the relevant contributions of other professionals involved in the patient's care.

Collected Pain Treatment History Information Entered into Health Record

Pain Treatment History:

Repeat PT referral has been placed. Patient was discharged from PT 6 months ago due to three no-show appointments. Patient reports she had transportation difficulties.

Past pharmacological treatments for pain: Naproxen (OTC) × 2 weeks: treatment resulted in stomach pain.

No history of interventional pain management approaches in the past

Patient reports she applies ice therapy to both knees when pain is elevated and limiting ADLs.

Example Collect Statement for Catherine T.

CT is a 76-year-old female who presents for pain management evaluation, reporting uncontrolled chronic bilateral knee pain with a confirmed diagnosis of OA. She is reporting pain levels that average 7/10 and range from 5/10 on good days to 10/10 on bad days, occurring three to four times per week. Pain is described as a stabbing sensation especially when walking or moving after periods of rest. Aching sensation occurs during rest, especially at night. Bad days occur approximately three to four times per week and pain increases with increased activity and movement after periods of rest longer than 30 to 60 minutes. Activity levels continue to decrease due to the higher pain levels. She previously was volunteering at the local library 3 times a week but now she is only able to tolerate volunteering one time a week due to high of levels pain. Sleep quality is rated as poor, waking up on average three times per night. She attributes her higher pain levels to the pain associated with OA of bilateral knees. However, she mentions her overall deconditioning and obesity due to poor diet and sedentary lifestyle are contributing to her overall pain levels. She is hoping that attending PT sessions will increase her strength and mobility; however, she struggles with transportation availability, so she is worried about attending multiple appointments. She also verbalizes that smoking could be worsening her pain as well although at this time she is not interested in smoking cessation treatment options nor reducing her current smoking. She reports a short trial of OTC naproxen to help control her pain. However, she discontinued this due to an increase in GERD symptoms when taking this agent. Currently, she reports she has not been taking any medications to help control her knee pain since she was waiting on this appointment with her doctor. She has been using ice treatments via bags of ice wrapped in a towel for 15 minutes when needed to help improve mobility approximately 2 times daily. She reports an allergy to adhesive tape and penicillin, both of which cause hives. Medical conditions include hypertension (controlled), Type 2 DM (controlled), allergic rhinitis (controlled), depression (not controlled), insomnia (not controlled), and GERD (controlled). Current labs are WNL. Prescription drug monitoring plan (PDMP) review is appropriate. Urine drug screen: No test on file. No history of drug or alcohol-related arrests. No aberrant drug behavior identified in chart review. Smoking 1 ppd × 60 years. No record of a controlled substance agreement on file.

Assessment of Collected Information

During the Assess step, the pharmacist reviews all subjective and objective information obtained during the Collect step to provide the best explanation of the patient's current health status. During this time, it is important to understand what type of conclusions you are working toward and to recognize how the information collected is related to the perception of pain control and the impact of pain on the patient's QOL and ADL. Many of the various healthcare concerns can be directly impacting each other and it is important to understand these dynamics when working to develop a proper treatment regimen for this patient. It is vital to use critical thinking standards during this step to ensure a full and complete assessment of the patient's situation. (See Table 1–1 and Chapter 1.) When assessing each current medical condition, it is important to consider the impact of other conditions, other medications, related patient treatment goals, and the patient's overall perception of pain. Additionally, completing a full medication review, ensuring each medication listed is linked to a current health-related problem, and making note of unnecessary drug therapy are important. Each medication should be assessed for efficacy, the patient's adherence patterns, current side effects, and any concerns the patient might have regarding each medication. Examples of patient concerns can include the cost of the medication, the dosing frequency, or administration problems such as difficulties swallowing large capsules. As the pharmacist focuses on the pain medication regimen, the assessment should include a review of previously prescribed medications and reasons for discontinuation. This full medication review provides the pharmacist with a more complete history when identifying drug therapy problems along with their contributing factors and their order of priority.

 KEY POINT

All healthcare issues identified in the collect phase must be assessed to determine what direct or indirect impact they can have on the patient's chronic pain.

 KEY POINT

Although using a numerical rating scale to assess pain is a start, it is very important for the pharmacist to ask detailed questions to assess all aspects of the pain the patient is currently experiencing.

ASSESS: Osteoarthritic Bilateral Knee Pain	
Conclusions	**Rationale: Information or Premise to Support the Conclusion**
Uncontrolled osteoarthritic bilateral knee pain	Reported pain ratings include average of 7/10, 5/10 on good days to 10/10 on bad days (three to four times a week). Goal pain rating: 2/10 along with improved QOL with better pain control. Activity levels have decreased as her ability to volunteer has decreased to 1 time per week in contrast to the three times weekly prior to pain escalation. She has become more sedentary and overall deconditioning has worsened. DoD pain supplemental questions demonstrate negative impact on overall QOL:
	Activity: 8/10; Sleep: 10/10; Mood: 7/10; Stress: 9/10
The patient has multiple contributing factors to her uncontrolled pain, including the following: inadequate pain management approach, poor diet, sedentary lifestyle, lack of transportation, nonadherence to PT or PT-based exercise routine, poor sleep quality, patient weight, smoking.	Patient currently only uses ice therapy to treat pain. Patient reports poor diet along with sedentary lifestyle, and pain interference with activity rating 8/10 on DVPRS supplemental questions. Patient has attended PT in the past but is not currently doing prescribed exercises. Lack of transportation options limits CT's ability to attend PT sessions. Sleep quality is reported as poor, rated 10/10 via DVPRS supplemental questions, which can contribute to worsening perception of overall pain control and pain-related outcomes.[29] Patient indicates pain has significantly affected her mood (7/10) and stress levels (9/10).
	Patient's current weight (196 lb); height 64 in. BMI: 33.6, which is considered Class 2 Obesity, which can worsen OA and subsequently increase OA-related pain leading to decreased QOL.[30] The patient is also smoking 1 ppd, which can also contribute to progression of OA and worsen overall pain.[30]

Critical Thinking Checks for Assessing This Patient's Osteoarthritic Bilateral Knee

To evaluate this patient's pain properly, it was needed to gather and fully consider all **relevant** and **significant** information needed, including her pain levels, her other conditions, therapeutic approaches, and their outcomes.

It was also necessary to assure that the **accuracy** and precision of this **information** was sufficient to support accurate reasoning.

Given the number of comorbid conditions, medications, and contributing factors to this patient's pain experience, a great **depth** of thought was needed to determine their relevance, significance, and interrelationships to fully explain their impact on her overall health and medication-related problems

To be **fair** and **objective**, it was important to be aware of potential biases for their negative impact on reasoning in this scenario, including framing, groupthink, implicit bias (weight, age, smoking history), and confirmation bias. I have objectively evaluated this information and formed conclusions without influence of my emotions or biases.

ASSESS: Depression, Insomnia, and Type 2 Diabetes	
Conclusions	**Rationale: Information or Premise to Support the Conclusion**
Uncontrolled mild depression with the following contributing factors: chronic pain, reduced QOL, reduced function, the passing of her husband 3 years ago, limited social interactions, and worsening insomnia.	Recent PCP note indicates patient completed a screening tool, which indicated mild depression. The patient is currently not prescribed an antidepressant. Chronic pain and the consequent negative impact on the patient's function and QOL may contribute to the patient's depression.[4,28] Other potential contributing factors include the loss of her husband 3 years ago, limited social interactions, and worsening insomnia.
Uncontrolled insomnia with the following potential contributing factors: pain, decreased activity levels, and depression	Patient reports chronic insomnia symptoms since childhood. However, symptoms have worsened. Worsening pain, worsening depression, decreased activity levels, and depression can have a negative impact on insomnia.[4,28]
Controlled Type II Diabetes	Hemoglobin A1C is currently 6.8%. Based on patient's current age and health status, her hemoglobin A1C goal is <7.0% to 7.5%, which translates into fasting and preprandial glucose levels averaging between 154 and 169 mg/dL.[31]

 KEY POINT

Chronic pain can result in a negative impact on the patient's overall activity and QOL, which could result in worsening depression symptoms.

Critical Thinking Checks for Assessing This Patient's Past Medical History

The information that I have was adequately **precise** to effectively draw conclusions about the patient's medical problems.

I have been thorough in summarizing all known contributing factors **significant** to the patient's medical problems.

In forming my conclusions, I have thought **deeply** by considering the interrelationships between the different medical conditions and my assessment of this patient's medical problems adequately address their complexity.

ASSESS: Drug Therapy Problems	
Conclusions	**Rationale: Information or Premise to Support the Conclusion**
Adverse Drug Reaction: Intolerance to naproxen	Worsening GERD symptoms began shortly after beginning a short trial of naproxen (220 mg po bid ×2 weeks) and they resolved shortly after its discontinuation. Other potential explanations for the worsening GERD symptoms include her obesity and cigarette smoking. However, these factors were stable at that time. In addition, she reported she has remained adherent to her omeprazole. There were no other identified new contributing factors that could have exacerbated GERD symptoms at that time.

Needs Additional Therapy: Pharmacological and nonpharmacological treatment indicated for OA-related pain	The patient has uncontrolled bilateral knee pain with multiple contributing factors and with no consistent therapeutic strategies other than ice therapy, which is inadequate on its own to manage this patient's pain.

 KEY POINT

It is important for the pharmacist to always assess all reactions to medications and identify even mild side effects since this could impact the patient's adherence to current medications.

Critical Thinking Checks for Assessing This Patient's Drug Therapy Problems

Before concluding that intolerance to naproxen was the likely cause of the patient's worsening GERD symptoms, other plausible hypotheses were considered. Compared to the competing hypotheses, naproxen usage had a stronger **logical** support for being the cause of the worsening GERD symptoms.

My assessment is expressed with sufficient **clarity, accuracy, and precision** to properly support the planning and implementation of therapeutic strategies and to be understood by other stakeholders.

ASSESS: Fall Risk Assessment

Conclusions	Rationale: Information or Premise to Support the Conclusion
Prevention assessment: Increased fall risk with the following contributing factors: bilateral knee pain, deconditioning due to reduced physical activity, inadequate PT due to inadequate transportation for keeping PT appointments	Fall risk assessment: Bilateral knee pain secondary to OA has decreased overall activity leading to further deconditioning. Because of unreliable transportation to attend PT sessions, she has not been engaging in strengthening exercises that could improve her condition. Fall risk due to deconditioning is possible. A general health risk assessment can identify other high-risk healthcare needs.

 KEY POINT

When pharmacists are working with older adults, assessing fall risk due to medications and other potential risk factors is very important.

Critical Thinking Checks for Assessing This Patient's Fall-Risk

In assessing this patient's fall risk, the most **significant** contributing factors to the patient's fall risk were identified and will be considered when developing and evaluating therapeutic alternatives.

Upon reviewing the patient's current medical history, it is important to understand how each of these conditions is related to pain management and the possible impact on each condition if not controlled. Considerations could include how each condition can impact the perception of pain, activity levels, or medication selections. During the patient interview, the pharmacist must work to gather more details regarding each of these disease states to fully understand the interrelatedness of each condition and their impact on her QOL.

ASSESS: Past Medical History	
Conclusions	**Rationale: Information or Premise to Support the Conclusion**
Hypertension: Currently controlled	Blood pressure readings provided in the EMR indicate a BP below target of <140/90.[31] Blood pressure control could be negatively impacted with an addition of an NSAID.[32,33]
GERD: Currently controlled	Based on information obtained during the patient's interview her symptoms associated with GERD are currently controlled. However, past history of a systemic NSAID (naproxen) exacerbated this condition and symptoms resolved upon discontinuation of the NSAID. A rechallenge with a nonselective NSAID could again lead to increased symptoms of GERD.
Depression: Mild depression diagnosed by PCP; no current treatment	Information gathered from the prior PCP note indicates the patient has been diagnosed with mild depression. Upon completion of medication reconciliation, it was determined CT is not taking an antidepressant at this time. Depression is commonly interrelated with insomnia and pain. The triad of these conditions can exacerbate each other when not treated.[4,34,35]
Insomnia: Currently uncontrolled and not treated	Information obtained from patient interview: Chronic insomnia symptoms since she was young. However, symptoms worsened following her husband's death 3 years ago. Insomnia has worsened with increased pain.

Critical Thinking Checks for Assessing This Patient's Past Medical History
Given that the patient has multiple conditions and medications that can potentially impact each other, and many potential contributing factors to these conditions, it was important to consider sufficiently **broad** information needed to evaluate interrelationships that will enable a **deep** understanding of the complexity of the patient's health, which will be important for therapeutic planning.

Given the complexity of this patient, who has several conditions and is taking several medications, it can be useful to create a concept map to help grasp some of the interrelationships that contribute to the complexity. (See **Figure 2-2.**) Understanding these interrelationships can be useful to create a comprehensive assessment of this patient, which is expressed in the Assess statement below.

Example Assess Statement for Catherine T.

CT is a 76-year-old female presenting for a pain management evaluation for her uncontrolled, chronic bilateral knee pain with a confirmed diagnosis of OA.

(1) Uncontrolled bilateral knee pain leading to decreased function, quality of sleep, and QOL.

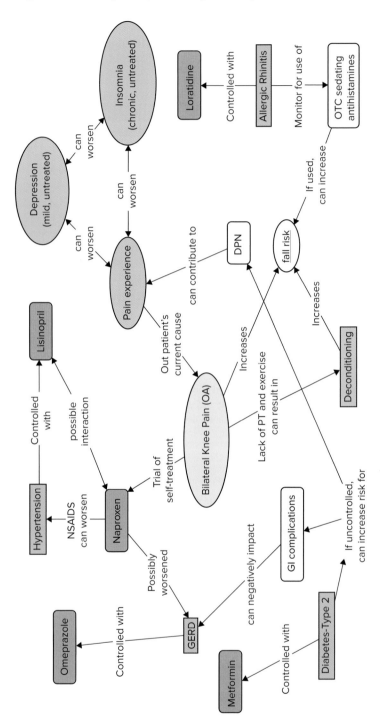

FIGURE 2-2. Concept map illustrating the interrelationships of CT's medications and conditions.

Reported pain ratings include average of 7/10, 5/10 on good days to 10/10 on bad days (three to four times a week). Goal pain rating: 2/10 along with improved QOL with better pain control. The patient currently only uses ice therapy to treat pain. A short trial of naproxen resulted in an ADR: worsening GERD symptoms, which resolved upon discontinuation of naproxen. The patient reports poor diet along with sedentary lifestyle and pain interference with activity rating 8/10 on DVPRS supplemental questions. The patient has attended PT in the past but is not currently doing prescribed exercises. Lack of transportation options limits the patient's ability to attend PT sessions. Sleep quality is reported as poor, rated 10/10 via DVPRS supplemental questions, which can contribute to worsening perception of overall pain control.[11] Patient indicates pain has significantly affected her mood (7/10) and stress levels (9/10).

Patient's current weight (196 lb) and height 64 in. BMI: 33.6, which is considered Class 2 Obesity, which can worsen OA and subsequently increase OA-related pain, leading to decreased QOL.[36]

The patient is currently smoking 1 ppd × 60 years. The patient is not interested in smoking cessation at this time (precontemplation stage). Cigarette smoking has been shown to increase pain intensity, which can translate into decreased ADLs and QOL.[30] Continued education on the health improvements of smoking cessation is indicated.

(2) Uncontrolled mild depression and insomnia: Currently not treated but under current monitoring by PCP. Depression and insomnia could be worsened by uncontrolled pain.[34,35]

(3) Controlled Type 2 Diabetes: Hemoglobin A1C is currently 6.8%. Based on patient's current age and health status, her hemoglobin A1C goal is <7.0% to 7.5%, which translates into fasting and preprandial glucose levels averaging between 154 and 169 mg/dL.[31]

Other Recent labs are reported as WNL, including CrCl and LFTs. The patient also smokes 1 ppd, which can also contribute to progression of OA and worsen overall pain.[30] The patient has not been evaluated for interventional pain management such as injection therapy. Risk assessment: No history of drug or alcohol-related arrests, no aberrant drug behavior identified in chart review. No record of controlled substance agreement or prescribing of controlled substances located in chart.

Drug therapy problems include the following:

- *Needs additional medication therapy:* Pharmacological treatment indicated for OA-related pain
- *Adverse drug reaction:* Intolerance to naproxen; patient stopped taking
- *Needs additional nonpharmacological pain management*

These conclusions drawn in the Assess step serve as the basis for the therapeutic decision-making that will occur in the Plan step, which will be described next.

Plan, Implement, and Monitor

PLAN: Goals	
Conclusions	Rationale: Information or Premise to Support the Conclusion
Goals include: 1. Improve pain symptoms in bilateral knees by reaching patient's pain goal of 2/10 within 4 to 6 weeks 2. Improve overall activity by increasing volunteer days by 1 day per week within 4 to 6 weeks 3. Within the next 4 to 6 weeks, improve overall QOL as measured by a 2-point reduction in each of the areas measured by the DoD assessment: activity, sleep, mood, and stress 4. Achieve a 5% weight loss over the next 6 months	Current pain rating (DoD pain assessment scale): 7/10 Low: 5/10 High: 10/10 three to four times a week. Goal: 2/10. Four to six weeks will provide adequate time to incorporate nonpharmacological and pharmacological treatment options for achieving average pain levels of 2/10 and achieving a 2-point reduction in each area measured by the DoD assessment. • Activity: currently 8/10; goal is to drop to 6/10 • Sleep: currently 10/10; goal is to drop to 8/10 • Mood: currently 7/10; goal is to drop to 5/10 • Stress: currently 9/10; goal is to drop to 7/10 Current BMI: 33.64 Class 1 Obesity based on current weight: 196 lbs, height: 64 in. Through diet changes and improvements in baseline activity, a 5% weight loss goal over 6 months is an achievable goal. Even a 5% weight loss can improve knee pain directly related to OA pain.[36]

 KEY POINT

The pharmacist should embrace the shared decision-making model when developing treatment goals. The patient's input in developing these goals is vital to promoting patient's buy-in to achieving these goals.

Critical Thinking Checks for Developing This Patient's Goals

The SMART goals were developed with a **clear** understanding by the patient of what is achievable for meeting her healthcare wants and needs.

The SMART goals set for this patient been **clearly** stated including their timeframe and expected outcomes.

The SMART goals were developed in consideration of the most **significant** factors affecting this patient's health and the most **significant** expected outcomes.

The SMART goals were developed with a **fair and objective** consideration and participation of the patient, without the undue influence of emotions or biases, and in a manner that empowers the patient to self-manage their health and health behaviors.

The SMART goals were developed with **deep** consideration of the complexities that could be involved in this patient's care.

The SMART goals make **logical** sense based on disease pathophysiology, a full assessment of the patient, clinical guidelines, potential therapeutic strategies, and what is realistically achievable for this patient.

 KEY POINT

Utilizing the SMART goal format helps ensure all elements of a proper goal have been considered and allows for easier monitoring and evaluation of success after the treatment plan has been initiated.

PLAN: Uncontrolled Bilateral Knee Pain Due to Osteoarthritis Nonpharmacological Treatment	
Conclusions	**Rationale: Information or Premise to Support the Conclusion**
Improve overall exercise as tolerated. Request for new PT appointment needed today. Identify transportation options to aid in adherence to appointments.	Working to improve overall activity slowly as tolerated by the patient can improve overall conditioning and could over time result in minor weight loss.
Ensure proper education on importance of PT and rationale behind attending PT sessions.	Continued education on the importance of attending PT to learn specific exercises that are safe for the specific patient will help prevent injury. Education on continued commitment to daily exercise and activity to improve overall conditioning is needed to help the patient understand the importance of this treatment aspect.
Increase daily physical activity as tolerated through PT and through volunteer work. Complete diet education program and adopt a healthier overall diet.	A 5% to 10% weight loss has been shown to reduce knee OA.[36] Incorporating a healthier lifestyle through a more balanced and healthy diet along with daily physical activity can help achieve these weight loss goals.
Refer to self-efficacy and self-management programs to begin after PT sessions.	Self-efficacy and self-management programs can help the patient learn new coping techniques for chronic pain. Additionally, programs that incorporate Cognitive Behavior Therapy-Insomnia (CBT-I) have shown to be very effective in improving depression, insomnia, and pain-related conditions.[37] A referral to a local program can be considered after PT sessions have completed to decrease concurrent appointments, since the patient reports transportation limitations.
Recommend completing a daily pain diary to track daily pain ratings, activity levels, and responses to medications. Document pain levels during rest and activity, side effects (if applicable), sleep quality, overall activity.	Pain diaries provide real-time tracking of pain rating scores based of the numerical ratings scales. Patients can report initial pain ratings when waking, after activity, after medications, and at bedtime to allow the clinician to observe trends over a period of time. Adverse effects from medications can be documented and activity and sleep quality. If the patient is prescribed short-acting opioids, documenting pain levels at time of dosing and 1 h following dosing can also aid in assessing effects of the regimen.
Continue ice therapy. Proper education on a safe way to use these treatment approaches is indicated.	Ice or heat have been shown to help improve the overall pain process.[38] For acute injuries there are more recommendations on when to use ice vs heat.[38] Heat or ice have been found to be effective in various painful chronic conditions such as OA. The patient can select ice or heat based on perceived efficacy.[38]

 KEY POINT

Education on benefits of weight loss through proper diet and increased physical activity can result in positive outcomes for all concurrent disease states.

KEY POINT

Incorporating various nonpharmacological treatment modalities can result in better overall pain control and could decrease the need for systemic medications and possible side effects that can occur from these medications.

Critical Thinking Checks for This Patient's Nonpharmacological Plan for Uncontrolled Bilateral Knee Pain Due to Osteoarthritis

The nonpharmacological recommendations were developed with a **broad, deep, and fair** consideration of all of the **significant** contributing factors and the complexity of this patient's health.

In developing my recommendations, I have thought **broadly** about different, complementary strategies that may be integrated into a comprehensive plan for this patient's care.

The nonpharmacological strategies for achieving the goals make **logical** sense based on disease pathophysiology, a full assessment of the patient, clinical guidelines, and available therapeutic strategies.

To achieve sufficient **precision** of communication about the nonpharmacological options to the patient, I identified details about the different options that are most **significant** for conveying.

Though medications are my expertise, in reasoning about the best nonpharmacological options for this patient's uncontrolled pain secondary to OA, I have the **accurate** and **clear** knowledge needed to make these recommendations.

PLAN: Uncontrolled Bilateral Knee Pain Due to Osteoarthritis Pharmacological Treatment	
Conclusions	**Rationale: Information or Premise to Support the Conclusion**
Topical Diclofenac 1% Gel: Apply 4 g to both knees qid	Due to the patient's history of worsening GERD with a trial of naproxen, utilizing a topical NSAID is a safer approach to limit side effects. Osteoarthritis guidelines recommend a topical NSAID as a first-line treatment option.[23] The topical gel formulation of diclofenac has 17 times lower systemic absorption compared to oral diclofenac,[39] resulting in lower risk of adverse effects, including GI toxicity.[40]
Acetaminophen 650 mg po q8h ATC	Efficacy is conditionally recommended by the ACR OA guidelines due to limited efficacy results in recent studies. Recent meta-analysis has demonstrated questionable efficacy when acetaminophen is used as monotherapy.[41]
	However, the risk of ADRs is lower compared to systemic NSAIDs when properly dosed. Acetaminophen could be added to the pain regimen with topical diclofenac and duloxetine if needed.[23]
Duloxetine 30 mg po daily for 7 days then increase to 60 mg po daily	Duloxetine is conditionally recommended by the OA ACR 2019 guidelines for the treatment of pain associated with OA as monotherapy or in combination with NSAIDs. Duloxetine is a level two recommendation for knee OA with depression in the 2019 OARSI guidelines.[42]
	CT has been diagnosed with depression and she is currently not on any agent to address her depressive symptoms. This agent can help with depression symptoms along with helping pain control via the descending pain pathway.[43]

Tramadol 50 mg po bid prn (to be considered at a later time if the other treatments are unsuccessful)	Tramadol is conditionally recommended by the OA 2019 ACR guidelines.[23] This agent is an opioid and due to concerns associated with opioids in regard to fall risk, addiction potential, etc., this agent is not an appropriate agent to recommend at this time. Trials of nonopioid treatment options would be a better option at this time.[23]

KEY POINT

Dosing of topical diclofenac is different depending on the area of the body. The upper body will receive a lower dose compared to the lower body.

KEY POINT

Although opioids such as tramadol can be used in managing chronic pain, it is suggested to utilize nonpharmacological and nonopioid treatment options as first-line treatment options due to the side effects and addiction risks commonly observed with opioid use.

Critical Thinking Checks for This Patient's Pharmacological Plan for Uncontrolled Bilateral Knee Pain Due to Osteoarthritis

Deeper thinking is involved to understand and address complexities associated with how depression, insomnia, and pain are interrelated. Initiating duloxetine, which is FDA-approved for OA-related pain could help with all three issues and help improve her QOL.[43]

In presenting the plausible therapeutic strategies, I assured that the patient **clearly** understood the benefits and risks of each option and was not overwhelmed with the information presented to her.

In consideration of the reasonable pharmacological options for managing this patient's OA pain, the recommended options are those that had the best **logical** arguments for goal achievement based on the patient assessment, SMART goals, and available options.

As described in Chapter 1, in therapeutic reasoning, the pharmacist engages the patient in setting goals for therapy and helps the patient choose among the best available strategies. Based on the pharmacist's knowledge, experience, and evidence-based practice, the pharmacist generates potential strategies, and develops arguments for and against them. Conclusions are drawn about the best strategies for the patient, which are those that have the best supporting argument for realistically meeting the patient's goals. One of the ways the logic of an argument can be represented is in the form of an argument map, which shows the premises supporting an argument. An example of a map supporting the argument for a recommendation of duloxetine for this patient is provided in **Figure 2-3.** The map shows part of the hidden underlying structure of the argument, beginning with conclusions drawn to create the Assessment, which support conclusions drawn for the SMART Goal, which underlies the premises–including one of the assumptions–that collectively help support the recommendation for duloxetine. Note that there are other ways of constructing argument maps.

Recommendation				
Duloxetine 30 mg po daily for 7 days then increase to 60 mg po daily				
Duloxetine can help with depression symptoms along with helping pain control via the descending pain pathway	Duloxetine is conditionally recommended by the OA ACR 2019 guidelines for the treatment of pain associated with OA	If duloxetine is helpful, an end result could include improving insomnia symptoms with improved pain control and lower depression symptoms	There are no contraindications to duloxetine for this patient	Assumption to verify: Medicare will pay for duloxetine
SMART Goal				
Within 4 to 6 weeks improve pain symptoms and reach patient set pain goal of 2/10, and improve overall QOL, as measured by DoD assessment questions, by 2 points				
Assessment				
Uncontrolled osteoarthritic bilateral knee pain with contributing factors that include the following: inadequate pain management approach, poor diet, sedentary lifestyle, lack of transportation, nonadherence to PT or PT-based exercise routine, poor sleep quality (insomnia), obesity, smoking, depression. Drug therapy problem: Needs additional therapy				

FIGURE 2-3. Argument map for duloxetine selection.

KEY POINT

Utilizing an argument map provides an opportunity to outline the thought process to justify a decision and also consider all possible assumptions made during this thought process.

PLAN: Uncontrolled Depression and Insomnia	
Conclusions	Rationale: Information or Premise to Support the Conclusion
Refer to PCP to re-evaluate depression and insomnia.	Continued monitoring of depression and insomnia symptoms by the PCP or other mental health providers is important. The pharmacist can verify appointments and confirm the patient is following up as scheduled. If the patient is missing appointments, identifying the reasons and educating the patient on the importance of these appointments can help improve attendance.

Provide extensive counseling on CBT-I, including sleep hygiene and behavioral strategies	CBT-I is a structured program that helps patients identify thoughts and behaviors which could be creating insomnia issues or worsening insomnia issues. Techniques of CBT-I include stimulus control, sleep restriction, sleep hygiene, relaxation training, sleep avoidance, and biofeedback techniques. CBT-I has been offered as face-to-face counseling, group therapy, telehealth, internet training, printed handouts, and cell phone applications.[44]
	Incorporating some of the behavioral strategies could prove beneficial in improving overall generalized insomnia issues.[45]

KEY POINT

It is important for the pharmacist to identify when a patient might need further assessment or treatment from the PCP. Providing the patient a complete rationale for the referral can help improve adherence to all appointments.

KEY POINT

Introducing nonpharmacological options such as CBT-I can help the patient learn self-management tools, which can prove helpful in managing multiple issues, such as insomnia and overall stress management, which can improve self-efficacy.

Critical Thinking Checks for This Patient's Nonpharmacological Plan for Uncontrolled Depression and Insomnia

In **fairness** to the patient and other stakeholders, I understood the roles of other providers in this patient's care and recognized when it was best to refer the patient for care by PCP when I was at the limit of my scope of practice.

Though medications are my expertise, in reasoning about CBT-I for this patient's insomnia, I have the **accurate** and **clear** knowledge needed to make this recommendation.

IMPLEMENT/MONITOR: Uncontrolled Bilateral Knee Pain due to Osteoarthritis	
Conclusions	Rationale: Information or Premise to Support the Conclusion
Implement: Educate patient on the importance of PT Confirm appointment for PT, identify community transportation options if needed	*Implement:* Physical therapy and follow-up exercises are important for long-term improvements in deconditioning.
Monitor: Monitor attendance, progress via PT notes, continue to encourage patient to attend PT appointments, and practice exercises as directed.	*Monitor:* Longitudinal education on the importance of attending PT appointments and continued dedication to completing PT exercises can aid in achieving the goal of improving overall activity.

Implement: Provide diet education focusing on healthy choices and monitoring daily food/calorie intake via free app. *Monitor:* Monitor the patient's evolving approach to incorporating healthier food choices. Monitor patient's weight at each visit.	*Implement/Monitor:* CT has indicated she is interested in improving her diet and minor slow changes can create a long-term improvement in food choices and quantity. It has been shown even a 5% weight loss can improve clinical outcomes in knee OA. Benefits continue to be seen with continued weight loss. Incorporating healthier food choices will aid in achieving the weight loss goals.[46]
Implement: Recommend: Diclofenac 1% gel: Apply 4 g four times daily on both knees using dosing card supplied in packaging. Education on proper use. • Measure 4 g of gel with supplied dosing card • Rub 4 g into one knee completely. Repeat process for the other knee • Repeat this process for both knees four times a day to ensure proper drug levels are maintained in the knee area. • Wash hands well following gel application. • Side effects are rare. If you experience any signs of a skin rash, contact your provider. • Onset of action could take up to 7 days although most patients report some relief in 1 to 2 days. *Monitor:* • Monitor for improvement in pain levels in both knees. • Monitor for worsening GERD symptoms or general stomach pain.	*Implement:* Utilizing the supplied dosing card will assure the patient receives the proper dosing with each application and will help maintain proper drug levels are maintained in the area of application. Following each application, the patient should be educated on the importance of washing her hands to remove medication from her hands. *Monitor:* Onset of action could be delayed up to 7 days. Monitor for pain reduction and any side effects including skin rash. Although very rare, side effects similar to those from oral naproxen can occur.

Implement: Recommend: duloxetine 30 mg po each morning for 7 days then increase to 60 mg po each morning. *Monitor:* • Monitor for common side effects including constipation, decreased appetite, dry mouth, nausea/vomiting, and somnolence. • Monitor for worsening depression or suicidal thoughts. If symptoms worsen, contact provider immediately. • Routine monitoring of renal and hepatic function indicated.	*Implement:* Dose titration for duloxetine is recommended to decrease risk of commonly reported side effects. Ongoing monitoring following dose titration is indicated to identify any commonly reported ADRs including nausea/vomiting, constipation, dry mouth, and somnolence. Reports of increased fall risk have been associated with duloxetine initiation in the elderly. Proper education on fall precautions indicated. *Monitor:* The most common side effects experienced by older adults in published studies include constipation, decreased appetite, dry mouth, nausea, and somnolence. These side effects were not determined to be severe in nature.[47] Additionally there is a small risk of increased falls upon duloxetine initiation.[48] Continued monitoring during dose titration and into full dose treatment is indicated. Duloxetine should not be used in patients with hepatic insufficiency or severe renal impairment or end-stage renal impairment. Routine monitoring of hepatic and renal impairment indicated.
Implement: Continue ice therapy as needed Education: proper use of ice; 15 to 20 minutes max three to four times a day on painful areas of the knees. Protect skin with light towel, skin should not have direct contact with ice Topics include: (1) how long treatment should last (15 to 20 minutes three to four times a day), (2) proper placement of ice/heat on the affected joint or injury, (3) If CT decides to switch to using heat therapy, discuss the dangers of heating pads and recommend a heat pack, which can be heated safely in a microwave oven. *Monitor:* Evaluate efficacy of ice therapy, proper use of ice, and any side effects associated with this therapy.	*Implement:* Ice therapy should be used only 15 to 20 minutes a day for a maximum of three to four times a day on painful areas of the knees. Use of ice for an excessive amount of time can increase the risk of vasoconstriction resulting in a reduction of vascular clearance of inflammatory mediators.[49]

Implement:	*Implement:*
Recommend completing a daily pain diary for the next month as medications are initiated. Document the following in the pain diary:	A pain diary helps capture snapshots of vital pain-related information between visits. Additionally, this information could be considered a little more accurate compared to information provided strictly from general recall during a clinic visit. This also provides a great educational tool for the patient to see trends in what improves or worsens pain. It can also help the patient recognize there is some improvement in activity, QOL, and pain levels as the full treatment approach is implemented.
• Pain rating via NRS upon waking	
• Pain rating via NRS at rest	
• Pain rating via NRS during activity and document type of activity	
• Side effects experienced from current pain regimen	
• Sleep quality: document if trouble falling asleep, staying asleep, etc. Also document reasons for awakening such as pain-related issues, bathroom needs, etc.	
• Document activity levels: exercise and description of exercise, increase in overall social or physical activity.	*Monitor:*
	Encouraging CT to bring in her pain diary with each follow-up visit is important to help monitor improvement in pain levels, reactions to medications, sleep quality, and activity levels.
Monitor:	
Encourage CT to bring in pain diary with each follow-up visit	

 KEY POINT

Pharmacists in this type of practice have the opportunity to continually educate and encourage the patient to attend PT appointments and complete the exercises on a regular basis even after PT has completed. Constant dedication to this practice can improve overall deconditioning.

 KEY POINT

Proper education on proper use of ice therapy should be completed and revisited during subsequent visits to ensure safety and efficacy.

 KEY POINT

Encouraging the use of a pain diary can help identify trends and possible unidentified contributing factors to current pain complaints.

IMPLEMENT/MONITOR: Depression and Insomnia	
Conclusions	Rationale: Information or Premise to Support the Conclusion
Implement: Direct patient to schedule an appointment with the PCP for further evaluation of depression symptoms. *Monitor:* At each follow-up visit, check frequency of follow-up appointments with providers and review PCP notes from previous evaluation(s).	*Implement:* Although we are recommending initiating duloxetine for OA-related pain, she might experience improvement in depression symptoms as well. It is important the patient is monitored for depression by the PCP to ensure she is improving in overall symptoms. *Monitor:* CT has reported she has had difficulty with transportation in the past and missed some PT appointments. It is important to verify she attends all follow-up appointments with all providers.
Implement: Recommend incorporating CBT-I practices to aid in treating chronic insomnia. Use of CBT-I printed educational materials, online resources, or free apps available for smartphones. Discuss which CBT-I approach CT is comfortable with trying and recommend she begin using this format and practice the recommended approaches. *Monitor:* Monitor for use of CBT-I educational tools and gradual implementation of these approaches. Monitor for improvement in insomnia symptoms.	*Implement:* Insomnia symptoms are chronic in nature and could be exacerbated by higher pain levels. CBT-I is considered a first-line nonpharmacological treatment. CT has transportation issues so utilizing printed material, internet training options, or app programs are recommended based on her comfort level. These programs will also include sleep hygiene education, which includes information on proper lifestyle habits including caffeine use in evenings, diet, exercise, environmental distractors, and age-appropriate expectations for sleep duration.[44] *Monitor:* Following up on efficacy of CBT-I approaches and overall sleep pattern is an important part of the continued assessment and also serves as an educational tool to help the patient identify behavioral changes that could be negatively impacting her sleep.
Implement: Educate patient on importance of smoking cessation. CT is considered in precontemplation at this time. *Monitor:* Interest in smoking cessation treatment options and any reduction in smoking frequency with ongoing education.	*Implement:* Patient is currently in the precontemplation stage of smoking cessation. Smoking can increase the severity of pain, which is another education point when discussing the health benefits of smoking cessation.[30] Continued education and follow-up is needed in hopes of transitioning patient from precontemplation to contemplation.[50] *Monitor:* Following up on smoking education counseling at each visit can help move a patient from precontemplation to contemplation state and possibly a successful smoking cessation plan.

Follow-up plan:	*Follow-up plan:*
1–2 months	Listing the topics for follow-up allows a clear guide for reassessment when the patient returns to the clinic.
Evaluation of:	
• Pain control after initiation of treatment regimen	
– Pain ratings based on NRS (upon waking, at rest, good days, bad days, during activity)	Following up within 1-2 months is a reasonable time frame to assess the achievement of the goals for this patient.
– Review baseline activity and assess if this has increased with improved pain levels	Reassessing the patient's pain ratings, baseline activity, and impacts of her pain are in accordance with her goals.
– Reassess overall impacts of pain by using the DoD/VA Pain Supplemental Questions	Assessing medication efficacy, safety, and adherence is a standard of practice for pharmacists.
• Assess efficacy, safety, and adherence to medications	Improvements in insomnia and mood are important outcomes for this patient's care.
• Assess if any improvement in insomnia or overall mood associated with previous depression symptoms	Although the patient is not interested in smoking cessation at this time, the negative impact of smoking on her health warrants an assessment of her interest in each visit with her.
• Assess interest in smoking cessation treatment options and approaches.	

 KEY POINT

Pharmacists should always screen for health-related social needs to identify any barriers that could negatively impact overall patient care.

 KEY POINT

Determining the proper follow-up time for a patient will be based on a variety of factors and should include shared decision-making with the patient.

Critical Thinking Checks for This Patient's Implementation and Monitoring Plan

In **fairness** to the patient, the implementation plan has been developed and communicated with an empathetic understanding of her perspectives and in a manner that assures she is empowered to self-manage her health and health behaviors.

The implementation plan was developed **fairly**, in full consideration that the patient can become overwhelmed with the actions needed for successful implementation, as there were several strategies that needed to be communicated in a relatively short encounter.

In developing and providing **clear** education to the patient, I carefully considered potential ambiguities, jargon, poor grammar, or other potential causes of unclear understanding by the patient.

The steps for implementing the strategies were **clearly** outlined and provided with enough clarity, accuracy, and details to facilitate their implementation by the patient.

To facilitate successful implementation of strategies that may be complicated for the patient, I have outlined and conveyed the most **significant** actions for strategy implementation.

In thinking **broadly** about this patient's care, I have determined that the physical therapist is a significant stakeholder for this patient's pain management and have **fairly** considered the integral contribution of PT to achieving the identified health outcomes.

CONCLUSION

Managing pain in any setting can be a very complex process, particularly with complex patients that have multiple pain conditions or comorbidities. The Pain Management Best Practices Inter-Agency Task Force recommends care should be individualized, multimodal, and multidisciplinary.[4] Pharmacists serve an important role in the multidisciplinary team when managing a patient's pain. Utilizing excellent critical thinking and clinical reasoning skills are vital when completing the necessary steps such as pain assessment, risk assessment, and treatment development. These skills will continue to develop and evolve as the pharmacist gains further experience with the unique variety of patients who present to the clinic on a daily basis.

Summary Points

- The experience of pain is a very individual personal journey, which will differ with each patient and which will require an individualized treatment plan.
- Utilizing the Pharmacists' Patient Care Process during a Medication Therapy Management session in a chronic pain clinic can help ensure a complete treatment plan is developed.
- Due to the subjectivity of pain, a comprehensive pain assessment should focus on physical, psychological, and social impacts.
- Collection of information during the MTM session should include a detailed chart review prior to the MTM session as part of the collaborative effort to provide patient-centered care in chronic pain management.
- Developing a professional rapport with the patient early in the MTM session is very important to help explore the patient's subjective experiences associated with chronic pain.
- Each stage of the PPCP offers opportunities to identify and complete education on important topics during the patient interview.
- When completing a medication review during the MTM session, it is important to review and consider all medications, not just the medications that have been prescribed for chronic pain management.
- When assessing a patient's current condition, consideration must be given to all other conditions, medications, related patient treatment goals, and the patient's overall perception of pain.
- Developing SMART goals with the patient's input provides a roadmap for future appointments for determining if treatment approaches have been successful.
- When treating acute or chronic pain, care should be individualized, include multimodal and multidisciplinary treatment approaches, and directly involve the patient in a shared decision-making model.
- Outlining the various treatment options in the Plan step of the PPCP can be very effective when determining what the best treatment is for the individual patient.

Abbreviations

ACE	Adverse Childhood Events
ACR	American College of Rheumatology
ADL	Activities of Daily Living

BMI	Body Mass Index
BPI	Brief Pain Inventory
CBD	Cannabidiol
CBT-I	Cognitive Behavior Therapy-Insomnia
CNS	Central Nervous System
CMP	Comprehensive Metabolic Panel
CrCl	Creatinine Clearance
DM	Diabetes Mellitus
DoD/VA	Department of Defense/Veterans Administration
DVPRS	Defense and Veterans Pain Rating Scale
ER	Emergency Room
ETOH	Alcohol
FDA	Food Drug Administration
GERD	Gastric Esophageal Reflux Disease
GHD	Generalized Anxiety Disorder
GI	Gastrointestinal
HbA1C	Hemoglobin A1C
IASP	International Association for the Study of Pain
LFT	Liver Function Test
MPQ	McGill Pain Questionnaire
MTM	Medication Therapy Management
NSAID	Nonsteroidal Anti-inflammatory Drug
NRS	Numerical Rating Scale
OA	Osteoarthritis
ORID	Opioid-Induced Respiratory Depression
ORT	Opioid Risk Tool
OTC	Over-the-Counter
PCP	Primary Care Providers
PCS	Pain Catastrophizing Scale
PDMP	Prescription Drug Monitoring Program
PHQ	Patient Health Questionnaire
PPCP	Pharmacists' Patient Care Process
ppd	Pack Per Day
PSEQ	Pain Self-Efficacy Scale
PT	Physical Therapy
PVD	Peripheral Vascular Disease
QOL	Quality of Life
THC	Tetrahydrocannabinol
WNL	Within Normal Limits

References

1. Raja SN, Carr DB, Cohen M, et al. The revised International Association for the Study of Pain definition of pain: concepts, challenges, and compromises. *Pain*. 2020;161(9):1976-1982.

2. Dahlhamer J, Lucas J, Zelaya C, et al. Prevalence of chronic pain and high-impact chronic pain among adults—United States, 2016. *MMWR Morb Mortal Wkly Rep*. 2018;67(36):1001-1006.

3. Greer N, Bolduc J, Geurkink E, et al. Pharmacist-led chronic disease management: a systematic review of effectiveness and harms compared with usual care. *Ann Intern Med*. 2016;165(1):30-40.

4. U.S. Department of Health and Human Services. *Pain Management Best Practices Inter-Agency Task Force Report: Updates, Gaps, Inconsistencies, and Recommendations.* 2019. Available at https://www. hhs.gov/sites/default/files/pmtf-final-report-2019-05-23.pdf. Accessed: August 15, 2022.

5. Persky AM, Medina MS, Castleberry AN. Developing critical thinking skills in pharmacy students. *Am J Pharm Educ.* 2019;83(2):7033.

6. Joint Commission of Pharmacy Practitioners. *Pharmacists' Patient Care Process.* 2014. Available at https://jcpp.net/wp-content/uploads/2016/03/PatientCareProcess-with-supporting-organizations. pdf. Accessed August 15, 2022.

7. Cleeland C. *The Brief Pain Inventory.* 1991. Available at http://www.npcrc.org/files/news/briefpain_ long.pdf. Accessed August 15, 2022.

8. Cleeland C. *The Brief Pain Inventory Short Form.* 1991. 2022. Available at http://www.npcrc.org/files/ news/briefpain_short.pdf. Accessed August 15.

9. Melzack R. The McGill pain questionnaire: from description to measurement. *Anesthesiology.* 2005;103(1):199-202.

10. McCaffery M, Beebe A. *Pain: Clinical Manual for Nursing Practice.* St. Louis, MO: Mosby; 1989.

11. U.S. Department of Veterans Affairs. *Defense and Veterans Pain Rating Scale.* Available at https:// www.va.gov/PAINMANAGEMENT/docs/DVPRS_2slides_and_references.pdf. Accessed August 15, 2022

12. Nicholas M. The pain self-efficacy questionnaire: taking pain into account. *Eur J Pain.* 2012; 153-163.

13. Spitzer RL, Williams JBW, Kroenke K, et al. *Patient Health Questionnaire-9 (PHQ-9).* Available at https://www.apa.org/depression-guideline/patient-health-questionnaire.pdf. Accessed August 15, 2022

14. Kroenke K, Spitzer RL, Williams JB. The PHQ-15: validity of a new measure for evaluating the severity of somatic symptoms. *Psychosom Med.* 2002;64(2):258-266.

15. Darnall BD, Sturgeon JA, Cook KF, et al. Development and validation of a daily pain catastrophizing scale. *J Pain.* 2017;18(9):1139-1149.

16. Felitti VJ, Anda RF, Nordenberg D, et al. REPRINT OF: Relationship of childhood abuse and household dysfunction to many of the leading causes of death in adults: the Adverse Childhood Experiences (ACE) study. *Am J Prev Med.* 2019;56(6):774-786.

17. Spitzer RL, Kroenke K, Williams JB, Löwe B. A brief measure for assessing generalized anxiety disorder: the GAD-7. *Arch Intern Med.* 2006;166(10):1092-1097.

18. Chung F, Yegneswaran B, Liao P, et al. STOP questionnaire: a tool to screen patients for obstructive sleep apnea. *Anesthesiology.* 2008;108(5):812-821.

19. Webster LR, Webster RM. Predicting aberrant behaviors in opioid-treated patients: preliminary validation of the opioid risk tool. *Pain Med.* 2005;6(6):432-442.

20. Wideman TH, Edwards RR, Walton DM, Martel MO, Hudon A, Seminowicz DA. The multimodal assessment model of pain: a novel framework for further integrating the subjective pain experience within research and practice. *Clin J Pain.* 2019;35(3):212-221.

21. Gatchel RJ, Peng YB, Peters ML, Fuchs PN, Turk DC. The biopsychosocial approach to chronic pain: scientific advances and future directions. *Psychol Bull.* 2007;133(4):581-624.

22. Block PR, Thorn BE, Kapoor S, White J. Pain catastrophizing, rather than vital signs, associated with pain intensity in patients presenting to the emergency department for pain. *Pain Manag Nurs.* 2017;18(2):102-109.

23. Kolasinski SL, Neogi T, Hochberg MC, et al. 2019 American College of Rheumatology/Arthritis Foundation Guideline for the Management of Osteoarthritis of the Hand, Hip, and Knee [published correction appears in Arthritis Care Res (Hoboken). 2021 May;73(5):764]. *Arthritis Care Res (Hoboken).* 2020;72(2):149-162.

24. Li Z, Lei X, Xu B, Wang S, Gao T, Lv H. Analysis of risk factors of diabetes peripheral neuropathy in type 2 diabetes mellitus and nursing intervention. *Exp Ther Med.* 2020;20(6):127.

25. Wang X, Perry TA, Arden N, et al. Occupational risk in knee osteoarthritis: a systematic review and meta-analysis of observational studies. *Arthritis Care Res (Hoboken).* 2020;72(9):1213-1223.

26. Smith TO, Dainty JR, Williamson E, Martin KR. Association between musculoskeletal pain with social isolation and loneliness: analysis of the English Longitudinal Study of Ageing. *Br J Pain*. 2019;13(2):82-90.

27. Bossenbroek Fedoriw K, Prentice A, Slatkoff S, Myerholtz L. A systematic approach to opioid prescribing. *J Am Board Fam Med*. 2020;33(6):992-997.

28. Kawai K, Kawai AT, Wollan P, Yawn BP. Adverse impacts of chronic pain on health-related quality of life, work productivity, depression and anxiety in a community-based study. *Fam Pract*. 2017;34(6):656-661.

29. Afolalu EF, Ramlee F, Tang NKY. Effects of sleep changes on pain-related health outcomes in the general population: a systematic review of longitudinal studies with exploratory meta-analysis. *Sleep Med Rev*. 2018;39:82-97.

30. LaRowe LR, Ditre JW. Pain, nicotine, and tobacco smoking: current state of the science. *Pain*. 2020;161(8):1688-1693.

31. American Diabetes Association. 12. Older adults: standards of medical care in diabetes-2021. *Diabetes Care*. 2021;44(Suppl 1):S168-S179.

32. Cheng HF, Harris RC. Cyclooxygenases, the kidney, and hypertension. *Hypertension*. 2004;43(3):525-530.

33. Huang HM, Huang CY, Lee-Hsieh J, Cheng SF. Establishing the competences of clinical reasoning for nursing students in Taiwan: from the nurse educators' perspectives. *Nurse Educ Today*. 2018;66:110-116.

34. Anderson KN. Insomnia and cognitive behavioural therapy-how to assess your patient and why it should be a standard part of care. *J Thorac Dis*. 2018;10(Suppl 1):S94-S102.

35. Andersen ML, Araujo P, Frange C, Tufik S. Sleep disturbance and pain: a tale of two common problems. *Chest*. 2018;154(5):1249-1259.

36. Kolasinski SL, Neogi T, Hochberg MC, et al. 2019 American College of Rheumatology/Arthritis Foundation Guideline for the Management of Osteoarthritis of the Hand, Hip, and Knee [published correction appears in Arthritis Care Res (Hoboken). 2021 May;73(5):764]. *Arthritis Care Res (Hoboken)*. 2020;72(2):149-162.

37. Roberts MB, Drummond PD. Sleep problems are associated with chronic pain over and above mutual associations with depression and catastrophizing. *Clin J Pain*. 2016;32(9):792-799.

38. Malanga GA, Yan N, Stark J. Mechanisms and efficacy of heat and cold therapies for musculoskeletal injury. *Postgrad Med*. 2015;127(1):57-65.

39. *Voltaren Gel (diclofenac sodium topical gel) 1% label (Rx label): Voltaren gel [product information]*. Endo Pharmaceuticals Inc., Malvern, PA. Available at https://www.accessdata.fda.gov/drugsatfda_docs/label/2016/022122s010lbl.pdf. Accessed August 15, 2022.

40. Honvo G, Leclercq V, Geerinck A, et al. Safety of topical non-steroidal anti-inflammatory drugs in osteoarthritis: outcomes of a systematic review and meta-analysis. *Drugs Aging*. 2019;36(Suppl 1):45-64.

41. da Costa BR, Reichenbach S, Keller N, et al. Effectiveness of non-steroidal anti-inflammatory drugs for the treatment of pain in knee and hip osteoarthritis: a network meta-analysis. *Lancet*. 2017;390(10090):e21-e33.

42. Bannuru RR, Osani MC, Vaysbrot EE, et al. OARSI guidelines for the non-surgical management of knee, hip, and polyarticular osteoarthritis. *Osteoarthr Cartil*. 2019;27(11):1578-1589.

43. Rodrigues-Amorim D, Olivares JM, Spuch C, Rivera-Baltanás T. A systematic review of efficacy, safety, and tolerability of duloxetine. *Front Psychiatry*. 2020;11:554899.

44. Soong C, Burry L, Greco M, Tannenbaum C. Advise non-pharmacological therapy as first line treatment for chronic insomnia. *BMJ*. 2021;372:n680. doi:10.1136/bmj.n680.

45. Rathbone AL, Clarry L, Prescott J. Assessing the efficacy of mobile health apps using the basic principles of cognitive behavioral therapy: systematic review. *J Med Internet Res*. 2017;19(11):e399.

46. McKee AM, Morley JE. Obesity in the elderly. In: Feingold KR, Anawalt B, Boyce A, et al., eds. *Endotext*. South Dartmouth, MA: MDText.com, Inc.; 2021.

47. Chen L, Gong M, Liu G, Xing F, Liu J, Xiang Z. Efficacy and tolerability of duloxetine in patients with knee osteoarthritis: a meta-analysis of randomised controlled trials. *Intern Med J*. 2019;49(12):1514-1523.

48. Nelson JC, Oakes TM, Liu P, et al. Assessment of falls in older patients treated with duloxetine: a secondary analysis of a 24-week randomized, placebo-controlled trial. *Prim Care Companion CNS Disord*. 2013;15(1):PCC.12m01419.

49. Olenak JL, Pezzino NC. Musculoskeletal injuries and disorders. In: Krinsky DL, ed. *Handbook of Nonprescription Drugs: An Interactive Approach to Self-Care*. Washington, DC: American Pharmacists Association; 2020.

50. Prochaska JO, Velicer WF. The transtheoretical model of health behavior change. *Am J Health Promot*. 1997;12(1):38-48.

51. Arbuck D, Fleming A. A pain assessment primer. *Pract Pain Manag*. 2020;20(4).

3

Ambulatory Care— Geriatric Care Cardiology

Nicole Early and Elizabeth Pogge

CHAPTER AIMS

The aims of this chapter are to:

- Discuss the roles of a systematic patient care process, clinical reasoning, and critical thinking in assessing and resolving medication-related problems as part of a collaborative effort to provide patient-centered care in hypertension management in an older adult.
- Illustrate common medication-related problems encountered in older adults using clinical reasoning and critical thinking techniques through utilization of the Pharmacists' Patient Care Process.

KEY WORDS

- Older adults • hypertension • polypharmacy • prescribing cascade • clinical reasoning
- clinical problem solving • medication-related problems

INTRODUCTION

Pharmacy practice in cardiology provides opportunity for managing chronic disease states such as hypertension, hyperlipidemia, anticoagulation, and heart failure (HF). Pharmacists working in a clinic to manage cardiovascular disease states often focus on patient education, appropriate medication selection, and patient safety.

Cardiovascular disease is the leading cause of death in the United States.[1] The American Heart Association reports that between 2015 and 2018, over 75% of adults, 60 to 79 years, had cardiovascular disease (defined as presence of hypertension, coronary heart disease, HF, or stroke).[2] Hypertension is common among older adults, afflicting more than half of US adults.[3] The incidence of hypertension increases with age, with a large percentage of older people having uncontrolled blood pressure.[4] With recent clinical guidelines on the management of high blood pressure recommending more stringent goals for older adults, healthcare providers are frequently faced with patients who have blood pressure readings that remain above goal despite being on multiple antihypertensive agents.[5] Older adults often pose a challenge to treat, with several potential barriers to care, including multiple comorbidities, heterogeneity in function, medication intolerances, polypharmacy, and lack of understanding regarding the importance of blood pressure-lowering.[6] The pharmacist can serve as part of an interprofessional team to help address these barriers to improve treatment of cardiovascular disease states in older adults.

 KEY POINT

Managing the pharmacotherapy of older adults is challenging as these patients often suffer from several comorbidities, which lead to use of multiple medications and increase the risk of side effects, drug interactions, and nonadherence.

OUR PRACTICE—AN OUTPATIENT PHARMACIST-RUN CARDIOVASCULAR RISK REDUCTION CLINIC

Our practice is an outpatient pharmacist-run clinic working under a collaborative practice agreement with a private cardiology practice, where pharmacists provide medication management services for blood pressure (hypertension and hypotension), HF, hyperlipidemia, smoking cessation, and polypharmacy (medication review). Pharmacists receive referrals from cardiologists and are asked to manage specific disease states through patient education, medication therapy management, monitoring, and follow-up. The pharmacists have prescribing authority, which can include medication initiation, discontinuation, and/or dose titration. Two of our three clinic locations are in retirement communities in the Phoenix Metropolitan area; therefore, most patients are over 65 years of age. This practice is staffed by two pharmacists who serve as professors at the nearby College of Pharmacy and is a training site for pharmacy residents and final-year pharmacy students.

UTILIZING CRITICAL THINKING SKILLS IN OUR PRACTICE

In this practice, critical thinking is utilized throughout the entire patient encounter. Patients who are referred often have multiple comorbidities and/or medication intolerances that can make first-line therapy ineffective or contraindicated. For example, a patient may present with a strong indication for statin therapy, but have a statin intolerance (eg, muscle-related symptoms, memory loss, or liver dysfunction), making an alternative treatment plan necessary. Shared decision-making is always practiced, with the patient being asked about goals, preferences, and values throughout the development of the treatment plan.

 KEY POINT

Shared decision-making allows patients to have input into plans, which can help patients achieve their specific goals.

As this site also serves as a training site for residents and students, critical thinking is utilized in the rotation teaching approach. For example, Socratic questioning— where students are asked a series of focused, open-ended questions—is used to probe the thinking of future pharmacists and to develop their skills for implementing critical thinking into their future practice.[7] As part of this practice, students are asked to provide their reasoning and/or evidence for their drug therapy recommendations. **Table 3-1** includes a list of questions that can be applied to assure that intellectual standards of critical thinking are met as the pharmacist provides ambulatory care services to older adults in a cardiology practice.

TABLE 3-1

Sample Standards-Based Questions That Can be Applied to Assure That Intellectual Standards for Critical Thinking Are Met as the Pharmacist Provides *Ambulatory Care Services to Older Adults in a Cardiology Practice*

Clarity (explicit, unambiguous, intelligible, free from confusion or doubt)	• What questions do I still have after reviewing previous provider notes about the patient? • Have I asked appropriate questions to gain insight into potential medication-related problems? • How will I clearly communicate medication changes to my patient and/or their caregiver? • Have I clearly and concisely documented the information gathered from and disseminated in the appointment?
Relevance (pertinent, applicable, germane)	• Is there additional information that I will need to gather from the patient or provider to address any concerns? • Which of the patient's concerns is most relevant to our discussion today? • What resources will I need to utilize to determine if the patient's complaint is related to a medication? • How will I keep the appointment on track so that I can gather and disseminate the most pertinent information?
Significance (important, nontrivial, necessary, critical, required, impactful)	• Are there any key details that are missing or need clarification before I develop an action plan? • What is most important to my patient (eg, longevity, quality of life)? • What limitations does this patient have that may impact their ability to follow through with changes? • How can I ensure the patient leaves the appointment with the necessary information and future next steps?
Objectivity (fact-based, unbiased)	• Have I allowed my biases to influence the questions that I asked when gathering information or developing my plan? • Have I avoided utilizing leading questions when gathering information? • What tools can I utilize to remain objective when assessing medication regimens? • Did I allow any irrelevant information to impact my decision making? • In developing a plan, have I utilized quality evidence-based medicine and avoided making changes based on emotions, biases, or feelings?

Fairness (unbiased, equitable, impartial)	• Have I created an environment where the patient feels comfortable sharing their opinions, thoughts, and preferences so we can work together to develop a patient-centered plan? • Have I listened to the patient's and/or caregiver's perspective with a nonjudgmental attitude? • Is the patient approaching this concern from a different point of view that I have not considered? • Have I made any premature judgments in the interest of moving the appointment along? • Have I considered the patient's and/or caregiver's viewpoint in developing a plan?
Accuracy (verifiable, valid, true, credible, undistorted)	• Are there any pieces of information that the patient verbally stated, where the nonverbal body language (or information gleaned from the chart or objective data) did not support that statement (eg, averting eye contact when reporting adherence with the medication regimen, or an unchanged lipid panel following statin initiation)? • If a disconnect occurs, in what other ways can I ask questions or are there other resources I can utilize to ensure information is accurate? • Am I using up-to-date, reliable resources when making a recommendation and developing my plan?
Precision (exact, specific, detailed)	• Do I have specific details to utilize when formulating a recommendation? • Would additional information better support my recommendation for a change in therapy? • When communicating with another provider, have I utilized pertinent details that reinforce the soundness of my recommendation?
Depth (roots, fundamentals, complexities, interrelationships, cause/effect, implications)	• When utilizing medication management tools and guidelines, have I considered the complexities of deprescribing agents and implications of those changes on the patient's symptoms and quality of life? • Have I considered the potential risks associated with the plan moving forward? • What will I monitor moving forward to determine efficacy of the plan? • Are there any psychosocial factors that must be addressed for patients to be able to implement changes?
Breadth (comprehensive, encompassing, alternative perspectives)	• What other life factors may be playing into the patient's ability to manage their disease state? • What strategies can I use to improve outcomes for the patient? • Who are the key stakeholders in helping this patient manage their condition? • What are alternative treatment options if the initial plan is not successful?
Logic (reasonable, rational, without contradiction, well-founded, sound)	• What other factors may be contributing to the current complaint? • Have I ensured that all decisions were logical in each step of the PPCP? • How will I determine if the implementation was successful?

 KEY POINT

Given the complexities of older patients, it is pertinent to utilize critical thinking to assess the risks and benefits of all decisions, including effects on other disease states.

APPLICATION OF THE PHARMACISTS' PATIENT CARE PROCESS IN OUR PRACTICE

The Pharmacists' Patient Care Process (PPCP) is applied for all patients who are referred to the pharmacist clinic. As with other practices, the first step is the Collect step, which begins with collecting information from the chart prior to the patient appointment, then via an in-person patient interview during the appointment. The patient interview always includes a thorough medication reconciliation and clarifies any previous medication intolerances or allergies. The interview will then be tailored to the patient's chief complaint. For example, in a hypertension patient appointment, additional patient interview questions will include a request for home blood pressure readings, in addition to questions pertaining to lifestyle factors that could influence blood pressure. During and after the patient interview, the pharmacist engages the PPCP Assess step which includes analyzing the patient's current therapy. After all information is collected and assessed, the pharmacist utilizes shared decision-making to develop a patient-specific plan for the patient in consideration of potential treatment options based on standards of care and the patient's preferences and goals.[6,8,9] Within this plan, appropriate monitoring and follow-up is developed. In the Implement step, each plan is written out for the patient to take home, with medication changes, lifestyle changes, and monitoring being included in each plan.[10] The Implement step also includes communicating the plan with other healthcare providers, including the patient's cardiologist, primary care provider, and other specialists when applicable.

THE COLLECTION OF PATIENT INFORMATION IN OUR PRACTICE

The Collect process begins with a chart review that will serve as the basis for the patient interview. This review is important to assess the patient's baseline disease states, cardiovascular risk, and medication-related concerns. **Table 3-2** includes examples of data that can be collected during a chart review, along with the rationale for collecting this data.

TABLE 3-2

Examples of Data That Can be Collected During Chart Review in Preparation for Patient Interview

Data to Collect During Chart Review	Rationale for Collecting Specific Data
Patient-specific characteristics: age, weight, comorbidities, current lab results (eg, renal/hepatic function, basic metabolic panel [BMP])	Patient-specific parameters are utilized to make appropriate medication selection and ensure proper dosing for medications. Weight trends can help identify unanticipated weight gain or loss.
Last office visit with the cardiologist that includes the pharmacist clinic referral to determine the main patient complaints, the focus of the appointment, and the cardiologist's recommendations during the last office visit	Determining the main reason that the patient is presenting to the clinic can help with focusing the interview to collect the most relevant information. Working under a collaborative practice agreement with many different disease states, the pharmacist should make sure that the appointment is focused on the appropriate disease states as requested by the cardiologist. The pharmacist should reiterate any recommendations provided by the cardiologist and can help identify nonadherence.

Current medications (including prescription medications, over-the-counter [OTC] medications, and supplements)	A complete list of medications is needed to determine the most appropriate additional therapy for the patient. Furthermore, agents that can worsen cardiovascular diseases (eg, non-steroidal anti-inflammatory drugs [NSAIDs] in HF) are identified for a discussion related to discontinuation.
Medication allergies or intolerances	Previous medication allergies or intolerances are necessary to determine if a re-challenge with a first-line agent can be considered, or if alternative options need to be explored.
Personal and family history of cardiovascular disease	For many cardiovascular diseases, the intensity at which the pharmacist treats a patient is based on baseline cardiovascular risk, which incorporates personal and family history of cardiovascular disease.
The cardiologist's treatment and goals of therapy	The pharmacist should make sure that their therapeutic plan aligns with the cardiologist's treatment plans and goals of therapy.
Previous (within the last 6 months) emergency room visits or hospitalizations	Reviewing recent hospital visits can help identify difficulties encountered in the past with treating this disease state (and other comorbidities) and prognosis of the patient.
Past medical history that could be a contributing factor to cardiovascular disease	Comorbid conditions are important for pharmacists to identify and assess, as some conditions, such as diabetes and chronic kidney disease, may worsen cardiovascular outcomes, guide selection of medications, and determine patient prognosis.
Insurance coverage	As many cardiovascular medications are brand names and therefore have high copays, it is important to consider insurance coverage. Due to fixed income in retirement, the overall cost of medications is often a significant barrier to care for older adults.

Information from the chart review will be utilized by the pharmacist to perform an effective patient interview. The patient interview serves to both reinforce information found in the chart review and gather additional necessary information that was not in the chart. Additionally, the interview is utilized to facilitate shared decision-making to create goals of care that consider patient-specific goals and preferences. Lastly, during the patient interview, patient education can occur to reinforce positive lifestyle factors and habits and correct detrimental ones.

Table 3-3 includes potential patient interview data that can be collected during a patient interview, which will be vital for fully assessing the patient and for developing a treatment plan.

In cardiovascular care, shared decision-making with the patient is often appropriate for clinical decisions that involve multiple reasonable options. In this context, it is important to note that patient preferences can vary from one patient to another, and they may change over time. An example of how preferences may change can be found in **Figure 3-1**.[6] This can occur frequently when treating cardiovascular disease in older adults, as many clinical situations are complex and dynamic and can have many potential solutions. Additionally, when working with older adults, life expectancy should always be considered to determine the intensity of treatment, which will help tailor the drug therapy plan. For example, in a patient with less than

TABLE 3-3

Patient Interview: Examples of Data That Can be Collected During the Patient Interview

- Self-reported health status, including complications, symptom management, and general well-being
- Verification of current medications listed in the chart, along with their dosing—including prescription medications, OTC medications, and supplements
- Adherence to medications
  - Does the patient use adherence aids or rely on someone to help manage current medications?
- Restrictions to instrumental activities of daily living (IADLs) that may affect disease states or the treatment plan
  - Is the patient able to open medication bottles or fill pill boxes?
- History of falls, hospitalizations, and emergency room visits
- Lifestyle habits, including diet, exercise, caffeine intake, tobacco use, sleep habits, and recreational drug use
- Type of home blood pressure monitor and home blood pressure readings for HF and hypertension clinic visits
- History of medication intolerances
  - Request (1) a description of what occurred with each medication, (2) how long before the intolerance developed, (3) how long before symptoms of the intolerance resolved upon stopping the medication, and (4) was the medication rechallenged and if so, what was the reaction
- Patient's goals for treatment
  - Consider goals of intensive risk reduction vs symptom control vs quality of life
- Insurance coverage, access issues, copayment costs, and patient-assistance programs used in the past

 KEY POINT

Reviewing the patient's goals of care is imperative when assessing for control and developing a plan. As patient's age, goals of care often change based on life expectancy.

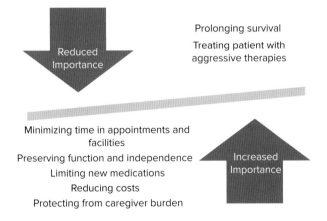

FIGURE 3-1. As patients age, their priorities will often change from a focus on aggressive treatment of disease and long-term survival to a focus on improved quality of life. (Adapted from Backman et al.[6])

3 years of life expectancy, statin therapy for primary prevention or intensive blood pressure lowering may not provide clinical benefit.[11,12]

When performing a patient interview, it is important to utilize open-ended questions to help ensure accuracy of gathered information. Furthermore, methods such as the teach-back method can be utilized to garner patient understanding of the topic.[13] Providing written education material (including medication changes) at a reading level of sixth to eighth grade is important to ensure understanding of the plan. Older adults commonly have comorbid memory concerns, so providing information using multiple methods can help improve understanding.[14]

An example of a cardiovascular management appointment provided in our practice is illustrated below with the analysis of the fictitious patient—Virginia H. She presents to the clinic with resistant hypertension (which can be defined as "blood pressure that remains above goal despite concurrent use of three antihypertensive agents of different classes taken at maximally tolerated doses, one of which should be a diuretic"),[5] comorbid HF with uncontrolled edema, and polypharmacy that has resulted in a prescribing cascade (which can be defined as "the situation in which a first drug administered to a patient causes adverse event signs and symptoms, that are misinterpreted as a new condition, resulting in a new medication being prescribed").[9] This case illustrates the reasoning that occurs during each PPCP step and will demonstrate the critical thinking utilized throughout. We will begin with an overview of Virginia H.'s case.

The Case of Virginia H.: Overview

Virginia H. (VH) is an 84-year-old female who was seen by her cardiologist for worsening lower extremity swelling with numbness and pain. The numbness and pain started 2 months ago in her ankles and is now traveling up her legs. She reported being unsteady on her feet and had a recent fall that resulted in shoulder pain. At her appointment, her blood pressure was elevated at 169/72 mm Hg with a pulse of 64 bpm. She also reported elevated blood pressure readings at home. Her cardiologist started her on hydrochlorothiazide 25 mg 2 weeks ago to help with her swelling and improve her blood pressure control. Upon failure to achieve her goal blood pressure, she was diagnosed with resistant hypertension, and she was referred to the pharmacist clinic for resistant hypertension and medication management. Below is the preliminary information about her past medical history and insurance coverage gathered during an initial chart review.

Past Medical History:
Chronic HF with preserved ejection fraction (HFpEF) (EF ~60%) × 10 years (uncontrolled current edema)
Hypertension × 30 years (uncontrolled)
Hyperlipidemia × 30 years (controlled)
Hypothyroidism (controlled)
Urinary incontinence (uncontrolled)
Injury-induced shoulder pain × 3 weeks (controlled)
Mild cognitive impairment
Insurance coverage: Medicare with supplemental part D

CLINICAL REASONING, CRITICAL THINKING, AND THE PPCP FOR THE CARE OF VIRGINIA H.

The following series of tables delineates the PPCP as it is applied for the provision of pharmacy care to VH. For each step, from Collect to Monitor, there is a description of the pharmacist's clinical reasoning along with examples of how the critical thinking standards can be applied to optimize the pharmacist's clinical reasoning. As with other chapters, clinical reasoning is described in terms of the conclusions drawn, along with case information or premises on which the conclusions are based. As a reminder, the critical thinking standards include clarity, relevance, significance, objectivity, fairness, accuracy, precision, depth, breadth, and logic, embodied in the mnemonic "Clear ROAD for Logic." (See Chapter 1.)

Collect

In this step, the pharmacist collects the subjective and objective information about the patient to gather relevant medical history, medication history, and clinical status of the patient. This step includes both information from the chart review conducted by the pharmacist in preparation for the visit and verified with the patient during the interview.

COLLECT: Current Medications and Immunizations	
Conclusions	Rationale: Information or Premise to Support the Conclusion
Perform a full and complete medication review with the patient during the hypertension consult. *(To be collected during the chart review and the interview)* Match each medication with its indication. Evaluate each medication for efficacy, current side effects, drug interactions, and adherence.	• While the focus will be on cardiovascular medications during the visit, evaluating all other medications allows me to gain an understanding of the complete medication regimen. • Confirming the indication for each medication will help identify potentially inappropriate medications. • By detecting and evaluating possible medication-related adverse effects and drug–drug interactions, pharmacists can play a valuable role in drug safety and can make recommendations for therapeutic alternatives. • A discussion related to adherence should focus on identification and reduction of barriers.
During the medication review, for each medication, reinforce the indication, purpose, proper dosing, use, and possible adverse effects that can occur. *(To be collected during the chart review and shared with patient during the interview)*	• Reinforcing medication indication, purpose, and proper use with the patient is important for optimal medication adherence. • The goal adherence rate for optimal medication efficacy is at least 80%; however, adherence to many chronic medications is around 50%.[15]
Determine if immunizations are up-to-date. *(To be collected during the chart review and the interview)*	• In older adults with cardiovascular disease, it is important to assure that the patient's immunizations are up-to-date, as they have an increased risk of complications and morbidity associated with vaccine preventable diseases.[16]

Critical Thinking Checks for the Collect Plan for This Patient's Current Immunizations and Medications
When reviewing medications for Virginia, I need to ensure that information is gathered in an **objective** manner with **accuracy** and **precision.** • For example, gathering accurate blood pressure readings and precise descriptions of VH's unsteadiness on her feet are necessary to determine optimal goals of care and if her current medications are appropriate.

- In older adults with cognitive impairment, it is important to assess if this impairment limits their ability to manage their medications. An accurate assessment of medication adherence is critical as logical conclusions drawn about therapeutic efficacy and safety rely on an accurate report of the patient's medication usage.
- Additionally, asking the patient to provide details about perceived side effects can help identify nonadherence issues associated with adverse drug reactions (ADRs).

Clear communication with the patient is crucial to ensure that information gathered and conveyed is clearly understood by both the patient and me.

- I must assure that I communicate with a vocabulary and phrasing that VH clearly understands.
- With older adults, I need to determine if there are any impairments in the patient's hearing. If there is a hearing impairment, it is crucial to speak clearly and loudly. Additionally, it can be valuable to limit ambient noises and allow the patient to see your face and lips when you are talking with them.[17]
- Changes in cognition may limit the patient's ability to comprehend and respond to questions asked.[18] For patients with cognitive impairment, ensure that information is presented in a direct manner, speaking both slowly and clearly. Provide information in written format for the patient and/or caregiver to take home and refer to. If the patient has a caregiver, include them in the discussion, while continuing to assure that the patient remains involved in the discussion throughout the interview.[14,19]

Given that the patient has several medical conditions, I need to operate out of **fairness** to her, respecting her autonomy, and ascertaining what concerns are most **significant** for her now and for her overall well-being. Given the complexity of the patient's case, I will ensure appropriate **depth** of thinking when considering benefits and potential risks for each therapeutic alternative, and their impact on other medical conditions.

- For example, for VH, it may be her acute problem with her leg swelling and associated pain that is most concerning for her, rather than her consistently elevated blood pressure readings or her urinary incontinence. In order to build rapport with the patient, I need to demonstrate that I will address her primary concern while also working towards resolving other identified problems important for her overall well-being.

Collected Current Medication and Immunization Information Entered Into Health Record

Current Medication Regimen:

Hydrochlorothiazide 25 mg po daily; Indication: hypertension and edema; the patient takes in the morning; ADR: urinary urgency (added 2 weeks ago)

Furosemide 20 mg po bid; Indication: edema, the patient takes in the morning and early afternoon; ADR: urinary urgency

Losartan 100 mg po daily; Indication: hypertension and HFpEF; the patient takes in the morning; no ADRs

Amlodipine 10 mg po daily; Indication: hypertension; the patient takes in the morning; ADR: lower extremity swelling

Carvedilol 25 mg po bid; Indication: hypertension and HFpEF; the patient takes in the morning and at bedtime; no ADRs

Hydralazine 50 mg po tid; Indication: hypertension; the patient takes in the morning and at bedtime; ADR: lower extremity swelling

Aspirin 81 mg EC po daily; Indication: no clear indication; the patient takes in the morning; no ADRs

Levothyroxine 175 mcg po daily; Indication: hypothyroidism; the patient takes in the morning 30 minutes before other medications; no ADRs

Atorvastatin 10 mg po daily; Indication: hyperlipidemia; the patient takes at bedtime; no ADRs

Oxybutynin ER 10 mg po daily; Indication: urinary urgency; the patient takes in the morning; ADR: dry mouth (added 4 weeks ago)

Diclofenac gel 1% apply 2 g (2.25 inches on dosing card) four times a day; Indication: shoulder pain, the patient applies 2.25 inches four times daily to her shoulder; no ADRs

The patient reports good adherence to her medications except the hydralazine in which she consistently misses the afternoon doses. She admits to occasionally missing her bedtime pills (atorvastatin, carvedilol, hydralazine) one to two times per month.

Current Immunizations:

Influenza vaccine: up-to-date

Pneumococcal vaccine: up-to-date

Zoster vaccine recombinant, adjuvanted (Shingrix®): completed

COVID-19 vaccine: up-to-date

 KEY POINT

In patients with polypharmacy, the risk of nonadherence increases. Assessing for adherence allows us to ensure that medication or dose changes are appropriately treating the condition.

COLLECT: Allergies, Vital Signs, Labs

Conclusions	Rationale: Information or Premise to Support the Conclusion
Verify the patient's medication allergies and document reaction to the medication. *(To be collected during the chart review and the interview)*	• Medication allergies along with the type of reaction should be confirmed in order to determine which medications may be considered and which should not be re-trialed.
Collect the patient's current vital signs, height and weight, and BMP. *(To be collected during the chart review and utilizes appointment vital signs)*	• Weight is important to determine if there are any significant weight changes. This could indicate fluid overload in HF. • Due to the impact of many cardiovascular medications on electrolytes, an updated BMP is crucial to ensure there are no electrolyte abnormalities. Additionally, the BMP will assess serum creatinine (SCr) levels and blood urea nitrogen (BUN) to determine if there have been changes in renal function or if dehydration is a concern. Many cardiovascular medications require renal dose adjustment or could contribute to dehydration.
Collect the patient's most recent fasting lipid panel and thyroid stimulating hormone (TSH). *(To be collected during the chart review)*	• This patient is on atorvastatin, so an updated lipid panel will help us determine if there are problems with efficacy or with adherence to her medication. • Thyroid function impacts the structure of the heart and cardiovascular hemodynamics. Excess or deficiencies in thyroid hormone can exacerbate cardiovascular disorders, including this patient's hypertension, hyperlipidemia, and HF.[20]
Collect both in-office BP results and the results she obtained at home via her blood pressure log along with technique and type of machine utilized. *(To be collected during chart review and interview)*	• Due to the potential for clinic blood pressure readings to be falsely elevated (white coat hypertension), home blood pressure readings allow the pharmacist to see how the blood pressure is in a relaxed state. White coat hypertension occurs in 15% to 30% of patients with elevated blood pressure readings and is more frequently seen in women and older adults.[21] • Inaccurate blood pressure readings can result from not using appropriate technique or using a nonvalidated blood pressure monitor.

Critical Thinking Checks for the Collect Plan for Virginia H.'s Allergies, Vital Signs, and Labs

When gathering information on allergies, it is important for me to obtain **precise** descriptions in order to **accurately** determine the true nature of the patient's response to the medications.

- For example, a review of the medical record showed that VH has a sulfa allergy, so it will be important for me to obtain details about her reaction to help determine if other agents with a sulfonamide moiety can be utilized. Due to structural differences, it is common for a patient with a sulfonamide antimicrobial allergy to not experience cross-reactivity with nonantimicrobial sulfonamide agents.[22] As most diuretics have a sulfonamide group, assessing a patient's sulfa allergy for nonantimicrobial reactions is important.

It is critical for me to focus on collecting the most **relevant** information on the patient's vital signs and labs and that blood pressure readings are **accurate**.

- When reviewing a patient chart, focusing on all the information available can be overwhelming and cause healthcare providers to overlook pertinent information. For VH, focusing on her weight over the past 1 to 2 months is important to assess how well her edema is controlled. Additionally, many hypertensive and HF agents can cause electrolyte dysfunction, dehydration, or kidney damage, making it important to focus on collecting information related to her kidney function (BUN/SCr) and electrolytes. For example, furosemide and hydrochlorothiazide can cause hyponatremia, hypokalemia, and hypomagnesemia, and hydrochlorothiazide can cause hypercalcemia, so it will be important to document the levels of these electrolytes.[5] Since VH has hyperlipidemia, it will be important to review her lipid panel, focusing on her triglycerides, high-density lipoprotein (HDL), and low-density lipoprotein (LDL) values. LDL is the primary focus, as this type of cholesterol is the primary cause of atherosclerosis, while high HDL is considered to be cardioprotective. Hypertriglyceridemia may lead to acute pancreatitis or increase very low-density lipoprotein (VLDL), which is atherogenic.[23]
- Since white coat hypertension is common among patients with hypertension diagnosis, maintaining a home blood pressure log is important when treating a patient's blood pressure, and I will discuss this with VH.[5]

Collected Allergies, Vital Signs, and Lab Information Entered Into the Health Record

Allergies: Sulfa—rash,[1] Ciprofloxacin—nausea/vomiting

Vital Signs: BP: 165/66 mm Hg; HR: 56 bpm

Labs: BMP: BUN 22, SCr 1.08, Na 143, K 4.2, Ca 9.5, glucose 97 mg/dL

Creatinine Clearance: actual body weight 61 mL/min; adjusted body weight 46 mL/min

Fasting Lipid Panel: TC 165 mg/dL, TG 147 mg/dL, HDL 35 mg/dL, LDL 85 mg/dL, VLDL 121 mg/dL

TSH: 0.1 mU/L

Height: 66 in; Weight: 221 lbs (205—1 year ago, 218—2 weeks ago); BMI: 35.8

---

[1]Patient reports a rash approximately 20 years ago when she took a sulfa medication. She states that she is unsure which medication this was, but she was taking it for an infection. Regarding her two current medications with sulfonamide moieties, furosemide and hydrochlorothiazide, she reports no allergy-related problem with over 5 years of furosemide therapy, and she has not experienced any rash since the addition of hydrochlorothiazide.

COLLECT: Social History	
Conclusions	Rationale: Information or Premise to Support the Conclusion
Gather a complete social history for the patient. *(To be collected during the chart review and the interview)*	Social factors—including dietary intake, alcohol and tobacco use, exercise habits, employment, insurance status, living environment, and marital status—can all have significant impacts on the patient's illness and medication experiences (as described in Chapter 1). They can also impact her ability to implement lifestyle changes and manage her cardiovascular disease.
Collect information on who lives with the patient. *(To be collected during the interview)*	Older adults reside in a variety of settings, including skilled nursing facilities, assisted living facilities, with family or independently. Depending upon the level of care provided by their facility or family, patients will have varying levels of responsibility for their medical care. Even those patients residing with family or in assisted living may have several hours of the day where they are alone in the residence.[24]
Collect information on instrumental activities of IADLs. *(Collected during the chart review and the interview)*	In older adults, it is important to assess IADLs to insure they are safe in their homes and are able to care for themselves. Older adults who have problems with their IADLs may be unable to adequately meet their basic needs, which can put them at risk for nutritional deficiency, falls, and accidental injury. When developing a plan for older adults, IADLs must be evaluated, since the care plan created may not be feasible if the patient is having difficulty with basic needs.[25]

Critical Thinking Checks for the Collect Plan for Virginia H.'s Social History

To gather the most **accurate** information needed to optimize my reasoning, **clear** communication with the patient and a **clear** understanding by me are critical. Additionally, it will be important to ascertain a **broad** array of psychosocial information that may be **relevant** to her health status.

- For example, VH has had a recent fall, has experienced worsening edema and has been diagnosed with resistant hypertension. I must collect information about psychosocial factors that may be contributing to these problems and to her overall health. For example, I will need to ask her about different factors that can impact her cardiovascular disease, such as her use of alcohol and caffeine, her dietary intake of sodium and saturated fat, and her physical activity and ability to exercise.[26]

Collected Social History Entered Into the Health Record

Denies alcohol and tobacco use, with no previous history of tobacco use

Denies current or past illicit substance use

Drinks 2 cups of decaffeinated coffee daily

Widowed × 5 years; retired; lives alone,[2] 2 sons who live on the East coast visit infrequently

Dietary habits: Wakes up late; eats 2 meals per day (11 AM and 5 PM), consumes mostly frozen meals, soups, and sandwiches. With each meal, she consumes meat, 2% milk, and cheese. She states she no longer cooks. Her dietary habits resulted in high saturated fat intake and high daily sodium consumption well above the recommended goal of 1500 mg/day.[5]

Exercise: Walks in the pool 2× per week for 30 minutes.

---

[2]She lives alone with very little outside help and is proud of the fact that she is able to live independently at her age.

COLLECT: Shared Decision-Making	
Conclusions	**Rationale: Information or Premise to Support the Conclusion**
Collect information about the patient's situation, lifestyle, baseline habits, values, ability, preferences, and attitude toward potential benefits and risks. *(Collected during the interview)*	Shared decision-making considers the patient's situation, lifestyle, baseline habits, values, ability, preferences, and attitude toward potential benefits and risks. It can be a valuable patient-centered therapeutic approach for older adults that should encompass medication management, self-care, and lifestyle changes.[6] Many clinical situations in cardiovascular care are not straightforward and entail multiple reasonable options, and older adults may have a different set of care goals compared to younger adults.[6] For example, when considering lifestyle changes, the patient's baseline habits, values, abilities, and preferences need to be taken into account in determining the feasibility and impact of these changes.
Collect information about the patient's current understanding and any potential misunderstanding of the disease states and the drugs available to treat the disease states. *(Collected during the interview)*	A patient's understanding about their medications and disease states can be critical for participation in their own care. With older adults, a clear understanding can be compromised by polypharmacy, multiple health problems, and the large amount of health information, including misinformation, available to patients through technology, advertisement, and the Internet. When collecting information from the patient related to their understanding, it is important to uncover any misinformation that can lead to nonadherence and inappropriate patient decision-making.
Collect information on potential challenges that affect older adults when implementing shared decision-making. *(Collected during the interview)*	There are several unique challenges that can affect older adults when implementing shared decision-making. For example, they may have difficulty sharing their goals of care due to cognitive impairment, physical limitations (eg, hearing loss, visual impairment, etc.), low health literacy, or cultural barriers. Additionally, older adults often experience situational complexity (eg, frailty, disabilities, polypharmacy, cost) and evidence gaps (underrepresented in clinical trials) that influence clinical decision-making.[6]

Critical Thinking Checks for the Collect Plan for Virginia H.'s Shared Decision-Making

To make the most appropriate recommendations, I will need to think **broadly** to collect a variety of information that can be important for shared decision-making. I need to be **fair-minded** and consider what is most **significant** to her in a manner that recognizes her autonomy, empowers her to participate in her care, and that honors her expressed desires for her care.

- A review of the chart shows that VH is receiving several medications for primary prevention of cardiovascular disease. It is important to assess how aggressive she would like to be with her primary prevention strategies to determine the best goals of care for her.
- While I am concerned about her systolic blood pressure being in the 160 mm Hg range, her major concern is related to how her edema is affecting her quality of life. She wants to prevent falling; therefore, we must use caution to avoid hypotensive events.
- As I discuss lifestyle changes with VH, I need to make sure that I gather her current lifestyle habits and how much she is willing to change. For example, if VH desires not to expend significant effort on food preparation, I will need to give her ideas for healthy options that she does not have to extensively prepare. When discussing exercise, I will need to consider that she has a difficult time walking and is a fall risk.

KEY POINT

By focusing on the patient's chief concern, we can help build rapport, which will make the patient more likely to adhere to the plan and return for future appointments.

Collected Shared Decision-Making Assessment Entered Into the Health Record

VH's main goal of care is to reduce her pain associated with her edema, which will in turn improve her quality of life. Her independence is important to her. She would like to stay in her own home as long as possible and continue to be able to drive. She feels she takes too many medications and would be interested in stopping anything that was deemed unnecessary. In terms of lifestyle changes, she reports that right now she is unwilling to make any significant changes to her activity level due to her edema-associated leg pain. She states she may be willing to work on her diet, but the changes must be easy to implement.

COLLECT: Cardiovascular Treatment History

Conclusions	Rationale: Information or Premise to Support the Conclusion
Collect information related to the patient's experience with cardiovascular disease states. Inquire how long she has had cardiovascular disease. *(To be collected during the chart review and the interview)*	Gathering a thorough history of cardiovascular treatment and an assessment related to the perceived importance of treatment can be helpful in determining therapy. When looking at cardiovascular disease, intensity of therapy may vary from provider to provider, especially among older adults. This can influence the patient's opinions related to intensive treatment.
Collect information related to home blood pressure monitoring, including technique and type of machine utilized. *(To be collected during the interview)*	Out-of-office blood pressure measurements are a valuable tool in the diagnosis and management of hypertension. There are often inconsistencies in many older adults between office and out-of-office blood pressure readings. This makes at-home monitoring important when determining treatment.[5] Proper technique with a validated automatic machine with appropriate cuff size for the upper arm is important for accurate blood pressure measurement.[5]
Collect information that may help identify potential barriers to optimal medical care. *(To be collected during the interview)*	Many barriers can be identified for optimal care. In older adults, the most common barriers are memory concerns, fixed income with high medical costs, and lack of awareness related to medication importance, all of which can lead to nonadherence.[25] Pharmacists can help identify barriers and develop solutions to address these barriers.[27]
Collect a full assessment of previous nonpharmacological and pharmacological hypertensive regimens. *(To be collected during the chart review and the interview)*	Previous cardiovascular regimens, including nonpharmacological therapy, are important to assess when developing a plan for treatment. When asking about previous therapy, it is important to consider why the therapy was discontinued as some medications may need to be re-trialed when treating cardiovascular disease. In older adults, assessing the dose in relation to adverse effects is important; some side effects are dose-related and could be prevented by starting at a lower dosage, and titrating slowly.

Collect information related to recent hospitalizations, emergency room visits, and falls. *(To be collected during the chart review and the interview)*	Recent hospitalizations, emergency room visits, and falls can help determine the intensity of treatment, identify areas of education, and guide clinical decision-making. Pharmacists can help identify medications that could lead to these negative outcomes and deprescribe.

 KEY POINT

Older adults are often on a fixed income, which limits their ability to pay medication-related copays and adhere to the prescribed therapy.

Critical Thinking Checks for the Collect Plan for Virginia H.'s Cardiovascular Treatment History

Obtaining a cardiovascular treatment history of the appropriate **depth** and **breadth** is critical to determine the patient's past experiences with medications and to help facilitate shared decision-making to determine the goals of care for this patient. Asking about past medication intolerances with the appropriate **accuracy** and **precision** will help inform future decisions related to this patient's care.

Collected Cardiovascular Treatment History Entered Into the Health Record

Hypertensive Treatment History:

- VH states her blood pressure has been elevated her entire life, and she states she "just runs a little higher than everyone else." She thinks she started her first blood pressure medication 30 years ago and reports being on many different medications. She is unable to recall the names of each of these medications and denies any antihypertensive medication intolerances. Her self-reported blood pressure goal is less than 160 mm Hg systolic. She denies any low blood pressure readings but reports occasional dizzy spells when she wakes up to urinate at night.

Heart Failure with Edema Treatment History:

- VH states she was diagnosed with HF approximately 10 years ago. It did not cause her any problems until approximately 5 years ago when she began to develop edema, for which she was prescribed furosemide. Her furosemide has been able to control her edema until approximately 1 year ago when it no longer completely resolved her swelling. She reports the swelling has continued to worsen over the past year and is affecting her ability to walk. This significantly affects her quality of life as she feels unsteady on her feet and had a recent fall.

Hyperlipidemia Treatment History:

- VH reports having high cholesterol for almost 30 years. She worked on her diet for several years, but her cholesterol remained high. At that time, she reports she "gave up" on lifestyle changes and decided that medications would be necessary. She has taken several different "statin" medications of unknown dosages and names. She denies any current problems related to her atorvastatin.

Example Collect Statement for Virginia H.

VH is an 84-year-old female who presents to the pharmacist clinic for cardiovascular risk reduction and treatment, and her chief complaint is persistent lower extremity edema, causing pain and numbness, which is affecting her quality of life and making her feel unsteady on her feet. She presents with multiple conditions, including

HF × 10 years, hypertension × 30 years, hyperlipidemia × 30 years, hypothyroidism, urinary incontinence, and mild cognitive impairment. Among her medications are hydrochlorothiazide 25 mg po daily (begun 2 weeks ago), furosemide 20 mg po bid, losartan 100 mg po daily, amlodipine 10 mg po daily, carvedilol 25 mg po bid, hydralazine 50 mg po tid, aspirin 81 mg EC daily, levothyroxine 175 mcg po daily, atorvastatin 10 mg po daily, oxybutynin ER 10 mg po daily, and diclofenac gel 1% topically four times a day.

Her lower extremity edema is 3+ pitting that has worsened over the past several months. Her shoes no longer fit, which makes it difficult for her to get out of the house. She is unsteady on her feet and is worried about falling. She reports one fall approximately a month ago. After this, she has been using a walker when she leaves her home. Her weight has increased by 3 lbs since her visit 2 weeks ago and 20 lbs in the past year. She reports some extra urination after taking the furosemide but not as much as she used to experience. She has not noticed any improvements in her edema since starting hydrochlorothiazide, and her blood pressure has remained above goal, leading to a diagnosis of resistant hypertension. Her in-office blood pressure is 165/66 mm Hg, and she states that her home blood pressure range from 150 to 180/70 to 80 mm Hg. She is unconcerned about her blood pressure and states it has been high for her whole life. She complains of occasional dizzy spells that occur when she wakes up in the middle of the night to urinate. She states that her urinary urgency has recently gotten worse over the last month, and her primary care provider started oxybutynin 4 weeks ago. She has not seen any efficacy from this medication and shares that she has to wear diapers to prevent leakage. She has been taking baby aspirin for many years based on a recommendation from her previous primary care provider.

She reports adherence to her medications, except she often forgets her midday dose of hydralazine due to doctors' appointments, social outings, or lunch dates. She utilizes a weekly pill box to help her remember her medications, but occasionally (one to two times per month) she misses her bedtime pills (atorvastatin, hydralazine, carvedilol).

When asked about her activities of daily living, she says she lives independently and takes care of her home, her bills, and her medications. She is well groomed today in the office. She has a walker with her and reports that she has been using it for the past month. She occasionally has trouble remembering details and attributes this to old age. She tries to exercise (walks in a pool) 2 days per week and eats mostly frozen meals, soups, and sandwiches that can be high in sodium.

She reports an allergy to sulfa (rash) and ciprofloxacin, which caused her to develop nausea and vomiting. The statuses of her medical conditions include hypertension (uncontrolled, resistant), chronic HFpEF with edema (uncontrolled), hyperlipidemia (controlled), urinary incontinence (uncontrolled), hypothyroidism (controlled), and mild cognitive impairment (controlled). Current labs are within normal limits. No current tobacco, caffeine, alcohol, or illegal drug use.

Assessment of Collected Information

The assessment phase is an important part of the PPCP process as this is where the pharmacist applies clinical reasoning and critical thinking skills to evaluate the collected subjective and objective information to create a comprehensive assessment that will form the basis for the patient-centered plan. Older adults are a heterogeneous population, with some patients in their 80s living independently, traveling, and working, while other 80-year-old adults may be completely reliant on a caregiver to perform their activities of daily living. When assessing the information collected from the patient, it is important to consider the patient's overall functional ability, goals of care, and ability to follow complex plans.

Polypharmacy (taking five or more medications) is common in older adults and is seen even more frequently among those who have cardiovascular disease.[28] Polypharmacy can often lead to patients being on potentially inappropriate medications due to drug–drug interactions or a prescribing cascade, which begins when a new medication is prescribed to treat an adverse drug effect of an existing medication.[29] It is during the assessment phase where pharmacists can play an important role in identifying potentially inappropriate medications and utilizing deprescribing in the Plan step to reduce these unnecessary or potentially harmful medications.[30]

A tool that can be utilized to help identify inappropriate medications is the American Geriatric Society's Beers' Criteria.[31] This criterion includes a list of potentially inappropriate medications for older adults, along with medications that should be used cautiously in those with certain disease states. Additionally, it includes common drug–drug interactions that should be avoided in older adults. While this tool is helpful in evaluating medications in older adults, it is important to consider that these medications are *potentially* inappropriate. This means there may be cases when these agents are warranted and should be recommended; however, if a medication included on this list being used by an older adult patient, it should serve as a reminder to do a thorough investigation.[32]

 KEY POINT

The Beers Criteria is a list of potentially inappropriate medications. There may be occasions when use of these medications is in the best interest of the patient; however, take the time to investigate the situation and ensure their use is appropriate.

During the Assess step, it is imperative to assess each medication, the dosing of that medication, along with the patient's current medical history to identify drug therapy problems. Common drug therapy problems that may be seen in older adults include unnecessary drug therapy, need for additional drug therapy, ineffective drug therapy, dosage too low, dosage too high, ADR, and nonadherence.[33] Each medication should be carefully assessed for these drug therapy problems, and a plan should be developed to address any identified concerns.

Older adults often experience more ADRs than their younger counterparts, making them more likely to have listed medication allergies in their chart.[34] This can render first-line medications inappropriate, leaving providers to utilize less effective second-line treatment options. Assessing each medication allergy is an important step to determine if a medication can be trialed in the future. Many listed chart allergies are intolerances and could be dose-related or related to the timing of when the medication was tried. The pharmacist can help identify true allergies and make recommendations related to utilizing other medications within the medication class to maximize the efficacy of the drug regimen. For example, it is common to have "statin medications" listed as an allergy in the chart; however, it is very uncommon for a patient to have a true "statin" allergy. Most patients will report an allergy to statins due to intolerance—most often muscle pain and/or weakness. When working with an older adult who recently had a heart attack, it is imperative to explore this intolerance and consider retrial with the patient's permission, due to the strong indication for statins in this patient population. Additionally, social factors such as dietary intake, alcohol and tobacco use, exercise habits, employment and insurance status, and living environment and marital status should be assessed as they can influence drug therapy recommendations.

 KEY POINT

When patients report allergies to medications, it is important to identify the specific reaction to identify alternative therapeutic options. It is important to consider that drug intolerances are not the same as allergies and may be tried again.

ASSESS: HFpEF with Uncontrolled Edema	
Conclusions	**Rationale: Information or Premise to Support the Conclusion**
Edema that is significantly impacting quality of life	VH has 3+ pitting edema on exam with associated pain and numbness. The edema is causing her to be unsteady on her feet, requiring use of a walker. Her shoes no longer fit. Her weight has increased approximately 20 lbs over the past year and 3 lbs in the last 2 weeks.
Drug therapy problem Ineffective drug: Furosemide may not be providing adequate diuresis	Loop diuretics are threshold dose medications that have a sigmodal dose-response effect.[35] An effective dose is defined by urine output of 3 to 4 L per dose. Furosemide oral absorption is about 50% and can vary between patients. This patient could be experiencing diuretic resistance; increasing the furosemide dosage or switching to an alternative loop could help overcome this resistance.[36]
The patient is not at risk for an allergic response to her current sulfonamide-containing medications based on her sulfa allergy	Loop diuretics (except ethacrynic acid) and all thiazide diuretics have a sulfonamide component. Since the patient is taking furosemide and hydrochlorothiazide without problems, she can likely use an alternative loop and/or thiazide diuretic without cross-reactivity with her allergy.
The patient is at risk for electrolyte abnormalities[36]	VH has been prescribed sequential nephron blockade with a thiazide and loop diuretic. This combination, given long term, increases her risk of electrolyte abnormalities including hyponatremia, hypokalemia, and hypomagnesemia. Additionally, this combination is not providing efficacy based on her reported symptoms.
This patient could benefit from additional therapy to reduce hospitalizations in HF	VH has HFpEF, so a focus should be on guideline-directed medical therapy and reducing BP to improve outcomes. Mineralocorticoid antagonists (MRA), sodium-glucose-cotransporter (SGLT2) inhibitors, angiotensin-receptor blockers (ARB), or sacubitril/valsartan therapy can decrease hospitalizations in HFpEF.[37] VH is currently on maximum dose ARB therapy. Several options could be done to optimize her HF regimen, including switching her ARB to sacubitril/valsartan, adding an SGLT-2 inhibitor, or adding an MRA.

The patient has multiple factors that may be contributing to her edema including medication adverse effects, limited mobility, comorbid disease states, and diet.	VH is on two antihypertensive agents (hydralazine and amlodipine) that can cause or worsen lower extremity edema. The risk vs benefit of each of these agents should be considered. Patient consumes a high sodium diet which could contribute to edema. Current HF guidelines recommend lowering sodium to reduce congestive symptoms.[37] Limited mobility will also worsen lower extremity swelling; patient should be encouraged to perform regular physical activity as able. Diclofenac is an NSAID. NSAIDs can block the effects of diuretics by inhibiting prostaglandins, leading to sodium and water retention or causing impairment in renal function or perfusion.[37] As this agent is topical, it has a lower risk of interfering with her diuretic regimen due to a limited systemic effect (average 6% systemic absorption).[38]

Critical Thinking Checks for Assessing This Patient's Heart Failure With Uncontrolled Edema

To evaluate VH's HF properly, it was needed to gather and fully consider all **relevant** and **significant** information needed, including her current medications, current disease states, and her personal goals and preferences.

- A proper assessment of VH's HF with uncontrolled edema includes a careful evaluation of her current and previous medications that were collected from the chart and from the patient interview. Her history of diuretic use is important when assessing her complaint of edema, with a focus on efficacy of her current diuretics.

Given the number of comorbid conditions, medications, and contributing factors to this patient's medication-related experience, **depth** and **breadth** of thinking was needed to determine their relevance, significance, and interrelationships to fully explain their impact on her overall health and medication-related problems.

- To develop an effective plan for resolving her edema, I must consider what previous treatments have worked and failed.
- For a complete assessment of her edema, her lifestyle should be considered. VH's high sodium diet and lack of physical activity are contributing to her edema. A detailed plan must include patient education that is relevant to her current IADLs.

It was necessary to assure that the **accuracy** and **precision** of the information gathered was sufficient to allow for effective reasoning.

- In addition to listening carefully to the patient during our discussion, I can utilize the medical record to identify any potential discrepancies that need to be resolved with further questioning. Additionally, I may find that there is some information the patient does not recall. In the event of missing information or discrepancies, I can review past provider records, reach out to the patient's pharmacy, or see if there is a caregiver who may recall additional details.

To be **fair** and **objective**, it was important to be aware of potential biases related to treating older adults. Throughout the collection process, I have objectively evaluated this information and formed conclusions without influence of my emotions or biases.

- For older adults, I need to consider ageist stereotypes and discrimination against older adults.[39] For this patient, her difficult-to-treat-edema has led providers to continue ineffective therapy. I need to be fair and objective while I develop her plan, and not allow potential bias based on her age or difficult-to-treat edema lead me to an unsupported conclusion that her edema is untreatable. Given that improving her persistent edema is her main concern, this should be my primary concern.

ASSESS: Hypertension	
Conclusions	Rationale: Information or Premise to Support the Conclusion
Patient has uncontrolled resistant hypertension[5]	VH is on three first-line medications for blood pressure (hydrochlorothiazide, losartan, amlodipine), along with two second-line agents (hydralazine and carvedilol). Her doses are maximized for each of these medications. She meets the definition of resistant hypertension[3]; therefore, she is a candidate for MRA therapy. Home blood pressure readings 150-180s/70-80s with an in-office reading of 165/66 mm Hg.
Drug therapy problem Ineffective drug: The addition of hydrochlorothiazide 2 weeks ago has not effectively lowered her blood pressure or reduced her edema	VH reports that she has not seen any improvements in her blood pressure readings or edema since starting hydrochlorothiazide.
Drug therapy problem Adverse drug reaction (potential): Amlodipine and hydralazine could be contributing to lower extremity swelling	Dihydropyridine calcium channel blockers, such as amlodipine, and arterial vasodilators, such as hydralazine, can cause or worsen lower extremity edema by causing vasodilation, and therefore may be contributing to factors for VH's edema.[40] This is known as vasodilatory edema and is dose-dependent. It is most common with arteriolar dilators (hydralazine), followed by dihydropyridine calcium channel blockers, and then alpha-blockers. Diuretics have little effect on vasodilatory edema as they merely diminish fluid retention but do not affect the vasodilatory mechanism of edema. ACEi/ARB therapy can help reduce vasodilatory edema via post-capillary dilation, which can normalize intracapillary pressures and reduce fluid in the interstitium.[40] Additionally, hydralazine is not first-line for hypertension and the patient has problems with adherence to hydralazine's three times per day dosing (see later on in the text). Therefore, it may be most appropriate to stop hydralazine. If edema is later determined to be related to amlodipine, we could attempt to lower the dosage as edema is a dose-related adverse effect.
Drug therapy problem Inappropriate adherence: Adherence to hydralazine is poor	Due to her lifestyle, VH is unable to comply with three times a day regimen. Other blood pressure medications manage blood pressure with once daily dosing.
Patient is undervaluing the importance of reducing her blood pressure	Virginia has self-reported that she is unconcerned about her elevated home and office blood pressure readings, stating it has been high for her whole life.
The patient has multiple factors that may be contributing to her hypertension, including excessive sodium intake, physical inactivity, comorbid disease states, and being overweight.	High sodium and low potassium diets are associated with elevated blood pressure.[5] Other treatable factors that can contribute to her hypertension include her weight (Weight: 221 lbs, BMI: 35.8), excessive dietary sodium (frozen foods, soups, and sandwiches), and low physical activity (due to edema-induced limited mobility).

---

[3]Resistant hypertension—Blood pressure that remains above goal despite concurrent use of three antihypertensive agents of different classes taken at maximally tolerated doses, one of which should be a diuretic.

KEY POINT

Consider if any medications may be contributing to a patient's complaint. If the medication may cause the adverse effect in question, it may be appropriate to discontinue the offending agent and identify an alternative therapy.

Critical Thinking Checks for Assessing This Patient's Hypertension

For a proper assessment of Virginia H.'s hypertension, previous medication regimens, current medication therapy, home blood pressure monitoring, and lifestyle factors need to be carefully assessed for **relevance** and **significance**. I utilized my knowledge related to the mechanisms of action for each medication, to gain a greater depth of understanding regarding the patient's current therapy and adverse effects.

- Current guidelines can be utilized to determine patient-centered goals for care and to assess current medication therapy for efficacy and safety.
- Several common adverse effects of antihypertensive medications are related to their mechanism of action. Examples include ACEi-associated cough caused by elevated bradykinin- and vasodilator-associated edema. Assessing medication dosing in relationship to medication adverse effects is imperative as often side effects are dose-related.

In order to **accurately** assess the effectiveness of her current therapy, I need to consider adherence with the medication regimen.

- Assessing adherence to antihypertensive therapy and utilizing methods to improve adherence (eg, reducing pill burden by combining medications or discontinuing medications with multiple daily doses) is an important part of antihypertensive management. Medications are most effective when taken as prescribed.

Lastly, I need to be **fair** and **objective** when establishing blood pressure goals, keeping in mind the patient's goals of care and overall health.

- VH's indifference related to her blood pressure could bias clinicians to not escalate or target appropriate blood pressure goals.

KEY POINT

We need to avoid bias due to older age and clinical inertia in older adult patients by adhering to guideline-recommended therapies when appropriate.

ASSESS: Primary Prevention of Atherosclerotic Cardiovascular Disease	
Conclusions	**Rationale: Information or Premise to Support the Conclusion**
The risk vs benefit of continued use of aspirin and statin therapy for primary prevention of atherosclerotic cardiovascular disease (ASCVD) should be evaluated Drug therapy problem Unnecessary drug therapy: aspirin	Aspirin 81 mg is not recommended for adults >70 years for the primary prevention of ASCVD.[26,41] VH is taking a statin for primary prevention of ASCVD. According to the 2018 cholesterol guidelines, shared decision-making should occur when determining if she should continue the statin medication.[23] Her current cholesterol panel is well controlled with an LDL of 85 mg/dL, and she is tolerating the statin with no ADRs.

| Patient could benefit from lifestyle changes for primary cardiovascular disease prevention | Several lifestyle changes can positively impact VH's ASCVD risk. The 2019 primary prevention guidelines recommend weight loss, a healthy diet with reduced sodium and increased potassium, physical activity, and moderate alcohol intake to reduce ASCVD risk.[26] |

Critical Thinking Checks for Assessing This Patient's Primary Prevention of ASCVD

I need to ensure that I have investigated the patient's risk for cardiovascular disease at the appropriate **breadth** and **depth** as this is a complicated situation, where it is difficult to apply primary literature to older patients with multiple comorbidities. I will also need to ensure I am **fair** and **objective** and that I avoid any age-related biases.

For older adults, determining the degree of ASCVD is a significant and relevant part of their past medical history, as this will categorize patients as secondary or primary prevention. Heart failure can oftentimes be categorized as ASCVD when it is ischemic in origin. For Virginia H., her HFpEF is nonischemic and is related to her long-standing hypertension. Assessing her past medical history from the chart and patient-reported history, it was determined that she falls in the category of primary prevention of ASCVD. For primary prevention in older adults, clinical trials and guidelines will provide the depth of knowledge needed to determine the appropriateness of medication therapy.

ASSESS: Other Drug Therapy Problems

Conclusions	Rationale: Information or Premise to Support the Conclusion
Adverse drug reaction: Exacerbation of urinary incontinence by furosemide and hydrochlorothiazide leading to a prescribing cascade	Loop diuretics increase urination which can cause or exacerbate urinary incontinence. This is a long-term side effect that demonstrates the efficacy of the medication.[42] Thiazide diuretics also cause increased urination upon initiation; however, patients often become tolerant of this side effect. Use of oxybutynin to treat urinary frequency demonstrates an example of a prescribing cascade, where it was added to treat a side effect. Furthermore, this agent could be contributing to her nighttime dizziness, which increases her risk of falling.
Ineffective drug: Oxybutynin for this patient's urinary incontinence Needs additional therapy for urinary incontinence	A recent meta-analysis found that behavioral therapy such as bladder training was statistically significantly more effective at reducing incontinence symptoms than anticholinergic agents in urgency urinary incontinence.[43] Patient reports oxybutynin has been ineffective after an adequate trial of 4 weeks; therefore, this agent should be stopped.
No current drug therapy problem related to patient's reported allergies to sulfa compounds and ciprofloxacin	For Virginia H., she reports a rash approximately 20 years ago when she took a sulfa medication. She states that she is unsure which medication this was, but she was taking it for an infection. In assessing her medications with her allergies, she reports no problem with furosemide (taking for 5 years), and no rash after the addition of hydrochlorothiazide 2 weeks ago. Therefore, she is not likely to be allergic to all sulfonamide medications. For her reported ciprofloxacin allergy, her reported nausea and vomiting indicate drug intolerance or adverse effects rather than a true allergy.

ASSESS: Additional Past Medical History	
Conclusions	Rationale: Information or Premise to Support the Conclusion
Pain (controlled)	VH has no current shoulder pain complaints related to her fall from 3 weeks ago. She reports using diclofenac gel four times daily.
Mild cognitive impairment	VH has mild age-related cognitive impairment. This is currently not significantly affecting her quality of life.
Hypothyroidism (controlled)	VH's TSH levels are within normal limits, indicating control and appropriate levothyroxine dosing and adherence.
Urinary incontinence (uncontrolled)	VH reports that her urinary incontinence is not controlled after an adequate trial of oxybutynin. She reports that her urinary urgency has recently gotten worse over the last month and that she wears diapers daily. Her incontinence is exacerbated by her use of diuretics (furosemide and hydrochlorothiazide).

Critical Thinking Checks for Assessing This Patient's Drug Therapy Problems and Past Medical History

My assessment is **logically** justified and was expressed with **clarity, accuracy,** and **precision** which allows for a patient-centered plan to be developed.

- Multiple drug therapy problems often lead to inappropriate prescribing and the prescribing cascade. It is **logical** that this patient may experience a prescribing cascade based on the addition of oxybutynin to control incontinence caused by furosemide and hydrochlorothiazide. Given that there are effective nonpharmacological approaches for incontinence and factoring the potential contributions to her edema by hydralazine and amlodipine, there is strong evidence to support deprescribing several agents for this patient.

In order to make the most appropriate plan, we must consider all comorbid conditions and medications at the appropriate **breadth** and **depth**.

- VH has several interrelated conditions and is experiencing polypharmacy. It is therefore critical for me to think broadly and deeply to grasp the complexity of the interrelationships between her conditions and her care, which include the drug interactions and side effects that she may experience.

Given the complexity of this patient, who has several concurrent conditions and is taking several medications, it can be useful to create a concept map to help grasp some of the interrelationships that contribute to the complexity. **Figure 3-2** shows a map that illustrates these interrelationships. It also depicts a common prescribing cascade that can be seen in this patient with a calcium channel blocker for hypertension-causing edema, the prescribing of a diuretic to help reduce this edema, and the patient receiving a prescription for oxybutynin due to worsening urinary urgency.[29] Using a concept map to depict interrelationships between conditions and medications can be useful for creating a comprehensive assessment of this patient, which is expressed in the Assess statement below.

Example Assess Statement for Virginia H.

Virginia H. is an 84-year-old female presenting to the pharmacist clinic for cardiovascular disease state management with a focus on worsening edema.

(1) HFpEF with uncontrolled edema that is affecting her quality of life.

Patient reports edema with associated pain and numbness. She complains of feeling unsteady on her feet, having to use a walker, and that her shoes no longer fit.

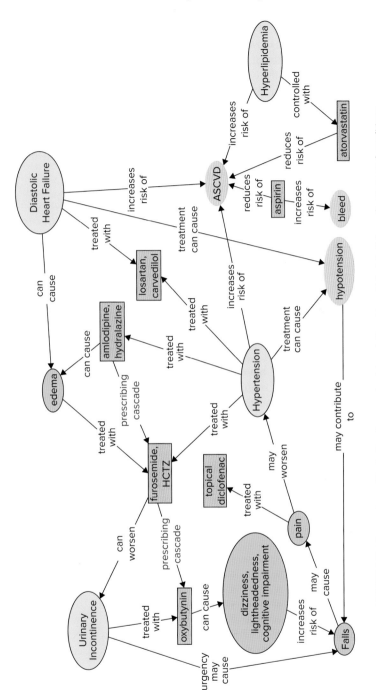

FIGURE 3-2. Concept map illustrating the complex interrelationships of Virginia H.'s medications and conditions.

This is impacting her quality of life as she is no longer able to be as active. Upon exam, the edema is 3+ pitting. Her weight has increased approximately 20 lbs in the past year, with an additional 3 lbs of weight increase over the past 2 weeks. She is taking furosemide 20 mg twice daily to treat this edema and reports that she is not urinating as much as she used to with this agent. Approximately 2 weeks ago, her cardiologist added hydrochlorothiazide to her furosemide. Since then, the patient has not noticed any improvement in her swelling. Sequential nephron blockade is not reducing VH's edema; therefore, the hydrochlorothiazide should be stopped. VH's high sodium diet, lack of physical activity, limited mobility, and her use of hydralazine and amlodipine are all potential contributing factors to her edema.

Loop diuretics are threshold dose medications that induce 3 to 4 L of fluid output with each dose. Patients can become diuretic resistant through multiple mechanisms, which make loop agents less effective.[44] One way to overcome diuretic resistance is to switch to an alternative loop diuretic. When picking an alternative loop, it is important to note that VH has a sulfa allergy. As she is taking furosemide without any problems, she will likely not have an allergic reaction to alternative loop agents such as bumetanide or torsemide.

VH's HFpEF could benefit from additional therapy with an MRA, such as spironolactone.

She could benefit from lifestyle counseling.

(2) Uncontrolled hypertension

VH reports uncontrolled home blood pressure readings in the 150-180s/70-80s with an office reading of 165/66 mm Hg. According to the 2017 ACC/AHA blood pressure guidelines and the 2022 HF guidelines, her blood pressure goal is <130/80 mm Hg.[5,37] She is currently taking three first-line blood pressure medications (amlodipine, losartan, hydrochlorothiazide) along with three second-line agents (hydralazine, carvedilol, furosemide), all at max doses. Her adherence is good with these medications, except hydralazine, where she reports missing the midday dose most days of the week. She is unconcerned about her elevated blood pressure, reporting that it has been high for over 30 years. Her amlodipine and hydralazine could be contributing to her persistent edema. She meets the definition of resistant hypertension and could benefit from the addition of MRA therapy.

VH's high sodium diet, low potassium diet, lack of physical activity, and weight are all contributing to her hypertension. She could benefit from lifestyle counseling.

(3) Primary prevention of ASCVD

VH's past medical history does not indicate clinical ASCVD; therefore, she meets the criteria for primary ASCVD prevention. She has been taking low-dose aspirin for years to prevent ASCVD. Updated practice guidelines no longer recommend aspirin for primary prevention in patients >70 years due to the increased risk of bleeding and lack of benefit seen in this patient population.[26,41] VH is receiving atorvastatin for primary ASCVD prevention. While her baseline cholesterol values are unknown, her current LDL value of 85 mg/dL indicates an appropriate response to therapy, as guidelines recommend adding on additional therapy in most patients if LDL remains above 100 mg/dL.[23] In this patient population, shared decision-making should occur when determining if she should continue the statin medication.[37]

VH's high sodium diet, low potassium diet, lack of physical activity, and weight are all contributing to her ASCVD risk. Lifestyle changes would be beneficial in reducing ASCVD risk.

Drug therapy problems for VH include the following:

- Adverse drug reaction: potential edema with hydralazine and amlodipine
- Adverse drug reaction: increased urination with diuretics
- Unnecessary drug therapy: aspirin 81 mg daily
- Ineffective drug: hydrochlorothiazide
- Ineffective drug: furosemide
- Ineffective drug: oxybutynin
- Inappropriate adherence: hydralazine
- Needs additional nonpharmacological therapy for urinary incontinence
- Needs additional pharmacological therapy for HF

These conclusions drawn in the Assess step serve as the basis for the therapeutic decision-making that will occur in the Plan step.

Plan, Implement, and Monitor

PLAN: Goals	
Conclusions	**Rationale: Information or Premise to Support the Conclusion**
Goals include: 1. Improve edema from 3+ to 2+ within 1 to 2 weeks. Eliminate her symptoms of pain, numbness, and unsteadiness. 2. Reduce blood pressure by 10 mm Hg in the next 4 weeks. 3. Reduce current dietary sodium by 1000 mg within the next 2 months with an optimal goal of <1500 mg/day. 4. Increase physical activity to 150 minutes per week over the next 3 months. 5. After reducing edema-associated weight gain, achieve a 5% weight loss over the next 3 months	1. Current edema is 3+ and is causing symptoms. Symptoms could be eliminated by improving edema. Most patients with edema will never have complete resolution of their symptoms but reducing the severity of symptoms is a realistic goal that can improve quality of life. 2. Goal blood pressure <130/80 mm Hg according to the most current hypertension and HF guidelines.[5,37] Upon utilizing shared decision-making with VH she is agreeable to a goal <130/80 mm Hg, but wishes to limit polypharmacy to reduce her fall risk. Blood pressure reduction should occur gradually in patients to limit symptoms of hypotension. Each additional blood pressure medication can reduce blood pressure by up to 10 mm Hg so this is an appropriate initial goal for this patient. 3. While restricting sodium to 1500 mg may be appropriate for some patients, guidelines have suggested that any reduction in sodium intake can reduce hypertension and congestive symptoms.[37] 4. This patient is limited in her mobility but is currently exercising in the pool for 60 minutes each week. Increasing this gradually to 150 minutes per week can help reduce her cardiovascular risk factors. 5. Reducing the weight in this patient is an important parameter to assess for improvement in edema if her excess weight over the past year is deemed to be related to fluid retention. Current BMI 35.8—obesity classification. After reducing extra weight associated with edema, a 3% to 5% weight loss (approximate goal weight 210 lbs at 3 months) can reduce cardiovascular risk.[26]

Critical Thinking Checks for Developing This Patient's Goals

Utilizing shared decision-making, SMART goals are developed for VH that are Specific, Measurable, Achievable, Realistic, and Timely. By using the SMART criteria, these goals are able to be understood by her. Due to the **breadth** and **depth** of information gathered and use of evidence-based medicine, SMART goals help set **clear** patient and provider expectations, while outlining the goals of care.

PLAN: Uncontrolled HFpEF with Edema

Goals:
1. Improve edema from 3+ to 2+ within 1 to 2 weeks. Eliminate her symptoms of edema-associated pain, numbness, and unsteadiness.
2. Reduce current dietary sodium by 1000 mg within the next 2 months with an optimal goal of <1500 mg/day.
3. Increase physical activity to 150 minutes per week over the next 3 months.

Conclusions	Rationale: Information or Premise to Support the Conclusion
Stop furosemide 20 mg po bid Start bumetanide 0.5 mg po bid	Due to patient not experiencing effective diuresis with furosemide, switching to an alternative diuretic is indicated.[36]
Start spironolactone 12.5 mg po daily	MRA therapy can reduce HF hospitalizations in patients with HFpEF.[37]
Reduce current dietary sodium by 1000 mg/day to an optimal goal of <1500 mg/day	A reduction in dietary sodium can improve congestive symptoms.[37]
Increase physical activity to 150 minutes per week	This patient is limited in her mobility but is currently exercising in the pool for 60 minutes each week. Increasing this gradually to 150 minutes per week can help reduce her cardiovascular risk factors. Increasing physical activity to a goal of 150 minutes per week can improve symptoms of HF.[37]
Elevate the lower limbs throughout the day and wear compression stockings if tolerated.	In VH's case, her HF is likely contributing to edema, which is addressed by diuretic therapy; however, in older adults, edema is commonly associated with venous insufficiency. Lower limb elevation and compression stockings, when tolerated, can help improve VH's symptoms.[45]

Critical Thinking Checks for This Patient's Uncontrolled HFpEF with Edema

In developing a treatment plan for Virginia H., I utilized **breadth** and **depth** to consider the risk vs benefits of each medication I was considering.

- When I develop a plan for older adults, it is important to consider polypharmacy. Can a new medication replace an existing medication, or do I need to add on additional therapy? If I am going to implement new drug therapy, I need to consider how this new drug will affect the other medications that the patient takes and their disease states. Education related to this medication is important. I need to make sure that VH understands how to monitor for efficacy and safety. Treatment benefits and risks should be **clearly** explained to the patient as part of the shared decision-making process. Using the teach-back method can be helpful to determine the patient's understanding of the new therapy.

When making lifestyle recommendations, they need to be **specific, relevant,** and **logical** to the patient.

- For VH who has limited mobility, it is important to suggest activities that she can perform, such as swimming or seated exercises. Furthermore, since VH does not cook, recommending frozen bags of vegetables or frozen nonprocessed meats could help her reduce her sodium consumption without causing a major inconvenience.

KEY POINT

When a patient does not have an adequate response to a medication, it may be appropriate to discontinue the medication and try an alternative agent, versus continuing the medication and contributing to polypharmacy.

PLAN: Uncontrolled Hypertension

Goals:
1. Reduce blood pressure by 10 mm Hg in the next 4 weeks.
2. Reduce current dietary sodium by 1000 mg within the next 2 months with an optimal goal of <1500 mg/day.
3. Increase physical activity to 150 minutes per week over the next 3 months.
4. After reducing edema-associated weight gain, achieve a 5% weight loss over the next 3 months

Conclusions	Rationale: Information or Premise to Support the Conclusion
Stop hydrochlorothiazide due to lack of efficacy	VH has seen no improvement in her edema symptoms or her hypertension since starting hydrochlorothiazide.
Start spironolactone 12.5 mg po daily for resistant hypertension	MRA therapy is first line for resistant hypertension, which is defined as being on three antihypertensives at maximum dose with uncontrolled blood pressure.[5]
Reduce dietary sodium by 1000 mg/day with an optimal goal of <1500 mg/day	Reducing dietary sodium can reduce systolic blood pressure by 5 to 6 mm Hg.[26]
Increase aerobic physical activity to 150 minutes per week	Increasing aerobic exercise to 150 minutes per week can reduce systolic blood pressure by 5 to 8 mm Hg.[26]
Reduce weight by 3% to 5%	Recommend a 3% to 5% reduction in body weight (goal weight 210 lbs at 3 months) in obese individuals to reduce hypertension. Every 1 kg reduction in body weight can reduce systolic blood pressure by 1 mm Hg.[26]

Critical Thinking Checks for Uncontrolled Hypertension

The foundation of this plan is to **clearly** educate VH on the importance of blood pressure lowering so she will want to work on controlling her hypertension.
• As the patient is on multiple antihypertensive agents currently, using medications that can control blood pressure and improve edema should be the initial goal. The spironolactone will not only lower blood pressure, but it also reduces the risk of HF hospitalization. Future changes may include use of alternative, more potent blood pressure medications, and combination medications to reduce pill burden and improve adherence for VH.

PLAN: Primary Prevention of ASCVD

Conclusions	Rationale: Information or Premise to Support the Conclusion
Stop aspirin	Recent clinical trial data recommends that adults >70 years do not take aspirin for primary prevention of ASCVD.[26] The 2022 US Preventative Services Task Force has concluded that initiation of aspirin for primary prevention in those 60 years or older has no net benefit.[41]

| Continue atorvastatin | Statins for primary prevention in older adults is controversial. There are few adults >70 years included in clinical trials, which limits our evidence of benefit; however, a few studies have shown that statin medications provide benefit in patients ≥75 years at ~2 years.[46–48] Additionally, one cohort study demonstrated an increased risk of cardiovascular hospitalization following statin discontinuation.[49] |
| Counseling patients on lifestyle changes to reduce ASCVD risk, including reducing sodium, weight loss, and physical activity | To reduce ASCVD risk, the DASH diet or Mediterranean diet can be utilized. Key components of these diets include replacing saturated fats with dietary monounsaturated and polyunsaturated fats, reducing dietary cholesterol, and limiting sodium. Other recommendations include reducing processed meats, refined carbohydrates, sweetened beverages, and trans fats. Other lifestyle changes include increasing physical activity to at least 150 minutes per week and weight loss of 3% to 5%.[26] |

Critical Thinking Checks for This Patient's ASCVD Risk

Developing a plan to reduce the patient's ASCVD risk will utilize an evidence-based, shared decision-making approach with an emphasis on **significance** to the patient.

- When developing a plan on how to reduce ASCVD risk, patient goals and preferences should be considered. This elderly female has an estimated 5-year mortality of around 25% to 30%, and this should be considered when evaluating primary prevention measures.[50]
- When making a plan for deprescribing, it is important to consider the patient's personal preferences. Patients may be more hesitant to discontinue OTC agents such as low-dose aspirin or supplements. **Clearly** explaining the potential harms and benefits can be helpful in providing education related to deprescribing.

I must discuss medication and lifestyle recommendations with appropriate **clarity** and ensure that changes are **logical** given the patient's current living situation.

- When making recommendations to stop primary prevention measures, patients may be resistant on the basis that they have been taking these therapies for years. It is important to provide appropriate patient education on why these agents are no longer recommended for primary prevention, including the reason behind this recommendation.
- In terms of lifestyle, VH could benefit from making several lifestyle changes. Reducing sodium in her diet, reducing her body weight by 3% to 5%, and increasing her physical activity could all reduce her ASCVD risk. A detailed plan must include patient education that is relevant to her current IADLs.

PLAN: Drug Therapy Problems	
Conclusions	Rationale: Information or Premise to Support the Conclusion
Stop hydralazine	Hydralazine could be contributing to lower extremity edema. Additionally, patient is not fully adherent with hydralazine, which is resulting in reduced efficacy.
Stop oxybutynin	Patient has seen no improvement in her symptoms with an adequate trial of oxybutynin. This medication is on the Beers® criteria for potentially inappropriate medications due to anticholinergic effects.[31]

Refer for nonpharmacological measures for urinary incontinence. Recommend reducing fluid intake before bedtime.	First-line treatment of urinary urgency is nonpharmacological management including bladder training, biofeedback, education, weight loss, and yoga.[43] Given her dizziness at night when she needs to urinate, we can also recommend reduced fluid intake before bed.

Critical Thinking Checks for This Patient's Drug Therapy Problems

- When a drug therapy problem is identified, it is important to consider what implications making a drug therapy change will have on all the patient's current disease states. This requires an analysis at the appropriate **depth** and **breadth**. For example, when deprescribing, I always try to anticipate how the medication will affect other disease states. I then develop a **logical** contingency plan in the event the patient complains of worsening symptoms after the agent is stopped.

When determining the appropriateness of VH's diuretic therapy, an argument map can be utilized to demonstrate the principles supporting an argument. An example of a map for supporting the argument to switch to an alternative loop diuretic for this patient is shown in **Figure 3-3**. The map

Recommendation

Stop Furosemide 20 mg Twice Daily. Start Bumetanide 0.5 Mg Twice Daily.

Loop diuretics are not "lazy." Each dose should induce 3 to 4 L of urine output.	Diuretic resistance is common with loop diuretics. This causes patients to not respond as well to the loop.	Furosemide has poor absorption (~50%) which can be variable among patients.	Switching to an alternative loop diuretic can help overcome diuretic resistance.	Assumption to verify: The patient is experiencing diuretic resistance.

SMART Goal

Within 1 week relieve edema symptoms, reduce weight by 2 to 3 lbs, and improve the patient's perception of their quality of life.

Assessment

Uncontrolled edema with contributing factors that include HF with preserved ejection fraction, high dietary sodium, sedentary lifestyle, and age. Drug therapy problem: Medication therapy no longer effective. Need alternative therapy.

FIGURE 3-3. Argument map for switching to an alternative loop diuretic.[36]

shows part of the hidden underlying structure of the argument, beginning with conclusions drawn to create the Assessment, which supports the recommendation for changing the loop diuretic.

 KEY POINT

The pharmacokinetics of loop diuretics are not linear. A threshold dose is needed to elicit an effective response (typically 3 to 4 L of urine output).

IMPLEMENT/MONITOR: HFpEF with Uncontrolled Edema and Uncontrolled Hypertension	
Conclusions	Rationale: Information or Premise to Support the Conclusion
Implement: Stop furosemide 20 mg twice daily. Start bumetanide 0.5 mg twice daily. Education: Take first dose upon waking and 2nd dose around 2 PM. *Monitor:* Monitor weight daily. Call the clinic with weight gain >2 lbs overnight or >5 lbs in 1 week Monitor lower extremity edema. Check BMP and magnesium in 1 week	*Implement:* Switching to an alternative loop diuretic will help overcome diuretic resistance to improve edema. Patients taking loop diuretics should be educated to take their last dose at least 4 h prior to bedtime to reduce nighttime urination. *Monitor:* Weight monitoring can be implemented at home to measure the effectiveness of loop diuretic therapy. BMP, with a focus on potassium, sodium, and renal parameters (BUN/SCr) should be monitored for 1 to 2 weeks after adjusting diuretics. Due to chronic diuretic therapy, a magnesium level should be drawn.
Implement: Stop hydrochlorothiazide 25 mg. Start spironolactone 12.5 mg take 1 tablet in the morning Education: The smallest strength tablet available is 25 mg so you will have to cut this tablet in half. *Monitor:* Monitor home blood pressure readings twice daily. Write down values in a blood pressure log and bring it to your next appointment. Call with systolic blood pressure readings consistently high (>180 mm Hg) or low (<100 mm Hg) Check BMP in 1 week Monitor for new-onset breast tenderness	*Implement:* Spironolactone is an effective treatment for HFpEF to reduce hospitalizations and reduce blood pressure in resistant hypertension. In older adults, this medication should be started at a low dose of 12.5 mg and labs monitored closely for hyperkalemia. *Monitor:* Home blood pressure monitoring can be done to assess the efficacy and safety of spironolactone. Spironolactone can cause hyperkalemia; therefore, a BMP should be drawn 1 week after initiation. Educate patients that spironolactone can cause breast tenderness.

Implement:	*Implement:*
Educate on the importance of reducing dietary sodium by 1000 mg/day with a goal to reduce to 1500 mg/day long term.	Dietary therapy, including reducing sodium and increasing potassium, can improve congestive symptoms and reduce blood pressure. VH should not be educated to increase potassium foods at this time due to the initiation of spironolactone, which can elevate potassium levels.
Provide dietary changes that can help reduce sodium, including limiting condiments, processed foods, canned foods, and frozen dinners. When processed foods are needed, purchase the low-sodium version, if available.	
Provide education on how to read food labels.	*Monitor:*
Monitor:	Dietary food logs can be helpful in determining a patient's adherence to dietary therapy, but they are cumbersome for older adults. As VH is not interested in making significant dietary changes, discussing the impact of sodium and adherence to reduced sodium intake are adequate monitoring parameters.
Monitor the patient's understanding of sodium's impact on blood pressure.	
Assess for adherence with reduced sodium diet.	
Implement:	*Implement:*
Increase physical activity to 150 minutes per week. Start by exercising in the pool for 30 minutes 3 days per week, with the goal to increase to 5 days per week.	Increased physical activity can improve symptoms of edema, reduce fatigue associated with HF, and reduce blood pressure.
Monitor:	*Monitor:*
Assess for adherence with exercise	A simple exercise recall is appropriate to determine adherence with this recommendation.

 KEY POINT

When making lifestyle suggestions, a patient's goals and ability to implement them must be incorporated into the plan.

IMPLEMENT/MONITOR: Primary Prevention of ASCVD	
Conclusions	**Rationale: Information or Premise to Support the Conclusion**
Implement:	*Implement:*
Stop aspirin	Aspirin is not recommended in VH for primary prevention
Monitor:	*Monitor:*
Self-reported aspirin use	When assessing OTC medication use, patient self-reported use is appropriate.
Implement:	*Implement:*
Continue atorvastatin 10 mg po daily	Utilizing shared decision-making, VH has decided to continue atorvastatin. She does not report any current adverse effects.
Monitor:	*Monitor:*
Fasting lipid panel in 1 year	Fasting lipid panel should be done yearly in patients on stable hyperlipidemia treatment.
Follow dietary and exercise recommendations in HFpEF and hypertension sections (see above)	

KEY POINT

Pharmacists play an imperative role in deprescribing efforts due to knowledge of guideline-recommended therapy, adverse effects, and interactions.

IMPLEMENT/MONITOR: Drug Therapy Problems

Conclusions	Rationale: Information or Premise to Support the Conclusion
Implement: Stop hydralazine when spironolactone is initiated. *Monitor:* Monitor home blood pressure readings twice daily. Call with systolic blood pressure readings consistently high (>180 mm Hg) or low (<100 mm Hg) Monitor lower extremity edema	*Implement:* Hydralazine should be discontinued to assess if it is contributing to lower extremity edema. By discontinuing hydralazine when spironolactone is initiated, we do not anticipate significant blood pressure elevations during the medication change. *Monitor:* When antihypertensive therapy adjustments are made, patients should be counseled to monitor their home blood pressure twice daily. Would expect improvement in edema with discontinuation of hydralazine.
Implement: Stop oxybutynin *Monitor:* Urinary urgency symptoms	*Implement:* Oxybutynin has not controlled VH's urinary urgency and she is complaining of dry mouth related to this medication and occasional dizzy spells. *Monitor:* When stopping oxybutynin, patients should be counseled to monitor for worsening of their urinary urgency symptoms.
Implement: Refer patient to primary care provider to discuss nonpharmacologic treatment options for urinary urgency *Monitor:* Urinary urgency symptoms	*Implement:* This visit focused on cardiovascular concerns related to hypertension and edema. While the oxybutynin was discontinued due to risk of adverse effects, referral for nonpharmacologic treatment options would be appropriate. Potential interventions include pelvic floor muscle training to strengthen the muscles and bladder training to hold urine for a longer length of time.[43] *Monitor:* Patient-reported incontinence episodes would be helpful for the primary care physician at follow-up appointment.

Critical Thinking Checks for This Patient's Implementation and Monitoring Plan

- Involving VH in the implementation section of her plan is critical as this is the section that she is most involved in. It should include **fair**, achievable steps that are **relevant** to her reported concerns and overall health. The implementation involves her managing her health at home and includes side effects she should watch for and monitoring that she should be implementing to determine if her new therapy is effective. The implementation plan should be **clear** and communicated in patient friendly terms. Written education material, including a detailed plan of the most **significant** aspects, should be provided for her at the end of the appointment. VH should be encouraged to ask questions related to the plan so the pharmacist can be reassured that she understands any medication and lifestyle changes that she should implement. Follow-up should be scheduled for 2 weeks with the pharmacist clinic to assure that she has been able to implement the plan, and further adjustments will be made at that time.

CONCLUSION

Cardiovascular care for older adults should be patient-centered; this is especially crucial given the complexity often seen in this patient population. The PPCP is a systematic clinical problem-solving tool that can be utilized to collect appropriate information, assess that information, and based on the assessment, work with the patient to develop a patient-centered care plan. Throughout the process, the pharmacist must apply excellent clinical reasoning and critical thinking skills and must consider patient preferences and utilize evidence-based medicine to make recommendations that optimize patient outcomes.

Summary Points

- Cardiovascular disease is prevalent in older adults; however, the management of these conditions is challenging due to comorbid disease states, polypharmacy, and variable life expectancy.
- Utilizing the patient care process when working with older adults allows the pharmacist to ensure a comprehensive treatment plan is developed.
- When collecting information from an older adult, multiple aspects should be considered, including a comprehensive chart review and a thorough patient interview that is tailored to the patient. Clear communication with the patient is crucial to ensure that information gathered and conveyed is clearly understood by both the patient and the pharmacist. The pharmacist should conduct the interview with a fair-minded approach, respecting the patient's autonomy, and determine the concerns that are most significant for her now and for her overall well-being. It is important to obtain precise descriptions of the patient's medication response in order to accurately determine their true nature. Additionally, it will be important to ascertain a broad array of psychosocial information that may be relevant to the patient's health status and that may be important to factor into therapeutic planning, implementation, and monitoring.
- When assessing an older adult with cardiovascular disease, it is critical to exhibit a broad mindset and consider all comorbid conditions, medications, and social history, in order to develop a comprehensive treatment plan. Appropriate depth and breadth of thinking are critical for the pharmacist to fully understand the complexities of the interrelationships to fully explain their impact on the patient's overall health and medication-related problems. To be fair and objective, it is important for the pharmacist to be aware of potential biases related to treating older adults and to evaluate information and form conclusions without the influence of emotions or biases. Assuring the assessment is logically sound and expressed with clarity, accuracy, and precision facilitates the development of the subsequent patient-centered plan.
- Incorporation of shared decision-making when developing the plan, with an emphasis on what is significant to the patient, can improve adherence and effectiveness. It is important to be fair and objective when establishing goals, keeping in mind the patient's own goals for their care and for their overall health, and it can be important to use the SMART criteria to construct goals to enable them to be understood by the patient. In developing a logical, evidence-based treatment plan for the patient, breadth and depth of thinking are required to consider interrelationships between the patient's conditions and medications,

and the risks versus benefits of each medication. Both medication and lifestyle recommendations are developed with the patient with clarity and fair-mindedness to help assure changes are appropriate and logical given the patient's current living situation.

- Due to the complexities of the older adult, it is imperative that the implementation plans are clear, and adequate monitoring and follow-up occur. Involving patients in the implementation of their plans is critical as this is the step they are most involved in. The implementation plan should be clear and communicated in patient friendly terms. Written education material should be provided, including a detailed plan of the most significant aspects for the implementation and monitoring of her therapeutic plan. The patient should be encouraged to ask questions related to the plan so the pharmacist can be reassured that any medication and lifestyle changes are well understood by the patient. An appropriate follow-up time should be clearly established to assure that patient was able to implement the plan with appropriate accuracy and precision, and to determine if further adjustments are needed.

Abbreviations

ACC/AHA	American College of Cardiology/American Heart Association
ACEi	Ace Inhibitor
ADR	Adverse Drug Reaction
ARB	Angiotensin Receptor Blockers
ASCVD	Atherosclerotic Cardiovascular Disease
BMI	Body Mass Index
BMP	Basic Metabolic Panel
BUN	Blood urea nitrogen
DASH	Dietary Approaches to Stop Hypertension
HDL	High Density Lipoprotein
HFpEF	Preserved Ejection Fraction
HR	Heart Rate
IADLs	Instrumental Activities of Daily Living
LDL	Low Density Lipoprotein
MRA	Mineralocorticoid Antagonists
NSAID	Nonsteroidal Anti-inflammatory Inhibitor
PPCP	Pharmacists' Patient Care Process
SGLT2	Sodium-Glucose Cotransporter
SCr	Serum Creatinine Levels
TC	Total Cholesterol
TG	Triglyceride
TSH	Thyroid Stimulating Hormone
VLDL	Very Low Density Lipoprotein

References

1. Centers for Disease Control and Prevention. *Heart Disease Facts.* U.S. Department of Health and Human Services; Updated February 7, 2022. Available at https://www.cdc.gov/heartdisease/facts.htm. Accessed March 11, 2022.
2. Virani SS, Alonso A, Aparicio HJ, et al. Heart disease and stroke statistics—2021 update: a report from the American Heart Association. *Circulation.* 2021;143(8):e254-e743.

3. Centers for Disease Control and Prevention. *High Blood Pressure.* U.S. Department of Health and Human Services; Updated September 27, 2021. Available at https://www.cdc.gov/bloodpressure/facts. htm. Accessed May 10, 2022.

4. Bowling CB, Lee A, Williamson JD. Blood pressure control among older adults with hypertension: narrative review and introduction of a framework for improving care. *Am J Hypertens.* 2021;34(3): 258-266.

5. Whelton PK, Carey RM, Aronow WS, et al. ACC/AHA/AAPA/ABC/ACPM/AGS/APhA/ASH/ASPC/ NMA/PCNA guideline for the prevention, detection, evaluation, and management of high blood pressure in adults: a report of the American College of Cardiology/American Heart Association task force on clinical practice guidelines. *Hypertension.* 2018;71(6):e13-e115.

6. Backman WD, Levin SA, Wenger NK, Gordon HJ. Shared decision-making for older adults with cardiovascular disease. *Clin Cardiol.* 2020;43(2):196-204.

7. Oyler DR, Romanelli F. The fact of ignorance: revisiting the Socratic Method as a tool for teaching critical thinking. *Am J Pharm Educ.* 2014;78(7):144.

8. Bays HE, Taub PR, Epstein E, et al. Ten things to know about ten cardiovascular disease risk factors. *Am J Prev Cardiol.* 2021;5:100149.

9. Orkaby AR, Onuma O, Qazi S, et al. Preventing cardiovascular disease in older adults: one size does not fit all. *Cleve Clin J Med.* 2018;85:55-64.

10. Joint Commission of Pharmacy Practitioners. *Pharmacists' Patient Care Process.* May 29, 2014. Available at https://jcpp.net/wp-content/uploads/2016/03/PatientCareProcess-with-supporting-organizations.pdf.

11. Yourman LC, Cenzer IS, Boscardin WJ, et al. Evaluation of time to benefit of statins for the primary prevention of cardiovascular events in adults aged 50 to 75 years: a meta-analysis. *JAMA Intern Med.* 2021;181(2):179-185.

12. Chen T, Shao F, Chen K, et al. Time to clinical benefit of intensive blood pressure lowering in patients 60 years and older with hypertension: a secondary analysis of randomized clinical trials. *JAMA Intern Med.* 2022;182(6):660-667.

13. Yen PH, Leasure AR. Use and effectiveness of the teach-back method in patient education and health outcomes. *Fed Pract.* 2019;36(6):284-289.

14. Linnebur SA, O'Connell MB, Wessell AM, et al. Pharmacy practice, research, education, and advocacy for older adults. *Pharmacotherapy.* 2005;25(10):1396-1430.

15. Lam WY, Fresco P. Medication adherence measures: an overview. *Biomed Res Int.* 2015;2015:217047.

16. Center for disease control and prevention. Vaccine information for adults: heart disease and stroke. Updated Feb 3, 2021. Available at https://www.cdc.gov/vaccines/adults/rec-vac/health-conditions/ heart-disease.html. Accessed May 11, 2022.

17. National Institute on Deafness and Other Communication Disorders. *Hearing Loss and Older Adults.* U.S. Department of Health and Human Services; Updated March 2016. Available at https://www.nidcd. nih.gov/sites/default/files/Documents/health/hearing/HearingLossOlderAdults.pdf. Accessed May 10, 2022.

18. Miller KE, Zylstra RG, Standridge JB. The geriatric patient: a systematic approach to maintaining health. *Am Fam Physician.* 2000;61(4):1089-1104.

19. Elliott RA, Goeman D, Beanland C, Koch S. Ability of older people with dementia or cognitive impairment to manage medicine regimens: a narrative review. *Curr Clin Pharmacol.* 2015;10(3):213-221.

20. Cappola AR, Desai AS, Medici M, et al. Thyroid and cardiovascular disease: research agenda for enhancing knowledge, prevention, and treatment. *Circulation.* 2019;139:2892-2909.

21. Franklin SS, Thijs L, Hansen TW, et al. White-coat hypertension: new insights from recent studies. *Hypertension.* 2013;62:982-987.

22. Giles A, Foushee J, Lantz E, Gumina G. Sulfonamide allergies. *Pharmacy (Basel).* 2019;7(3):132.

23. Grundy SM, Stone NJ, Bailey AL, et al. 2018 AHA/ACC Guidelines on the management of blood cholesterol: A repots of the American College of Cardiology/American Heart Association Task Force on Clinical Practice Guidelines. *Circulation.* 2019;139:e1082-e1143.

24. Nilsen ER, Hollister B, Soderhamn U, Dale B. What matters to older adults? Exploring person-centered care during and after transitions between hospital and home. *Clin Nurs.* 2022;31:569-581.

25. Graf C. The Lawton Instrumental Activities of Daily Living (IADL) Scale. *Try this: Best Practices in Nursing Care to Older Adults*. 2008;108(4):59.

26. Arnett D, Blumenthal RS, Albert MA, et al. American College of Cardiology/American Heart Association Task Force on Practice Guidelines. 2019 ACC/AHA guideline on the primary prevention of cardiovascular disease: a report of the American College of Cardiology/American Heart Association Task Force on Clinical Practice Guidelines. *J Am Coll Cardiol*. 2019;74(10):e177-e232.

27. Lauffenburger JC, Isaac T, Bhattachary R, et al. Prevalence and impact of having multiple barriers to medication adherence in nonadherent patients with poorly controlled cardiometabolic disease. *Am J Cardiol*. 2020;125(3):376-382.

28. Sheikh-Taha M, Asmar M. Polypharmacy and severe potential drug-drug interactions among older adults with cardiovascular disease in the United States. *BMC Geriatr*. 2021;21(1):233.

29. Savage RD, Visentin JD, Bronskill SE. Evaluation of a common prescribing cascade of calcium channel blockers and diuretics in older adults with hypertension. *JAMA Intern Med*. 2020;180(5):643-651.

30. Krishnaswami A, Steinman MA, Goyal P, et al. Deprescribing in older adults with cardiovascular disease. *J Am Coll Cardiol*. 2019;73(20):2584-2595.

31. 2019 American Geriatrics Society Beers Criteria Update Expert Panel. American Geriatric Society 2019 Updated AGS Beers Criteria for potentially inappropriate medication use in older adults. *J Am Geriatr Soc*. 2019;67(4):679-694.

32. Steinman MA, Beizer Jl, DuBeau CE, et al. How to use the American Geriatrics Society 2015 Beers Criteria—a guide for patients, clinicians, health systems and payors. *JAGS*. 2015;63:e1-e7.

33. Steele KM, Ruisinger JF, Bates J, et al. Home-based comprehensive medication reviews: pharmacist's impact on drug therapy problems in geriatric patients. *Consult Pharm*. 2016;31(10):598-605.

34. Davies EA, O'Mahony MS. Adverse drug reactions in special populations - the elderly. *Br J Clin Pharmacol*. 2015;80(4):796-807.

35. Islam MS. The art and science of using diuretics in the treatment of heart failure in diverse clinical settings. *Adv Exp Med Biol*. 2018;3:47-65.

36. Novak JE, Ellison DH. Diuretics in states of volume overload: core curriculum 2022. *Am J Kidney Dis*. 2022;80(2):264-276.

37. ACC/AHA Joint Committee Members. 2022 AHA/ACC/HFSA Guideline for the Management of Heart Failure. *J Card Fail*. 2022;S1071-9164(22)00076-8.

38. GSK HealthPartner. *Voltaren Arthritis Pain Safety Profile*. Available at https://www.gskhealthpartner.com/en-us/pain-relief/brands/voltaren/products/arthritis-pain-safety/. Accessed June 14, 2022.

39. Wyman MF, Shiovitz-Ezra S, Bengel J. Ageism in the health care system: providers, patients, and systems. In: Ayalon L, Tesch-Romer C, eds. *Contemporary Perspectives on Ageism. International Perspectives on Aging, volume 19*. Cham: Springer; 2018:193-212.

40. Messerli FH. Vasodilatory edema: a common side effect of antihypertensive therapy. *Am J Hyper*. 2001;14:978-979.

41. US Preventive Services Task Force, Davidson KW, Barry MJ, et al. Aspirin use to prevent cardiovascular disease: US Preventative Services Task Force Recommendation Statement. *JAMA*. 2022;327(16):1577-1584.

42. Ekundayo OJ, Markland A, Lefante C, et al. Association of diuretic use and overactive bladder syndrome in older adults: a propensity score analysis. *Arch Gerontol Geriatr*. 2009;49(1):64-68.

43. Balk EM, Rofeberg VN, Adam GP, et al. Pharmacological and nonpharmacologic treatments for urinary incontinence in women: a systematic review and network meta-analysis of clinical outcomes. *Ann Intern Med*. 2019;170(7):465-479.

44. Gupta R, Testani J, Collins S. Diuretic resistance in heart failure. *Curr Heart Fail Rep*. 2019;16(2):57-66.

45. Cabrera VJ. Edema. In: Sydney E, Weinstein E, Rucker L, eds. *Handbook of Outpatient Medicine*. Cham: Springer; 2018:299-307.

46. Ridker PM, Lonn E, Paynter NP, Glynn R, Yusuf S. Primary prevention with statin therapy in the elderly: new meta-analyses from the contemporary JUPITER and HOPE-3 randomized trials. *Circulation*. 2017;135:1979-1981.

47. Shepherd J, Blauw GJ, Murphy MB, et al. Pravastatin in elderly individuals at risk of vascular disease (PROSPER): a randomised controlled trial. *Lancet*. 2002;360:1623-1630.

48. Orkaby AR, Driver JA, Ho YL, et al. Association of statin use with all-cause and cardiovascular mortality in US Veterans 75 Years and older. *JAMA*. 2020;324:68-78.

49. Giral P, Neumann A, Weill A, et al. Cardiovascular effect of discontinuing primary prevention at the age of 75: a nationwide population-based cohort study in France. *Eur Heart J*. 2019;40:3516-3525.

50. ePrognosis. *ePrognosis Calculators*. Available at https://eprognosis.ucsf.edu/. Accessed May 12, 2022.

4

Ambulatory Care—Type 2 Diabetes Management

Bradley Phillips and Michelle Farland

CHAPTER AIMS

The aims of this chapter are to:
- Discuss the roles of a systematic patient care process and clinical reasoning in assessing and resolving medication-related problems as part of a collaborative effort to provide patient-centered care in type 2 diabetes mellitus (T2DM) management.
- Incorporate the elements of the Pharmacists' Patient Care Process (PPCP) in a simulated patient case while outlining critical thought processes and clinical reasoning as it relates to the care of a person with T2DM.

KEY WORDS

• Type 2 diabetes • critical thinking • clinical reasoning • medication optimization • chronic disease state management • Pharmacists' Patient Care Process • patient-centered care

INTRODUCTION

Providing care for patients with diabetes mellitus (DM) requires a multifactorial approach and is ideally conducted in an interdisciplinary practice. The World Health Organization describes diabetes as "a chronic disease that occurs either when the pancreas does not produce enough insulin or when the body cannot effectively use the insulin it produces."[1] The primary concern of the resultant hyperglycemia is the negative impact on nerves and blood vessels. These negative impacts result in chronic complications of diabetes, including microvascular complications (eg, retinopathy, nephropathy, neuropathy) and macrovascular complications (eg, transient ischemic attack, cerebral vascular accident, myocardial infarction).

According to the American Diabetes Association (ADA), Standards of Medical Care in Diabetes 2023, the diagnosis of DM is made following a fasting plasma glucose (≥ 126 mg/dL), 2-hour oral glucose tolerance test (≥ 200 mg/dL following 75 g anhydrous glucose), random plasma glucose (≥ 200 mg/dL with classic symptoms of hyperglycemia such as polyuria, polydipsia, polyphagia), or A1C ($\geq 6.5\%$).[2] Confirmation of the diagnostic test is needed in the absence of unequivocal hyperglycemia.

Over 37 million Americans have a diagnosis of diabetes, with about 90% having type 2 diabetes mellitus (T2DM). The cost of diabetes care in the United States has risen significantly in recent years, with a 26% increase between 2012 and 2017. In 2017, the estimated cost of diabetes was $327 billion (US dollars), with direct medical costs contributing $237 billion and reduced productivity contributing $90 billion.[3]

Diabetes management requires active participation from the patient in many aspects of their lives, and accordingly, it requires healthcare providers to actively engage in the biopsychosocial model when applying a multifactorial approach to providing care to each patient. Therefore, the ADA recommends "people with diabetes can benefit from a coordinated multidisciplinary team that may include and is not limited to diabetes care and education specialists, primary care and subspecialty clinicians, nurses, registered dietitian nutritionists, exercise specialists, pharmacists, dentists, podiatrists, and mental health professionals."[4]

 KEY POINT

Diabetes is a multifactorial disease state and requires a team approach to care. An interprofessional team is desirable to provide support needed by the patient, while keeping in mind that the patient is at the center of this team, not simply a receiver of information and treatment.

OUR PRACTICE—AN OUTPATIENT INTERDISCIPLINARY ENDOCRINOLOGY PRACTICE

Our practice is an outpatient interdisciplinary endocrinology service that is embedded within an academic health system. The healthcare providers within the practice include endocrinologists (attendings and fellows), advanced practice registered nurses (APRNs), dieticians, pharmacists, social workers, and nurses. We also collaborate closely with the diabetes self-management education program within the health system that is led by nurses and dieticians. Within the practice, pharmacists accept referrals from endocrinologists, APRNs, and dieticians. The patient population at this practice spans the entire age spectrum of adulthood (18 years and older) and includes all types of diabetes (eg, type 1 DM, type 2 DM, type 3c DM, latent autoimmune diabetes of adulthood, gestational diabetes, posttransplant diabetes). The pharmacists focus on providing care to patients with diabetes and blending medication adjustments to achieve glycemic control with self-management education that is individualized for each patient. Pharmacists typically evaluate and monitor patients who have not met glycemic goals and require frequent follow-ups for medication adjustments and individualized education/reinforcement. Pharmacists see patients between visits with the endocrinologists and APRNs. Patients are provided reminder phone calls for their upcoming appointments with the pharmacist and instructed to bring in all medications they are currently taking or the most up-to-date detailed list.

UTILIZING CRITICAL THINKING SKILLS IN OUR PRACTICE

Critical thinking is essential when caring for patients with diabetes for the entire cycle of the Pharmacists' Patient Care Process (PPCP). The process starts with the collection of information, which is obtained from numerous sources, including the patient/caregiver, electronic health records, and glucose monitoring devices.

Pharmacists must review the information provided and determine patterns of blood glucose values, influencing factors contributing to those patterns, and impacts of the patterns on the patient's daily activities. Safety is of utmost importance in diabetes, which takes the form of avoiding hypoglycemia and minimizing hyperglycemia. Diabetes management also incorporates the use of high-risk medications (eg, insulin) that have potential to cause significant harm to the patient when used improperly. During the treatment of diabetes, there are three primary factors that impact the blood glucose level at any given time: medications, diet, and physical activity. These factors can be heavily influenced by the patient's psychological and social factors (eg, health beliefs, mood, personal choices, access to healthcare, access to healthy food, social support, and health literacy). A multifactorial approach is needed when providing care to patients with diabetes, because a change to one aspect of the care plan has potential to significantly impact many aspects of patients' lives. Identification of blood glucose patterns and care plan development must be individualized, as the interpersonal response to treatment varies significantly due to the number of influencing factors that can alter the blood glucose at any given time. Critical thinking is therefore essential to all aspects of the PPCP when caring for people with diabetes. **Table 4-1** delineates some of the questions pharmacists in this practice can ask themselves to help assure effective critical thinking through the application of the intellectual standards of critical thinking: clarity, relevance, significance, objectivity, fairness, accuracy, precision, depth, breadth, and logic—embodied in "Clear ROAD to Logic" mnemonic described in Chapter 1.

 KEY POINT

Identification of glucose patterns for individual patients is critical to developing a treatment plan that fits the patient's needs. The three primary factors that influence glucose patterns include medications, diet, and physical activity.

TABLE 4-1

Sample Standards-Based Questions That Can Be Applied to Assure That Intellectual Standards of Critical Thinking are Met as the Pharmacist Provides Care for People with Type 2 Diabetes

Clarity (explicit, unambiguous, intelligible, free from confusion or doubt)	• Has the type of diabetes been clearly described to ensure understanding of the pathophysiology of disease? • Is the blood glucose monitoring (BGM) or continuous glucose monitoring (CGM) data of sufficient duration or values to identify patterns in glucose levels? • Does the documented medication information reflect the actual use of medications (eg, drug, dose, frequency) as reported by the patient? • Has all information been collected to ensure clarity of glucose patterns identified (eg, food intake, physical activity, organ function [eg, heart, kidney, liver])? • Does the patient clearly understand their role in their diabetes management in a way that empowers them to be agents of their own care?

Relevance (pertinent, applicable, germane)	• What information have I obtained that is most relevant to assessing glycemic control? • What information have I obtained that is most relevant to assessing the presence/risk of micro- and macrovascular complications of diabetes? • Have I evaluated all contributing factors (comorbid conditions, medications, lifestyle choices, etc.) related to the patient's diabetes?
Significance (important, nontrivial, necessary, critical, required, impactful)	• Have I compared the disease outcome measures to the treatment targets of national guideline standards? • Have I obtained insight from the patient to identify his/her primary concerns and desires for the treatment plan? • When reviewing BGM or CGM data, have I focused mostly on pattern recognition as opposed to individual data points?
Objectivity (fact-based, unbiased)	• When interviewing the patient to collect information, have I asked questions in a manner that does not impose judgment so that I am able to obtain the most objective information possible? • Am I able to identify when information documented in the electronic health record (EHR) about the patient includes presumptions of behavior patterns instead of objective elements (eg, If the patient reports adherence, do I suspect nonadherence?) • Have I formed any preconceived notions or introduced biases upon review of the patient's medical information?
Fairness (unbiased, equitable, impartial)	• Have I identified the patient's preferences related to food choices, so not to impose specific eating patterns on the patient he/she may not find to be enjoyable? • Have I considered the patient's preferences and health beliefs to assist with developing a treatment plan that will be accepted by the patient to meet their desires? • Have I identified when I am imposing my own preferences into recommendations for lifestyle modification or my own health beliefs into the treatment plan? If so, have I taken steps to prevent this from occurring in the future? • Have I taken the same steps to improve access to healthcare services for each patient I interact with?
Accuracy (verifiable, valid, true, credible, undistorted)	• How can I verify the information collected from the patient is accurate? • Is there any collected information lacking the accuracy needed to perform an appropriate assessment? • Am I utilizing the most appropriate resources to develop an evidence-based diabetes treatment plan for my patient?
Precision (exact, specific, detailed)	• What information provided by the patient requires further probing questions to obtain specific details needed for appropriate assessment? • How can I phrase my questioning to the patient to obtain a detailed social history needed for assessment? • How detailed should the information I provide to educate the patient be? Did I consider the patient's health literacy when developing an education approach?

Depth (roots, fundamentals, complexities, interrelationships, cause/effect, implications)	• What are the modifiable and nonmodifiable risk factors contributing to the patient's diabetes? • Are there areas of the patient's care plan that are considered out of my scope of practice and require a multidisciplinary approach to effective care? • What are possible financial implications of my treatment plan that would be a direct cost to the patient?
Breadth (comprehensive, encompassing, alternative perspectives)	• Does my treatment plan effectively manage all comorbid disease states relating to the patient's diabetes? • Besides the patient, who else needs to be involved in the patient's treatment plan (caregivers, specialty providers, etc.)? • What are alternative therapy options to consider if my first-line options are not feasible?
Logic (reasonable, rational, without contradiction, well-founded, sound)	• Does my treatment plan sound reasonable and easily understandable by the patient? • Am I able to defend my treatment rationale using evidence-based literature and guidelines? • Did I provide appropriate rationale to support my treatment plan?

APPLICATION OF THE PPCP IN OUR PRACTICE

The PPCP is essential for pharmacists to provide patients with appropriate treatment tailored to their diabetes management. The Collect step starts before the patient interview and consists of a thorough review of the patient's medical record. This review allows the pharmacist to obtain an overall health status for the patient while focusing on diabetes-related objective information that is either required to be used later in the PPCP or encourages further questioning during the patient interview. This step continues with the patient interview where more subjective and objective information is collected, which is vital to diabetes management as patient-reported information (eg, food intake, physical activity, blood glucose) is used to develop treatment plans. Once all pivotal information is collected, the pharmacist assesses both objective and subjective data. The full assessment of the collected information in the Assess step provides the pharmacist with benchmarks for chronic disease state control and determines if the patient is meeting the currently established goals of therapy. The conclusions drawn about the patient's medication-related clinical status and the nature of the patient's drug therapy problems in the Assess step transition the pharmacist into the next step of the PPCP to develop a patient-centered care plan.

 KEY POINT

The Collect step begins with a thorough review of the patient's medical record, which enables the pharmacist to obtain an overall health status for the patient while focusing on diabetes-related objective information that can help determine questions to ask during the patient interview and will be needed for subsequent PPCP steps.

The Plan step will be based on a culmination of all assessments made thus far to create a roadmap of how the patient is going to achieve goals of therapy. This step begins with reiterating established goals with or without adjustments made based on the patient's current clinical status or desires. It can also include new goals to be created in collaboration with the patient and healthcare team (eg, for new patients or based on new assessments). This could include goals for both pharmacological and nonpharmacological interventions discussed with the patient and healthcare team. Within the Plan step, multiple pathways of the existing treatment plan and potential new strategies are considered and placed into the context of the needs, abilities, support, desires, values, and beliefs of the patient. Arguments for and against alternative strategies are developed, culminating in the selection of strategies that have strong supporting rationale. The plan is then discussed with the endocrinologist and the patient to make the final determination of the plan details, thus transitioning the process into the Implement step. The final step, Follow-up: Monitor and Evaluate, establishes appropriate follow-up and monitoring parameters determined by the finalized treatment plan. With diabetes being a chronic disease state, the PPCP is repeated at subsequent follow-up visits and progression through the PPCP steps is a continuous process as both disease state and treatment plans will change throughout the treatment course of T2DM.

 KEY POINT

In the Plan step, the existing treatment plan and potential new strategies are considered. Arguments for and against alternative strategies are developed, culminating in the selection of strategies that have strong supporting rationale.

THE COLLECTION OF PATIENT INFORMATION IN OUR PRACTICE

Patient information is collected from different sources to ensure all viable information is obtained and nothing pertinent is missing prior to the next step. A comprehensive review of the medical record is performed to collect any applicable objective information, such as the patient's medical history, disease progression, laboratory data, and medication history. **Table 4-2** includes examples of information that is routinely collected for the management of T2DM with accompanying rationales expressing the importance of why the information is collected. After reviewing the medical record, the pharmacist is able to establish a baseline of the patient's health status prior to the interview, to identify areas of improvement for initial visits or evaluate progress made since the previous visit.

TABLE 4-2

Examples of Data That Can Be Collected During Chart Review in Preparation for Patient Interview	
Data to Collect During Chart Review	**Rationale for Collecting Specific Data**
Patient Characteristics (age, height, weight)	These factors are used to make evidence-based therapy selections and determine appropriate dosing of medications. This information is also incorporated into the calculation of the patient's atherosclerotic cardiovascular disease (ASCVD) risk.

Allergies (with reaction)	Documentation of allergies is required to ensure patient safety when making therapy recommendations. Allergic reaction descriptors can help determine if it is a true allergic reaction or side effect of a medication, which can determine if therapy options can be rechallenged, or if further therapy options should be considered due to reaction severity.
Pertinent Laboratory Data (including, but not limited to, CMP, A1C, fasting lipid panel, TSH, urine microalbumin-to-creatinine ratio)	Laboratory data is used to assess disease state control and organ function status. It also can establish a baseline to identify possible adverse drug reactions of the treatment plan affecting organ systems. This information is also used to determine appropriate dosing of medications and calculation of ASCVD risk.
Past Medical History	T2DM management has an emphasis on cardiovascular risk reduction. In addition, comorbid chronic conditions need to be evaluated for overall cardiovascular risk. Comorbid conditions are also taken into consideration as treatment options for T2DM could affect other conditions such as cardiovascular risk reduction through blood pressure control. Knowing the patient's past medical history could lead to efficacious therapy options targeting multiple disease states or it can help determine contraindications to therapy. Presence or absence of microvascular complications of T2DM (eg, nephropathy, neuropathy, retinopathy) also influence decisions made regarding treatment goals for glycemic control.
Insurance Coverage	Medication affordability can be a common barrier to therapy options. Knowing the patient's insurance coverage helps to determine possible therapy options and options that can be eliminated with cost being a factor.
Immunizations and Medications (Prescription and nonprescription/supplements)	As multiple years can span between immunizations, the medical record is a good source to determine if patients are appropriately immunized. A thorough and complete medication list should be collected that includes both prescription and nonprescription medications. This list is used to check for drug-drug or drug-disease state interactions that currently exist for the patient or would be taken into consideration when implementing the treatment plan. Being aware of the medications the patient has used in the past and the reason for discontinuation will assist with developing a medication treatment plan.
Recent Hospitalizations and Transition of Care	A review of the patient's medical record would reveal any additional medical encounters that may have occurred between visits (eg, hospitalizations, emergency department or urgent care visits, outpatient visits with other healthcare providers). This is pertinent, as changes could have occurred outside of the clinic setting that will affect how the patient is evaluated and treated. Changes relating to newly diagnosed disease states, disease state status, laboratory data, or medications would need to be taken into consideration. The patient may also require additional education related to acute changes that may have occurred.

| Previous Office Visits | Prior encounters with the patient would be collected and reviewed for continuity of care and tracking progression of disease state control. Reviewing prior data of blood glucose control can also assist with interpreting the data the patient presents with during the present encounter with a pharmacist. Being knowledgeable of the anticipated changes that should occur to the blood glucose patterns based on the plan that was implemented at the most recent office visit will help to identify questions that need to be addressed with the patient if those changes are not observed. |

The Collect step continues with the patient interview where more subjective and objective information is obtained. The interview with the patient, and caregiver if applicable, provides an opportunity to collect information that may not be present in the medical record and settle any gaps of information determined prior to speaking with the patient. It also serves to confirm previously collected information from the medical record and provides the opportunity for further clarification and validity. **Table 4-3** lists examples of information that can be collected during the patient interview to confirm existing data or add value as newly collected information.

 KEY POINT

The accuracy of information collected is critical to decision-making for patients with diabetes.

TABLE 4-3

Patient Interview: Examples of Data That Can Be Collected During the Patient Interview

- Duration of disease states
  - T2DM and comorbid conditions
- Social history
  - Employer, relationship status, alcohol, tobacco, illicit substances, social support to assist with implementation of treatment plan
- Family history
  - First-degree relative information (most pertinent)
- Typical food intake
  - 24-hour dietary recall
  - Detailed food diary
  - Identifying who shops for food and prepares meals in the home
  - Planning for celebrations and holidays
- Physical activity
  - Type of activity, including intensity
  - Frequency and duration of activity
  - Duration of time sedentary
- Medications and allergies
  - Current prescription medications
  - Previous antihyperglycemics used and reason for discontinuation
  - OTC medications and supplements
- Adherence to therapy
  - Frequency of/reason for missed doses
  - Adherence aids and/or strategies used

- Patient acuity/health literacy
  - Newest Vital Sign (NVS)[5,6]
  - Rapid Estimate of Adult Literacy in Medicine (REALM)
  - Test of Functional Health Literacy in Adults (TOFHLA)[7]
  - Numeracy skills are of high importance when developing intensive insulin regimens
- Patient monitoring data
  - BGM or CGM
  - Frequency and pattern identification of hypoglycemia and hyperglycemia
  - Methods used to manage hypoglycemia and hyperglycemia
  - Blood pressure/heart rate
- Impact T2DM has on mood and wellbeing
  - Patient-identified areas of frustration
  - Methods used to reduce stress
- Symptoms of microvascular complications of T2DM:
  - Peripheral neuropathy: sensory exam (eg, 10-g monofilament neurological exam of the foot; vibration sensation using a 128-Hz tuning fork, or ankle reflexes); presence of symptoms of numbness/tingling of lower extremities; calluses or ulcers on feet from visual inspection[8]
  - Autonomic neuropathy: nausea following food consumption; dizziness upon standing; frequent falls
  - Retinopathy: changes in vision; history of most recent dilated retinal exam
- Vaccine history
- Frequency of dental exams
- Patient's perspective on areas for improvement in glycemic control to assist with improving quality of life
- Patient willingness to implement improvements in health status based on their abilities, interest, and motivation to change

This background knowledge of T2DM and our practice is applied below with an in-depth analysis of a fictitious case of a patient with T2DM who presents to our clinic for a routine follow-up visit. This analysis will illustrate the reasoning that occurs during each PPCP step and will demonstrate how critical thinking can be applied to optimize the reasoning process in each step. The primary goal of this analysis is to enable the reader to grasp how the PPCP, clinical reasoning, and critical thinking can combine to optimize patient-centered care for a T2DM patient.

The Case of Carlos P.: Overview

Carlos P. (CP) is a 64-year-old man who presents to the endocrinology clinic for a routine follow-up visit for T2DM. He was first diagnosed with T2DM at the age of 52. He was referred to the pharmacy service within the clinic to further assist with blood glucose control, medication management, and education. His antihyperglycemic medications include metformin, empagliflozin, insulin glargine, and most recently linagliptin, which he started in the last 6 months. He confirmed that he is taking medications for other indications and was able to bring all of them to the visit. His spouse will also be joining him as she is equally invested in his care. CP stated that he would like to speak with the pharmacist, as lately, he has been having difficulties controlling his blood glucose. Today, he presents with his glucometer and reports that his blood glucose values continue to be elevated; however, he denies any symptoms of hyperglycemia.

Past Medical History: T2DM, myocardial infarction (MI) 14 months ago, hypertension (HTN), dyslipidemia, hypothyroidism, chronic kidney disease (CKD) Stage 3b, obesity (class I).

CLINICAL REASONING, CRITICAL THINKING, AND THE PPCP FOR THE CARE OF CARLOS P.

The following series of tables breaks down the PPCP (Collect, Assess, Plan, Implement/Monitor) with conclusions and corresponding rationales pertaining to the provision of care for CP. For every conclusion made during each step of the PPCP, there is clinical reasoning emphasizing the value of the information and justifying the conclusion being made. The critical thinking standards are applied as the PPCP is broken down to divulge a pharmacist's critical thought processes and considerations within this patient care setting.

Collect

As previously described, the Collect step requires obtaining information through both medical record review and the patient interview with CP. Information, both subjective and objective, is collected from these sources to provide understanding of CP's current health status. Pharmacists are also able to collect information through the use of examinations during the visits, such as any point-of-care testing or evaluation for microvascular complications. Oftentimes, information collected during chart review is confirmed or denied with the subsequent patient interview. The pharmacist will distill all collected information into succinct and sufficiently detailed information to be used for assessment in the next step of the PPCP.

COLLECT: Medications/Immunizations	
Conclusions	Rationale: Information or Premise to Support the Conclusion
Perform a thorough medication reconciliation. *(Collected during the chart review and the interview)*	• As the medication specialist within a medical team, pharmacists are responsible for ensuring that CP is on appropriate medications with matching indications. • Even though the emphasis for the visit will be placed on medications for T2DM and associated complications, all medications will be reviewed for indication, safety, efficacy, and adherence. • If CP reports any information that might be a medication side effect or adverse reaction, the pharmacist must be able to recognize if any of his current medications may be a contributing factor.
Review previous antihyperglycemic medications. *(Collected during the interview)*	• Identifying medications CP has previously tried for T2DM management helps to determine future treatment options. • This helps to identify previous adverse drug reactions or intolerances that may require avoidance of certain medication classes.

| Immunization status. *(Collected during the chart review and the interview)* | • With T2DM considered an immunocompromised condition, it is recommended that CP obtains the appropriate immunizations to stay healthy.[9] People with T2DM have an increased susceptibility to some infectious diseases and require vaccinations outside of the routine adult immunization schedule (eg, pneumococcal pneumonia, influenza, hepatitis B, COVID-19).[4,10] |

 KEY POINT

It is important to confirm how the patient is actually taking the medication rather than relying solely on the prescribed instructions.

Critical Thinking Checks for the Collect Plan for Carlos P.'s Medications/Immunizations

When performing the medication reconciliation with CP, **accuracy** is key. When possible, there should be another source to confirm the information that he is providing about his medications and immunizations. Additional sources of validation could consist of the medication bottles, the caregiver, or prescription refill history. However, for this to happen, there needs to be **clear** communication with him, either during or prior to the visit, on how the medication reconciliation will be performed and what is needed for appropriate validation. With this in mind, the confirmed medication list provided can be more **precise** with exact drug instruction details including drug name, dose, route, and frequency.

• CP is able to recall all of the medications he is currently taking and reported no adverse drug reactions. The medication doses, routes, and frequencies were able to be visually confirmed with the medication bottles and reporting from his spouse. He was commended for bringing in his medications and stated that the reminder call from the clinic instructed him to bring in all of his medications, both prescription and nonprescription. CP's spouse also indicated that she takes pride in helping him remember to take his current medications. He stated that he is up-to-date on all recommended immunizations, which was able to be confirmed through documentation in the medical record.

Drug therapy selection for T2DM management involves a process of **reasoning** to identify the best options from among many viable options for the patient. Therefore, **breadth** is essential to encompass not only the antihyperglycemic medications that CP is currently taking, but also those he has previously tried with the reason for discontinuation. This will help in later steps of the PPCP to identify or rule out available therapy options.

• CP reported all of his antihyperglycemic medications, which were able to be confirmed in the medical record. He stated that he previously used glipizide; however, it was discontinued when insulin was initiated to reduce the risk of hypoglycemia. With this information, the pharmacist can conclude that sulfonylureas, the medication class containing glipizide, may not be the most appropriate option due to risk of hypoglycemia with concomitant insulin.

 KEY POINT

When performing medication reconciliation with patients, accuracy is critical, and when possible, there should be other sources to validate the information that patients provide about their medications and immunizations.

Collected Medications/Immunizations Information Entered into Health Record

Current medication regimen:

- Metformin 1000 mg by mouth twice daily when awakening and with dinner (bid); Indication: T2DM; adverse drug reaction (ADR): none reported
- Empagliflozin 25 mg by mouth once daily; Indication: T2DM; ADR: none reported
- Insulin glargine U-100 32 units subcutaneously daily at bedtime (HS); Indication: T2DM; ADR: none reported
- Linagliptin 5 mg by mouth once daily; Indication: T2DM; ADR: none reported
- Aspirin 81 mg by mouth once daily; Indication: MI; ADR: none reported
- Atorvastatin 20 mg by mouth once daily HS; Indication: Dyslipidemia; ADR: none reported
- Metoprolol succinate 50 mg by mouth once daily; Indication: MI/HTN; ADR: none reported
- Lisinopril 40 mg by mouth once daily; Indication: HTN; ADR: none reported
- Levothyroxine 75 mcg by mouth once daily; Indication: Hypothyroidism; ADR: none reported

Past antihyperglycemic medications:

- Glipizide

Current immunizations:

- Influenza vaccine: up-to-date
- Pneumococcal vaccine: up-to-date
- Hepatitis B: up-to-date
- All other routine vaccinations: up-to-date

COLLECT: Allergies, Labs, Vital Signs

Conclusions	Rationale: Information or Premise to Support the Conclusion
Allergies to medications/environment, with reaction(s). *(Collected during the chart review and the interview)*	• Allergies to medications and environmental factors should be confirmed with CP from the medical record review and the interview. • These could pose limitations to therapy depending on the severity of the reaction to a medication or medication class. • If therapy options become too limited, pharmacists can consider rechallenging medications with less severe reported reactions or considering a medication within the same class that may have a decreased chance of reaction occurrence.
Baseline laboratory data to evaluate overall health status. *(Collected during the chart review)*	• Baseline laboratory data is used to evaluate organ systems that can be negatively affected by long-standing T2DM, such as the kidneys, liver, and pancreas. • Also used to monitor trends through the course of therapy that may be altered through medication changes and disease state progression
Collect laboratory data pertinent to chronic disease states. *(Collected during the chart review)*	• Data pertaining to T2DM is collected to evaluate disease state control and progression of the disease state. Examples include albumin-to-creatinine ratio (to assess for microvascular complications (nephropathy)) and A1C. • Cutoffs are also used to help determine appropriate therapy, such as elevated A1C values requiring injectable therapy or cardiovascular risk scores requiring appropriate statin therapy. • Due to a diagnosis of hypothyroidism and being treated with levothyroxine, a thyroid stimulating hormone (TSH) level is acquired to measure thyroid function.

| Vital signs and home monitoring factors: blood pressure, heart rate, blood glucose, weight/height. *(Collected during the chart review and the interview)* | • Lifestyle management is an important aspect of chronic disease state control, especially T2DM. By collecting vital signs and data that CP monitors at home, pharmacists are able to evaluate trends and efficacy of lifestyle recommendations between visits.
• Blood glucose values must be thoroughly reviewed to determine if and when CP experiences hyperglycemia or hypoglycemia, as this may affect therapy options.
• This information can also be used to instill autonomy in CP and to reward his efforts toward chronic disease state control.
• Since he is taking lisinopril, metoprolol succinate, and empagliflozin, vital signs are necessary as these medications may reduce blood pressure and/or heart rate. |

Critical Thinking Checks for the Collect Plan for Carlos P.'s Allergies/Labs/Vital Signs

Precision and **accuracy** are essential when confirming medication allergies. Being as specific as possible when describing allergic reactions can help differentiate mild from severe reactions. There should be no doubt as to what medications should be avoided due to severity of the reaction.

Labs and vital signs are objective information and often difficult to dispute their accuracy. Questions of accuracy can occur when blood glucose values do not correlate to the collected A1C, leading to the need for more detailed questioning to determine the discrepancy. However, it should be explained to CP the **significance** of obtaining specific labs in a fasted state to ensure the **accuracy** of the results. For any self-reported information such as blood glucose, it is important to confirm the **accuracy** with which he is collecting this information in order for it to be credible. This would provide **clarity** from him on his understanding of how to appropriately obtain this information.

• CP stated that he has no known drug allergies (NKDA). to any medications he has tried. Therefore, the pharmacist should not have to deviate from the decided treatment plan based on medication allergies. Except for his self-reported blood glucose values, his labs were received through venous blood draw. He is able to accurately describe the steps he takes when using his glucometer, which confirmed appropriate use of the device.

When analyzing the available information, laboratory data that are **relevant** to CP's chronic disease states or that may be affected by drug therapy should be emphasized. This does not mean that irrelevant information should be ignored, but rather it should be addressed, if needed, outside of our intended visit for T2DM management. When considering relevant information, the pharmacist must be able to determine what is most **significant** and how it is significant, which can be a challenge considering the **depth** of understanding required due to the complexities of the relationships between T2DM, therapy options, and other disease states.

• The comprehensive metabolic panel obtained for CP came back within normal limits except for elevated blood glucose and altered, but stable values related to kidney function (to be discussed in the Assess step). With this information, medications will be evaluated for appropriate dosing based on current organ function. For reasons mentioned in the previous table, other relevant information about CP was obtained that will need to be assessed for their **significance** to his T2DM and its management, and his overall health, including A1C, albumin-to-creatinine ratio, fasting lipid panel, blood pressure and heart rate, TSH, and his weight.

Collected Allergies/Labs/Vital Signs Information Entered into Health Record

Allergies:
- No known drug allergies (NKDA)

Comprehensive metabolic profile (CMP):
- 2 months ago: within normal limits (WNL), except for blood glucose 150 mg/dL, SCr 1.7 mg/dL, estimated glomerular filtration rate (eGFR) 44 mL/min/1.73 m^2
- 8 months ago: WNL, except for blood glucose 186 mg/dL; SCr 1.72 mg/dL, eGFR 44 mL/min/1.73 m^2
- 12 months ago: WNL, except for blood glucose 212 mg/dL, SCr 1.8 mg/dL, eGFR 42 mL/min/1.73 m^2

Pertinent labs:
- A1C 8.9% (2 months ago); 9.2% (8 months ago); 10.2% (12 months ago)
- Urine albumin-to-creatinine ratio 100 mg/g
- Fasting lipid panel: total cholesterol (TC) 203 mg/dL, high-density lipoprotein (HDL) 30 mg/dL, triglycerides (TG) 190 mg/dL, low-density lipoprotein (LDL) 135 mg/dL
- TSH: 0.8 mIU/L

Vital signs:
- BP 138/85 mm Hg, heart rate 64 bpm
- Weight 215 lb
- Height: 67 in
- BMI: 33.7 kg/m^2

Blood glucose values (downloaded from CP's glucometer): testing one to four times per day:
- Fasting BG average: 170 mg/dL (range 140-236 mg/dL)
- Prelunch BG average: 192 mg/dL (range 173-268 mg/dL)
- Predinner BG average: 204 mg/dL (range 164-283 mg/dL)
- Bedtime average: 216 mg/dL (range 157-298 mg/dL)

COLLECT: Medical History

Conclusions	Rationale: Information or Premise to Support the Conclusion
Past medical history. *(Collected during the chart review)*	• Past medical history is used to evaluate the presence of disease states that frequently co-occur with T2DM (eg, micro- or macrovascular complications; hypothyroidism). It is also used to investigate potential limiting factors to medications, as some have contraindications to therapy based on medical history (such as medullary thyroid cancer or pancreatitis for glucagon-like-peptide-1 receptor agonists). • Can also be used to guide recommendations for lifestyle modifications (such as protein intake, sodium intake, or types of physical activity CP can initiate).
Family medical history. *(Collected during the interview)*	• Family medical history is used to screen for chronic disease states with genetic components that CP may be at increased risk for developing. • Family history can contribute to CP's cardiovascular risk and therapy considerations (such as a family history of premature ASCVD). It can also be used to help determine exclusions to therapy, similar to past medical history.

Critical Thinking Checks for the Collect Plan for Carlos P.'s Medical History

The past medical history gathered from the medical record review should be **accurate** and **broad**, encompassing all diagnoses and conditions. These should be confirmed with the CP and as well as additional information surrounding the disease states such as time and circumstances of diagnoses and progression of disease states. The information obtained via medical record review or patient interview should be **precise**. If a patient reports a heart problem, this could mean a host of possibilities such as coronary artery disease, heart failure, or a heart attack in which all have different associated risks and considerations. Knowing the exact confirmed diagnosis helps the pharmacist evaluate the appropriateness of the patient's medications. Family history can be **relevant** to the management of T2DM, as it can support the pharmacist's evaluation of disease risk. This also applies to familial health history, as immediate family member health history can be applicable to explaining CP's health history.

- CP's medical chart has a detailed record of his past medical history. He is also able to confirm this list of disease states and any specific information such as when he experienced the heart attack and the age he was diagnosed with T2DM. This timeline is beneficial to ensure he is on the appropriate medications and assessing risk due to longstanding T2DM. The longer the duration of T2DM, the higher the risk may be for micro- and macrovascular complications. The reported family history is relatable to his medical history as these chronic disease states (T2DM, HTN, dyslipidemia) have familial components.

 KEY POINT

Knowing the duration of the patient's diabetes and history of disease control is helpful to determine the likelihood of both short- and long-term complications of diabetes.

Collected Past Medical/Family Information Entered into Health Record

Past medical history:
- T2DM (diagnosed at age 52)
- ASCVD s/p (status post) MI (14 months ago)
- HTN
- Dyslipidemia
- Hypothyroidism
- CKD Stage 3b
- Obesity (class I)

Family medical history:
- Mother—T2DM, HTN, obesity
- Father—HTN, dyslipidemia, MI (at age 47)

COLLECT: Social History

Conclusions	Rationale: Information or Premise to Support the Conclusion
Occupational status. *(Collected during the interview)*	• Activity levels throughout the day can vary tremendously based on the person's occupation. This will need to be taken into consideration when providing lifestyle recommendations. We also need to consider the feasibility of lifestyle recommendations in our treatment plan to reflect CP's needs and schedule (eg, working night shifts)
	• Many times, with occupations that have a higher activity level, there is risk for the patient to experience hypoglycemia at work and therefore a plan to manage this should be discussed to reduce his risk of experiencing a severe hypoglycemic episode.

	• Patient acuity and educational level can be inferred from conversing with CP which can enable tailoring of how information is presented to him during his visit to foster understanding. Pharmacists should anticipate that many patients will require educational reinforcement across the continuum of the lifespan of T2DM regardless of occupation, and therefore should determine the amount of education completed and health literacy of the patient.
Marital status/ support. *(Collected during the interview)*	• Assistance at home is an important consideration for pharmacists when making treatment recommendations. If CP can stay accountable or overcome barriers to therapy with the help of a strong support system, treatment options that otherwise may not be manageable by him alone can be considered.
Substance use. *(Collected during the interview)*	• Patients should limit alcohol consumption to the recommended amount of two drinks per day for males and one drink per day for females.[11] Chronic alcohol consumption over the recommended limit could affect therapeutic considerations depending on the degree of liver function, requiring additional monitoring or alterations in drug therapy. Alcohol can also lead to hypo- and hyperglycemic changes in blood glucose.
	• Collecting information about CP's smoking history can provide an opportunity for the pharmacist to counsel him on smoking cessation to improve cardiovascular disease risk and overall health status for patients, for example, by using the 5 A's approach—ask, advise, assess, assist, arrange.[12]
	• Illicit substance use would also be collected from CP, as certain substances could pose difficulties for chronic disease state control, for example through elevations in blood pressure, heart rate, and cardiovascular risk.

 KEY POINT

Patients will require reinforcement of diabetes and treatment-related knowledge throughout the course of the disease.

Critical Thinking Checks for the Collect Plan for Carlos P.'s Social History

Elements of a patient's social history are personal and sometimes difficult to discuss. Empathizing and building a trusting relationship with patients that conveys **fairness** and is free from any biasing assumptions or attitudes, encourages the patient to be **objective** and honest when elaborating on specific information. This, in turn, helps to ensure the collection of **accurate** information needed to develop an appropriate assessment and treatment plan.

• For example, a benefit of a trusting relationship is the avoidance of social desirability bias in which a patient reports what they believe is socially acceptable rather than reporting negative behaviors they actually engage in, such as substance use. This would also be an appropriate opportunity to emphasize any patient confidentiality agreements made when CP was established with the clinic service.

• CP has developed a trusting relationship with the endocrinologist and pharmacists at our clinic, as we have been managing his T2DM for quite some time. Due to this positive, trusting relationship, he is genuine and honest when relaying information during his visit. He has been living with his spouse for the last couple of years and feels loved and supported by her. He also enjoys his job and has positive relationships with his coworkers. CP stated that he has friends with past histories of substance abuse and therefore does not partake in any recreational drug or alcohol consumption.

KEY POINT

To help assure accuracy of information collected from the patient, the pharmacist can engage the patient with a fair-minded approach that builds an empathetic, trusting relationship that shows fairness toward the information divulged and is free from any biasing assumptions or attitudes. This approach can provide a rapport that encourages the patient to be objective and honest when elaborating on specific information.

Collected Social History Information Entered into Health Record

Social history:

- Lives at home with spouse
- Works as manager at a local retail store
- Denies tobacco, alcohol, and illicit substances

COLLECT: Lifestyle Habits

Conclusions	Rationale: Information or Premise to Support the Conclusion
Diet. *(Collected during the interview)*	• Recollection of diet is important to identify improvements and can assist in controlling disease state markers such as blood pressure and glucose. A detailed list, or food diary, is preferred in order to make isolated recommendations for dietary improvements. • Dietary habits can also be factors to consider when determining appropriate therapy, especially within the realm of T2DM. Pharmacists need to be cognizant of reported dietary habits and patterns that can be addressed to decrease glycemic risk when making recommendations.
Exercise. *(Collected during the interview)*	• Exercise, specifically aerobic exercise for a defined period of time, can assist with disease state control. With an emphasis on exercise, we need to ensure CP's blood glucose is stable prior to physical activity to avoid safety concerns such as hypoglycemia. • Exercise is not limited to stereotypical activities performed in designated establishments such as a gymnasium. Pharmacists need to inquire more deeply into aerobic activities that could be considered moderate to vigorous such as activity while working, hobbies, or household work.

Critical Thinking Checks for the Collect Plan for Carlos P.'s Lifestyle Habits

The pharmacist should be on a quest to discover causes and factors associated with a patient's suboptimal lifestyle habits. For example, CP may have difficulties eating healthy foods or exercising at certain times of the day due to time constraints or pressure-laden responsibilities, and as a result, resort to unhealthy habits. Pharmacists should treat their patients' responses with **fairness** and understanding in order to establish trusting relationships that promote **objectivity** and openness for both the patient and the pharmacist. For example, instead of having patients conform to strict lifestyle recommendations, a trusting relationship provides an atmosphere for considering flexible options that best meets the patient's needs and routines. **Precision** and **accuracy** of lifestyle information is helpful as the pharmacist can focus on specifics of where improvements can be made, while considering the needs and desires of the patient.

- CP brought in a 24-hour dietary recall that includes an appropriate level of detail to make assessments on their dietary habits. He is currently skipping breakfast, which may be explained by his work hours or other priorities. His diet is significant for quick and easy meals, which could be explained by difficulties finding time for healthy meal planning. His diet is lacking food groups recommended for T2DM control such as fruits, nonstarchy vegetables, and whole grain options. He is also having difficulties with portion control and consumption of sugary beverages. He has provided some helpful details on his physical activities at home and at work.

Collected Lifestyle Habits Information Entered into Health Record

24-hour dietary recall: (consumes two meals/day):

- Breakfast: none, skips this meal 6 to 7 days/week
- Lunch [1 pm]: sandwich (2 slices white bread, turkey, cheese, lettuce); potato chips (1 "grab bag" size; 1.75 oz); Coke (12 oz)
- Dinner [7 pm]: three slices cheese pizza; salad (lettuce, carrots, tomato, bell pepper, ranch dressing); Coke (12 oz)
- Snacks: rarely consumes snacks, but usually includes peanut butter crackers or nuts.
- Beverages: coffee with Splenda/creamer, regular soda, water
- No recent changes in diet. Open to adjustments to improve BG control.

Physical activity:

- Walking while at work (approximately 90 minutes daily, 5 days/week), no other intentional physical activity
- Splits household work responsibilities with spouse and mows the lawn twice a month

COLLECT: Barriers to Therapy

Conclusions	Rationale: Information or Premise to Support the Conclusion
Adherence. *(Collected during the interview)*	• Prior to making therapy adjustments or initiations, information about adherence to current therapy must be collected and evaluated to avoid inappropriate prescribing. Through counseling and education on the impact their medications can have on their T2DM, therapy escalation can be avoided. • Adherence can be selective to a specific medication and not always generalized to all medications. It is important to identify this "selective nonadherence" to identify the reason for nonadherence before creating additional interventions. • If there are issues with adherence, the pharmacist should delve deeper into reasons for nonadherence as these will play a role in treatment plan development.
Affordability. *(Collected during the interview)*	• If there is difficulty affording medications, this could eliminate treatment options that tend to be more cost prohibitive and can streamline more affordable options. • Conversely, if medication affordability is not an issue, it provides treatment options to consider without cost concerns. • Knowing CP's insurance carrier can provide formulary coverage information on preferred therapy options through his insurance. • If CP is not able to afford healthy food options, such as nonstarchy vegetables and lean protein, he may be relying on more affordable options, which are oftentimes refined or processed foods high in carbohydrates. Affordable dietary options will need to be considered to meet his needs.

Health literacy. *(Collected during the interview)*	• The progression of T2DM management often involves complex treatment regimens, requiring adjustments to medications, medication doses, food choices, and physical activity. Many times, these decisions also change day-to-day based on the blood glucose patterns the patient identifies and do not only occur under the direction of healthcare providers.
	• Inadequate health literacy could pose a barrier to a patient's understanding of their disease states, complications, treatment options, and ability to make appropriate day-to-day decisions to maintain glycemic control.
	• The Newest Vital Sign (NVS) is a tool that can be administered during a patient encounter in a brief period of time to assess health literacy and numeracy. The tool presents patients with a nutrition label followed by a series of questions associated with interpreting information contained on the nutrition label. Scores on the NVS range from 0 to 6, with higher scores indicating greater health literacy. This instrument is applicable to identifying skills needed for people with T2DM as they are often required to interpret nutrition labels and display mathematical skills for appropriate administration of treatment.

 KEY POINT

To overcome barriers to care, consider the patient's health beliefs, values, abilities, needs, and access when designing a treatment plan.

Critical Thinking Checks for the Collect Plan for Carlos P.'s Barriers to Therapy

Clarity and **precision** of patient-reported medication usage is important to assure an **accurate** assessment of adherence and to determine measures (eg, pill boxes, timers) to improve adherence if needed. The timing of missed doses can be **relevant** for explaining discrepancies in laboratory work or possible adverse effects experienced. For example, missing a couple doses of their antihyperglycemic medication over the last couple of months is unlikely to have a significant impact on their A1C versus not using their medications for the last month. Barriers to therapy should be considered and assessed prior to making any further medication therapy recommendations to see if it can be corrected through education, counseling, and adherence.

• CP is occasionally having difficulty taking his medication at bedtime. Nightly activities, such as watching television, is his outlet to unwind after a stressful workday. This is an opportunity to talk about either the use of adherence aids to foster nighttime adherence or possibly shifting medication administration to a more appropriate time within his schedule. As of now, he is missing evening doses of metformin, insulin glargine, and atorvastatin once weekly, which will be assessed for their relevance and addressed with him.

Collected Barriers to Therapy Information Entered into Health Record

Medication adherence:

• Reports adherence to most medications with occasional missing of bedtime medications if he falls asleep watching television, which occurs once weekly.

Medication affordability:

• He can afford medications currently prescribed and denies treatment costs being a financial burden.

Medication insurance:

• Private insurance supplied by employer

Health literacy scores:

• NVS—4

Example Collect Statement for Carlos P.

CP is a 64-year-old man presenting to clinic today to meet with a pharmacist for T2DM. He has been having difficulties managing his T2DM for the last 12 years. Past medical history includes T2DM, ASCVD s/p MI, HTN, dyslipidemia, hypothyroidism, CKD Stage 3b, and obesity (class I). Family history is significant for T2DM, HTN, obesity, dyslipidemia, and MI (father at age 47). His current antihyperglycemic medications are metformin, empagliflozin, insulin glargine, and linagliptin. CP stated that he previously used glipizide; however, it was discontinued with initiation of insulin glargine to avoid hypoglycemia. He does not have any current issues with medication affordability. He reports being adherent to most medications and not currently using any reminder aids to help with adherence. However, he misses his bedtime medications about once per week. He reports NKDAs to medications or to environmental factors and is up-to-date on all recommended vaccinations.

CP lives at home with his spouse who is very supportive. He provided a 24-hour food diary at today's visit. He has made improvements in his diet; however, he admits to unhealthy dietary habits such as skipping breakfast and eating unhealthy and highly processed meals for dinner consisting of fast foods (eg, pizza) and sugar-sweetened beverages (eg, soda). He is also finding it difficult to decrease his soda intake. He stated that it is difficult planning meals for the day and that his spouse does most of the grocery shopping and cooking. He is currently a manager at a local store, which requires a mix of standing and walking during his shift. He performs limited physical activity, mostly obtained during his normal work responsibilities, but has no other intentional physical activities. He denies any use of alcohol, tobacco, or illicit substances.

CP's CMP is within normal limits except for elevated blood glucose and serum creatinine. The albumin-to-creatinine ratio is elevated at 100 mg/g. Kidney function is diminished, but stable from baseline. TC, TG, and LDL levels are elevated, whereas HDL is decreased. Body mass index (BMI) is 33.7 kg/m^2 and he admits has been having difficulty losing weight and keeping it off. Blood pressure today is 138/85 mm Hg with a heart rate of 64 bpm. CP confirmed that these values are similar to when he intermittently checks at home. He remembered to bring his glucometer in and reports testing his blood glucose about one to four times per day. Average blood glucoses are 170 mg/dL fasting, 192 mg/dL prelunch, 204 mg/dL predinner, and 216 mg/dL at bedtime. He has noticed that his blood glucose levels have improved over time; however, he most recently noted that they seem to be staying the same. He denies any symptoms of hyper- or hypoglycemia, peripheral neuropathy, or acute vision changes. CP's main goals are to get blood glucose under control, lose weight, and remain healthy for his loved ones.

Assessment of Collected Information

Assess is the next step of the PPCP where all information collected from the previous phase is evaluated. Both subjective and objective information gathered from the chart review and patient interview are analyzed. This includes medication indications, effectiveness, safety, and adherence. This information enables the pharmacist to draw conclusions on chronic disease state control, risks, and drug therapy problems. Most likely, the pharmacist has already created hypotheses surrounding the patient's health status during the Collect step; however, they are able to be either accepted or rejected upon further review of the information. When making disease state assessments, it is important to recognize that most chronic disease states are intertwined and overlap with each other and thus must not be viewed in isolation. Therefore, it is important to have a basic understanding of these disease state processes to understand the complexities needed to draw sound conclusions. For example, poor dietary and exercise habits can be factors contributing to obesity, elevated blood glucose in T2DM, or elevated blood pressures in hypertension. The pharmacist needs to be able to make these connections when assessing the information and developing a treatment plan. As a foundational part of their practice, pharmacists must also investigate and evaluate the potential overlap between the patient's medications and their disease states and take primary responsibility on the healthcare team for analyzing the patient's medications for their effects on underlying disease state processes and for determining the next steps of drug therapy.

 KEY POINT

Many disease states commonly occur together and therefore cannot be assessed and treated in isolation. Diabetes commonly co-occurs with HTN and dyslipidemia before other diabetes-related complications develop.

ASSESS: Type 2 Diabetes—Glycemic Control	
Conclusions	Rationale: Information or Premise to Support the Conclusion
Uncontrolled blood glucose and A1C, due to poor dietary and exercise habits and inadequate medication therapy	• CP's reported blood glucoses are above the recommended ADA goals of 80 to 130 mg/dL for fasting blood glucose and <180 mg/dL 2-hour postprandial.[2] • Based on his age, comorbidities, support system, and motivation for controlling his T2DM, an attainable A1C goal would be <7%. With the current A1C being 8.9%, he is above our target goal. To assess T2DM control, accurate goals of therapy must be established. A baseline goal of <7%, per ADA guidelines, indicates disease state control. However, patient factors, such as risk of hypoglycemic events, duration of the disease, life expectancy, pertinent comorbid conditions, vascular complications, available support system, and most importantly patient preference, can make this goal either more or less stringent to create a real-world attainable goal with an emphasis on safety.[13,14] For CP there are many factors to consider when determining his A1C goal. Some factors that would lean toward a more stringent goal would be a lack of hypoglycemia history reported, long life expectancy, and a highly motivated and readily available support system. However, his history of long-standing T2DM, relevant comorbidities, and established vascular complications would warrant a less stringent goal. With all factors taken into consideration, a baseline goal of <7% is appropriate.

Needs additional drug therapy to achieve glycemic control	• Except for missing his evening dose of insulin glargine once a week, CP is adherent to the current antihyperglycemic regimen. The medications he currently takes span various mechanisms of action and complement one another for disease state control. Given his history of ASCVD, treatment goals should incorporate glycemic control and secondary prevention of ASCVD. Medications that assist with both of these domains should be strongly considered.[15,16] While lifestyle modifications can help to achieve glycemic goals, they alone are unlikely to reach treatment targets. Emphasizing compliance with the once weekly missed dose of basal insulin (glargine) would be beneficial, but is also unlikely to be enough to reach target goals. In addition, medication causes of hyperglycemia are not present, such as concurrent use of corticosteroids, phenytoin, or estrogen. Therefore, additional drug therapy is needed to achieve glycemic goals and secondary prevention of ASCVD.
Poor dietary and exercise habits	• Poor dietary habits are a contributing factor to elevated blood glucose as the patient is consuming foods high in trans and saturated fats, and carbohydrates, especially with dinner and sugar-sweetened beverages. • The pharmacist may need to evaluate exercise further as CP's occupation may be positively contributing to exercise, but it still may be below the recommended target of 150 minutes of moderate-to-vigorous aerobic exercise at least 5 days/week with incorporation of strength/balance training 2 to 3 days/week.
Immunizations are current	• It is recommended with a diagnosis of T2DM to obtain annual influenza, pneumococcal, and hepatitis B vaccinations in addition to routine adulthood vaccinations.[10] • Immunization recommendations involve consideration of not only immunocompromised disease states (T2DM in this case), but also patient age and comorbid conditions. CP is currently up-to-date with all reported vaccinations, based on his age and current disease states. We will need to educate him on recommended vaccinations as he continues to age.

 KEY POINT

When determining if additional drug therapy is needed to achieve glycemic control, assess current medication use including efficacy, safety, mechanism of action, adherence, affordability, and the patient's preferences.

Critical Thinking Checks for Assessing Carlos P.'s Type 2 Diabetes—Glycemic Control

As self-reported blood glucoses are a major driving force in assessing disease state control and course of therapy, **clarity** with how patients measure their blood glucose ensures **accuracy** of their self-reporting through confirmation of appropriate collection and testing methods and should be assessed at all initial visits and periodically thereafter. If patients are unsure of how to check their blood glucose or are checking them incorrectly, the reported blood glucose values may be too unreliable to accurately evaluate. If blood glucose is not being checked as often as recommended, this would present an opportunity for the pharmacist to explain the **significance** of checking blood glucose, as it is a major driving force in determining the next steps of treatment, whether it be escalation or de-escalation of therapy.

To draw the most **logical** conclusions about CP's T2DM control and need for additional therapy, significant **depth** and **breadth** of thought is required.

- There are several factors, including his hypoglycemia history, life expectancy, motivation and support system, comorbidities, and vascular complications, which led to the conclusion of <7% as a proper A1C goal for him, on which the conclusion of uncontrolled T2DM was based. There are also several considerations, including his concurrent conditions and the impacts of his diet and adherence patterns, which led to the conclusion of the need for additional therapy. It is important to grasp the complexities of the interrelationships of these factors to develop an integrated understanding that enables the drawing of sound and comprehensive conclusions on CP's glycemic control.

ASSESS: Type 2 Diabetes—Microvascular Complications	
Conclusions	**Rationale: Information or Premise to Support the Conclusion**
Nephropathy is present as evidenced by urine albumin-to-creatinine ratio being elevated	• Albuminuria is a sign of kidney damage, as albumin, due to its size and charge, does not normally diffuse in large amounts through the glomerular filtration system, but can pass into the urine if the kidneys are damaged, as in diabetic nephropathy. A level <30 mg/g is considered normal, whereas a level ≥30 mg/g is considered high urinary albumin excretion. CP currently has high albuminuria with an albumin-to-creatinine ratio of 100 mg/g. • Treatment of albuminuria consists of using an angiotensin-converting enzyme inhibitor (ACEi) or angiotensin receptor blocker (ARB) therapy to slow kidney disease progression.[17] CP is currently taking an ACEi (lisinopril).
Need for referral to determine additional microvascular complications	• Other common microvascular complications of long-standing T2DM include neuropathy and retinopathy. CP denies vision changes and neuropathic symptoms; however, referral to appropriate healthcare practitioners is still warranted for proper evaluation.

Critical Thinking Checks for Assessing Carlos P.'s Type 2 Diabetes—Microvascular Complications

Using appropriate pharmacological therapy for albuminuria requires a **depth** of understanding why ACEi/ARB therapy is recommended as medications in these classes have been shown to reduce urinary albumin excretion and delay progression to end-stage kidney disease.[18,19] It also requires an understanding of the potential effects of implementing either of these drug classes on other disease states such as HTN. Knowing the **breadth** of related microvascular complications that can occur from T2DM helps determine appropriate screening and monitoring parameters. Accordingly, retinopathy, nephropathy, and neuropathy (peripheral and autonomic) should be discussed at patient encounters and referred to specialty providers for further evaluation and assessment.

ASSESS: HTN/CKD Progression	
Conclusions	Rationale: Information or Premise to Support the Conclusion
Uncontrolled hypertension	• CP's blood pressure is 138/85 mm Hg. He stated that his blood pressure at home when he checks is around the same. As blood pressure is above the recommended goal of <130/80 mm Hg, his blood pressure is uncontrolled.[16,20,21]
CKD Stage 3b	• CKD is classified through eGFR ranging from normal function to kidney failure and presence of albuminuria.[22] • As CP's eGFR is 44 mL/min/m² with an albumin-to-creatinine ratio of 100 mg/g, his kidney function is considered to be moderately to severely decreased with moderately increased albuminuria.[22]
Needs additional therapy to achieve target blood pressure and to prevent progression of Stage 3b CKD	• CP is adherent to the current antihypertensive medications. The medications he currently takes span various mechanisms of action and complement one another for disease state control. In addition, reducing sodium intake can assist with decreasing blood pressure. His current treatment regimen does not meet criteria for considering resistant HTN and further exploration of secondary causes of HTN is not warranted.[23]
Metformin dose too high	• Detrimental medications, or ones that may require adjustments based on kidney function, need to be identified to prevent adverse effects and/or inappropriate treatment. Metformin has potential to accumulate with decreases in kidney function and could result in lactic acidosis.[24] When the eGFR is >30 mL/min/1.73 m², yet below 45 mL/min/1.73 m² the maximum dose of metformin should be 1000 mg daily (divided into two doses). When the eGFR is <30 mL/min/1.73 m², metformin should be discontinued.
Empagliflozin and lisinopril are appropriate to continue	• Empagliflozin and lisinopril require monitoring for efficacy and safety related to kidney function. At this time, both medications are appropriately dosed based on CP's current kidney function.

 KEY POINT

Re-evaluate existing medications to determine safety and efficacy of use when kidney function changes.

Critical Thinking Checks for Assessing Carlos P.'s HTN/CKD Progression

As blood pressure levels are needed to determine the course of therapy in HTN/CKD, there needs to be **clarity** and **precision** with how CP takes his blood pressure. Like blood glucose mentioned previously, technique on obtaining blood pressures should be assessed at the initial visit and periodically for established patients to ensure **accuracy** of the reported data and determine disease state control.

- Pharmacists need to take into consideration the **breadth** of evidence that supports a blood pressure goal of <130/80 mm Hg as there are many different guidelines used to determine blood pressure goals. Choosing a blood pressure goal may not always be a straightforward decision, as different sources could recommend different goals of therapy. It is up to the pharmacist to weigh the risks vs benefits amongst conflicting goals to determine the most appropriate option.

- Various sources of guideline-based evidence are applicable to determining a blood pressure goal for CP. ADA guidelines recommend targeting a blood pressure <130/80 mm Hg as his 10-year ASCVD risk score is ≥15%.[16] The American College of Cardiology (ACC) and American Heart Association (AHA) recommend a goal of <130/80 mm Hg for the general patient population and, in the case of our patient, for secondary prevention of cardiovascular events.[20] Since CP has CKD with presence of albuminuria, the Kidney Disease Improving Global Outcomes (KDIGO) guidelines recommend a goal of <130/80 mm Hg.[22] After reviewing all applicable evidence, the recommended blood pressure goal for him is <130/80 mm Hg.

ASSESS: Cardiovascular Disease Risk	
Conclusions	Rationale: Information or Premise to Support the Conclusion
Atorvastatin dose too low: Current use of moderate-intensity statin therapy when high-intensity therapy is indicated	• Lipid levels are required to assess disease state control. TC, HDL, TG, and LDL are not within the desirable ranges for disease state control. These levels are used to evaluate current therapy and determine if further treatment is needed. • Statin intensity is a categorization used to classify the expected decrease in LDL upon initiation of the medication and dose. The patient's current statin therapy, atorvastatin 20 mg by mouth once daily, is moderate intensity. High-intensity statin therapy (those that lower the LDL ≥50% from baseline) is indicated for patients with T2DM who have a history of ASCVD (eg, MI), or if the 10-year risk for ASCVD is ≥20%.[25]
Elevated cardiovascular risk	• Lipid levels are a key element in determining CP's risk for developing ASCVD within the next 10 years. This, in combination with other factors, establish the gravity of this risk as a score above 20% is considered to be very high and warrants appropriate statin therapy. His 10-year ASCVD risk is 36.6%, which is well above this threshold. • However, ASCVD risk calculation is not as pertinent to determine appropriate therapy for CP as he has already experienced a cardiovascular event (an MI) placing him at an elevated cardiovascular risk warranting secondary prevention with statin therapy. • Family history of premature ASCVD (first-degree relative <55 years in males and <65 in females) is another risk factor for CP due to his father's history of MI at age 47.[25]

Critical Thinking Checks for Assessing Carlos P.'s Cardiovascular Disease Risk

Pharmacists need to have a **logical** understanding of factors that could affect the results of a cholesterol panel. For example, consider a patient who reports adherence with healthy diet and exercise, but who has an elevated cholesterol panel that has been relatively controlled up until recently. Factors such as sampling error, medications, or nonfasting state could all be reasonable explanations for an elevated cholesterol panel. Pharmacists should be **objective** and **fair** by analyzing for possible lurking variables that may be causing the elevation rather than allowing **implicit biases** to lead the pharmacist to believe patients report false information about their lifestyle habits. This analysis requires a **breadth** of knowledge to understand all potential lifestyle factors that should be considered before inquiring more deeply about what patients believe are healthy lifestyle choices. Pharmacists understand the **significance** between the connection of elevated cholesterol and cardiovascular disease risk. However, this may not be apparent to patients since uncontrolled dyslipidemia itself is not noticeable through signs or symptoms. **Clear** communication should be provided to CP to help him understand this fact and to emphasize the importance of controlling cholesterol levels through both pharmacological and nonpharmacological approaches.

ASSESS: Hypothyroidism	
Conclusions	**Rationale: Information or Premise to Support the Conclusion**
Controlled hypothyroidism	Goals of therapy include normalization of TSH with suppression of symptoms if present. As CP's TSH is within normal range (0.45-4.12 mIU/L) with the absence of hypothyroidism symptoms (fatigue, cold intolerance, weight gain, bradycardia), therapy adjustments are not needed at this time.[26]

Critical Thinking Checks for Assessing Carlos P.'s Hypothyroidism

There are interconnected relationships between CP's T2DM and comorbid conditions that could present factors negatively affecting his health outcomes.[27,28] **Deep** and extensive **breadth** of thinking is required to understand how these disease states affect each other. For assessing disease state control, there needs to be a **logical** explanation of how one disease state may be affecting the other through underlying pathophysiological processes (in this case, the connection between thyroid disorders and T2DM). These explanations may lead to recommendations in the treatment plan to target these processes to achieve disease state control. Conversely, knowledge of the interrelationships can enable the pharmacist to conclude that a condition may not be negatively affecting health outcomes, such as in our patient's case where his thyroid disorder is controlled and less likely to be affecting his T2DM.

KEY POINT

In patients with T2DM, there are often interconnected relationships between a patient's T2DM and comorbid conditions that could lead to negative health outcomes for the patient. This requires the pharmacist to possess a deep and extensive breadth of understanding of how these disease states affect each other.

ASSESS: Health Literacy/Numeracy/Concordance to Treatment Plan	
Conclusions	Rationale: Information or Premise to Support the Conclusion
Adequate health literacy	• NVS scores range from 0 to 6 with the following breakdown classifications: high likelihood of limited health literacy (score: 0-1), possibility of limited health literacy (score: 2-3), and adequate health literacy (score: 4-6) • When provided the NVS, CP scored a 4 and is therefore determined to have adequate health literacy.

Critical Thinking Checks for Assessing Carlos P.'s Health Literacy/Numeracy/Concordance to Treatment Plan

It is important for pharmacists to assess the health literacy of patients and to provide an appropriate level of **clarity** when educating and counseling them. There are population risk factors to consider that may suggest a lower level of health literacy for certain patients such as those of advanced age, low educational level, or low socioeconomic status. However, it is important for pharmacists to remain **fair-minded** and **objective** when conversing with patients as the level of conversation may require adjusting away from the patient's anticipated health literacy level. This requires tactful consideration of how patients interact during the visit through body language, lack of questioning, or limited responses, as credentials (eg, educational degrees earned) do not always equate to a patient's health literacy level. It is recommended to conduct your visits and provide educational material at a sixth-grade level or lower to account for possible health literacy issues.[29]

In CP's situation, there are numerous medical conditions that demonstrate interrelationships that are important to note. These interrelationships contribute to the complexity of the thought process used to complete an assessment of his health conditions and identify how the potential treatment of one medical condition can influence another. **Figure 4-1** demonstrates these relationships, which are also summarized in the Assess statement created for CP.

Example Assess Statement for Carlos P.

CP is a 64-year-old man presenting to the endocrinology clinic for continued management of his T2DM and related comorbid conditions.

1) Uncontrolled T2DM:

   a. CP's A1C of 8.9% is above the recommended target goal of <7%. His fasting blood glucose average is 170 mg/dL, which is also above the recommended goal of 80 to 130 mg/dL. His antihyperglycemic medications consist of metformin, empagliflozin, insulin glargine, and linagliptin. He reported poor dietary habits and lack of aerobic exercise, which is contributing to elevated blood glucose. He reports adherence with most medications; however, he admits to missing bedtime medications once weekly. He stated that he has no difficulties affording his medications at this time and is up-to-date on all recommended immunizations. He has a diagnosis of microalbuminuria with an albumin-to-creatinine ratio of 100 mg/g and is currently being treated with lisinopril. CP cannot recall the last time he has been to any specialty provider such as an

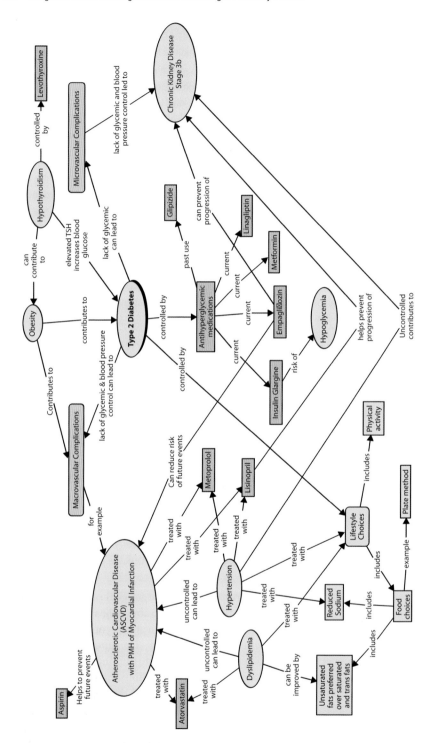

FIGURE 4-1. Concept map illustrating the interrelationships of CP's medications, lifestyle choices, and conditions.

ophthalmologist or podiatrist, but follows up with his primary care provider annually.

b. **Drug therapy problems include:**

   i. Metformin dosage too high based on current kidney function

   ii. Needs additional drug therapy to achieve glycemic control

   iii. Inappropriate adherence with medications administered in the evening, though frequency of missed doses not likely to be sole reason for lack of disease control

2) Uncontrolled HTN/Stage 3b CKD:

a. Blood pressures are averaging 130s/80s mm Hg at clinic visits and at home, which is above the recommended goal of <130/80 mm Hg. CP confirmed his ability to correctly monitor his blood pressure at home. He reports poor dietary habits, food content high in sodium, and absence of physical activity outside of work. He does not consume any alcohol, tobacco, or illicit substances. He consumes regular soda throughout the day and one cup of coffee in the mornings; however, it is after he checks his blood pressure. The most recent eGFR is 44 mL/min and has been consistently less than 45 mL/min meeting the criteria for Stage 3b CKD. He is currently taking metoprolol succinate, empagliflozin, and lisinopril for blood pressure reduction and renal protection. Except for metformin, all medications are appropriately dosed per renal function at this time.

b. **Drug therapy problems include:**

   i. Needs additional drug therapy to achieve blood pressure control and to reduce risk of progression of CKD

3) ASCVD Risk Reduction:

a. CP is considered elevated risk for a recurrent ASCVD event because he experienced an MI and is receiving treatment for secondary prevention. His 10-year ASCVD risk percentage, although not as clinically necessary for therapy determination for secondary prevention, is 36.6% and considered high risk. His family history is also significant for premature ASCVD as his father experienced an MI at age 47.[25] He is currently taking empagliflozin, aspirin, atorvastatin, and antihypertensives for cardiovascular risk reduction, which aligns appropriately with post-MI treatment recommendations. The dose of atorvastatin is considered subtherapeutic as therapy warrants a high-intensity statin to achieve a 50% reduction in LDL due to cardiovascular history/risk.

b. **Drug therapy problems include:**

   i. Dosage too low for atorvastatin. Current dose is a moderate intensity dose: CP qualifies for a high-intensity dose

4) Controlled Hypothyroidism:

a. The most recent TSH of 0.8 mIU/L is within the desired range of 0.45 to 4.12 mIU/L.[26] CP is adherent with his levothyroxine, which he takes in the morning. As TSH is within goal and he reports no hypothyroidism signs or symptoms, this condition is controlled.

PLAN: Goals	
Conclusions	Rationale: Information or Premise to Support the Conclusion
Glycemic goals include: 1. Reduce A1C to <7% within the next 12 months. 2. Reduce the fasting blood glucose to consistently be between 80 to 130 mg/dL and the postprandial blood glucose to consistently be <180 mg/dL within the next 6 months. 3. Reduce weight by 5% to 10% within 12 months.	1. Reducing the A1C to below 7% will assist in avoiding long-term consequences of T2DM, such as the development of microvascular (neuropathy, nephropathy, and retinopathy and macrovascular (heart attack, stroke) complications.[30–32] The A1C is a measure of the average blood glucose over the prior 2 to 3 months, so changes in this value will lag behind changes in the blood glucose. 2. Achieving fasting and postprandial blood glucose targets consistently will result in achievement of the A1C target of <7%. The fasting and postprandial blood glucose change more rapidly than the A1C, and therefore can be used to tailor the treatment regimen in shorter intervals than relying solely on the A1C. 3. Weight loss can improve glycemic control and insulin sensitivity.[33] Improving glycemic control can then result in delaying onset or progression of microvascular complications of diabetes.
HTN/CKD goals include: 1. Reduce the blood pressure to <130/80 mm Hg within the next 3 months. 2. Delay progression in kidney function decline for as long as possible.	1. Reducing the blood pressure will assist with preventing future cardiovascular events such as MI and stroke. 2. Controlling the blood pressure will also assist with stabilizing kidney function and with preventing further decline in function. However, this alone will not be sufficient as there are other factors relevant for preventing kidney function decline, including glycemic control and appropriate medication therapy (eg, ACEi and SGLT2i to help delay progression).
ASCVD goals include: 1. Secondary prevention of ASCVD events for as long as possible. 2. Reduce LDL by at least 50% from baseline (before drug therapy was initiated).	1. Measures for secondary prevention of ASCVD events include chronic disease state control and preventative medication therapies. 2. One intermediate target used to identify if current medication therapy is effective is change in LDL from baseline (defined as prior to initiation of lipid-lower medications, such as statins). If this goal is not achieved and the LDL remains above 70 mg/dL, additional drug therapy options may be considered.[25,34]
Hypothyroidism goals include: 1. Maintain TSH 0.45 to 4.12 mIU/L without symptoms of hypo or hyperthyroidism[26]	1. The goal is to maintain a euthyroid state to prevent onset of symptoms of hypothyroidism (indicating treatment needs to be increased) or hyperthyroidism (indicating treatment needs to be decreased).

KEY POINT

Management of diabetes extends beyond glycemic control. It is important to consider monitoring and management of complications related to the function of associated systems, such as cardiovascular, nervous, renal, and ophthalmic systems.

Plan, Implement, and Monitor

Critical Thinking Checks for Developing Carlos P.'s Treatment Goals

The treatment goals developed for CP need to be specific, measurable, achievable, realistic, and timely (SMART). These are the elements to incorporate when creating goals for patients. These goals were created using a **depth** and **breadth** of understanding of his chronic disease states and what is needed to acquire positive outcomes. This is accomplished through the use of only **relevant** evidence-based guidelines to determine individualized goals for him. There should be **clarity** and a sense of **fair-mindedness** when presenting these goals to CP so that he understands what to work toward and instill autonomy for chronic disease state control. Also, the **significance** of not obtaining these goals and the long-term effects of uncontrolled chronic disease states should be discussed with CP.

KEY POINT

SMART goals are created with a depth and breadth of understanding of the patient's chronic disease states and what is needed to acquire positive outcomes.

PLAN: Type 2 Diabetes—Glycemic Control

Goals:
1. Reduce A1C to <7% within the next 12 months.
2. Reduce the fasting blood glucose to consistently be between 80 and 130 mg/dL and the postprandial blood glucose to consistently be <180 mg/dL within the next 6 months.
3. Reduce weight by 5% to 10% within 12 months.

Conclusions	Rationale: Information or Premise to Support the Conclusion
Initiate semaglutide 0.25 mg SC once weekly	There are numerous therapy options to consider when managing T2DM and it is important to consider all options while narrowing down to the most appropriate choice. CP is currently using a biguanide (metformin), sodium-glucose cotransporter 2 inhibitor (SGLT2i) (empagliflozin), basal insulin (insulin glargine), and dipeptidyl-peptidase 4 inhibitor (linagliptin). Therefore, alternative medications within these drug classes would not be an option as that would be considered a duplication of therapy and would increase the risk for adverse effects from the medication class. Besides insulin glargine, which is titrated based on blood glucose values, all other current antihyperglycemics are at their maximum dosages and therefore cannot be increased.
	He previously used a sulfonylurea (glipizide); however, this was discontinued when basal insulin was initiated to decrease risk of hypoglycemia. As this risk is a class effect, other sulfonylureas would not be an appropriate option.

Like sulfonylureas, meglitinides (repaglinide and nateglinide) carry a greater risk of hypoglycemia compared to other noninsulin antihyperglycemics and should be avoided at this time.

Alpha-glucosidase inhibitors (acarbose and miglitol) were not considered at this time due to their limited efficacy to lower the A1C and tolerability issues (eg, gastrointestinal intolerances such as flatulence and diarrhea).

Colesevelam and bromocriptine were also not considered due to lack of efficacy in A1C lowering and they are not included in the treatment algorithm by the ADA.

Adding bolus insulin (eg, rapid-acting insulin such as insulin aspart or insulin lispro) would be effective to control prandial blood glucose elevations; however, it would also increase the risk of hypoglycemia, weight gain, and possibly the treatment cost/burden to CP.

Titrating the basal insulin CP is currently taking could be a convenient option as he is already administering it once daily. One strategy consists of providing a titration schedule to increase the dose periodically to achieve a target fasting blood glucose. This approach is independently done by the patient using the parameters provided by the healthcare provider. However, this strategy requires extensive education, counseling, and patient understanding of the titration schedule required to control fasting blood glucose.

Initiating a thiazolidinedione (eg, pioglitazone) could be an appropriate option as it is inexpensive, well tolerated, improves insulin resistance, and has been shown to provide additional cardiovascular disease prevention.[35] In the 2023 ADA guidelines, it is considered a third-line agent in patients with T2DM and ASCVD after first initiating an SGLT2i and Glucagon-like Peptide Receptor Agonists (GLP-1 RA). Pioglitazone could also be considered in the future if CP develops nonalcoholic fatty liver disease (NAFLD).

When considering a medication that maximizes both A1C and cardiovascular risk reduction potential, the most appropriate option at this time would be a GLP-1 RA. ADA guidelines recommend GLP-1 RA's as first-line therapy for patients with ASCVD, high risk of ASCVD events, and/or CKD making this medication class the most appropriate for CP.[16] Cardiovascular risk reduction is not a class effect amongst GLP-1 RAs as an agent with proven benefit in reducing cardiovascular disease should be selected, which includes semaglutide SC, liraglutide, and dulaglutide.[36–38] Any one of these options would be appropriate and many factors may come into play when choosing the right one, or possibly eliminating this class as an option, with the main factors being affordability and frequency of administration. To minimize the number of self-administered injections, liraglutide was eliminated due to its once-daily administration, while both dulaglutide and semaglutide are once weekly. From here, it may be the subtle nuances in medication attainability/affordability that would elevate one option over the other. Regardless, either semaglutide or dulaglutide, in the absence of barriers to therapy, seems to be the most appropriate therapy for CP due to their once weekly administration, A1C reduction, cardiovascular protection, and their ability to delay the progression of CKD.

Semaglutide is available in both oral and subcutaneous dosages forms. The subcutaneous form was chosen for this patient, because it has stronger evidence to support its use to prevent ASCVD and this patient has demonstrated comfort and adherence with the SC route with his insulin therapy.

Discontinue linagliptin	Linagliptin is a dipeptidyl peptidase-4 inhibitor. Dipeptidyl peptidase-4 is the enzyme that degrades endogenous GLP-1. With the initiation of a GLP-1 RA, which is not degraded by dipeptidyl peptidase-4, this class of medications has an overlapping mechanism of action and will not result in any net benefit. Therefore, it should be discontinued.
Continue insulin glargine and empagliflozin	CP is currently able to tolerate insulin glargine and empagliflozin. Both contribute to improved glycemic control while empagliflozin has the added benefit to reduce risk of future ASCVD events and delay progression of CKD.[39,40]
Reduce metformin dose to 500 mg BID	Due to Stage 3b CKD, with eGFR below 45 mL/min/m^2, the dose of metformin should be decreased by 50% to a maximum dose of 500 mg BID to reduce the risk of lactic acidosis.[24] Elevated metformin concentrations, which can occur when eGFR is below 45 mL/min/m^2, can inhibit mitochondrial respiration, which leads to increased plasma lactate levels.[41] Lactic acidosis is usually caused by a combination of elevated plasma lactate concentrations plus an additional event or disease that also increases risk, such as cirrhosis, sepsis, or hemodynamic instability. These conditions can be unpredictable; therefore, the risk of lactic acidosis is reduced by reducing metformin concentrations through dose reduction when the eGFR is below 45 mL/min/m^2. Lactic acidosis is an important adverse effect to avoid because the mortality rate following diagnosis is 50%.
Encourage weight loss	Weight loss of 5% to 10% can assist with improving glycemic control and insulin sensitivity.[33] This can be accomplished with education focused on food intake and physical activity.

 KEY POINT

Treatment considerations for glycemic control need to be individualized for each patient. While following the most current guidelines is a starting point for considering potential treatment options, those options then need to be critically reviewed to identify the one(s) that will be most appropriate for the specific patient. Multiple elements will contribute to this individualization such as comorbid conditions, glycemic patterns, treatment goals, patient preferences, and treatment burden.

Critical Thinking Checks for Carlos P.'s Type 2 Diabetes—Glycemic control

Appropriate therapy cannot be determined without a **depth** and **breadth** of understanding of the different treatment choices, as there are many medications available for treating T2DM and many complexities to consider, including the interrelationships among this patient's medications and disease states as shown in **Figure 4-1**. Pharmacists need to think with great **precision** in determining and considering the **relevant** details needed for decision-making about the many plausible therapeutic options. Treatment plans require individualization for patients, as there is no "one size fits all" option for managing T2DM. Providing patient-centered care, with a deep underlying knowledge and following guideline recommendations and principles of evidence-based medicine, can help ensure the therapeutic decision-making is **objective** and free of bias or preconceived preference toward one drug or drug class. This can enable the pharmacist to make the most **logical** and optimal decision for the patient. Even if guidelines and the assessment of the patient information leads to the most appropriate treatment options, they may not be feasible options for the patient. To determine feasibility for the patient, there should be **clarity** of communication with patients about all viable options and the communication should be **fair-minded** to ensure patient understanding and instill a sense of autonomy of their role in their own care.

KEY POINT

In the Plan step, appropriate therapy is best determined with a depth and breadth of understanding of the many different treatment choices for T2DM and complexities to consider, including the complexity and dynamics of the relationships between the patient's medications and disease states.

Figure 4-2 represents the thought processes utilized to determine appropriate medication options and achieve glycemic control for CP. The diagram begins with the assessment of the current problem, followed by a review of the current medications CP is prescribed. Knowing that additional medication therapy is needed, it also considers the advantages and disadvantages of all available medication options to achieve glycemic control. The conclusions made through consideration of advantages and disadvantages are included. Future considerations are also incorporated into the conclusions to demonstrate the conditions in which certain medication treatment options would be preferred. The decision tree concludes with the final determination of the medications that will be recommended to continue, discontinue, or to initiate.

PLAN: Type 2 Diabetes—Microvascular Complications	
Conclusions	Rationale: Information or Premise to Support the Conclusion
Refer patient to specialty providers	It is recommended for patients with T2DM to have an initial dilated eye exam at the time of diagnosis performed by either an optometrist or ophthalmologist. If there is no evidence of retinopathy and blood glucose is well controlled, then screening should be considered every 1 to 2 years. For neuropathy, all patients with T2DM should be assessed at initial diagnosis, followed by annual evaluations by a healthcare provider.[8]

Critical Thinking Checks for Carlos P.'s Microvascular Complications

Pharmacists need **depth** and **breadth** of understanding of how uncontrolled T2DM affects certain vascular systems. It is important to understand these effects to determine appropriate preventative care, which in our case is targeted on nephropathy, neuropathy, and retinopathy. Patients oftentimes do not associate changes in vision or neuropathic pain with uncontrolled T2DM or may not realize those are possible complications. There should be **clarity** when explaining the **significance** of being routinely monitored for these microvascular complications. That way, he can detect early signs and symptoms of these complications and stay vigilant with physician follow-up.

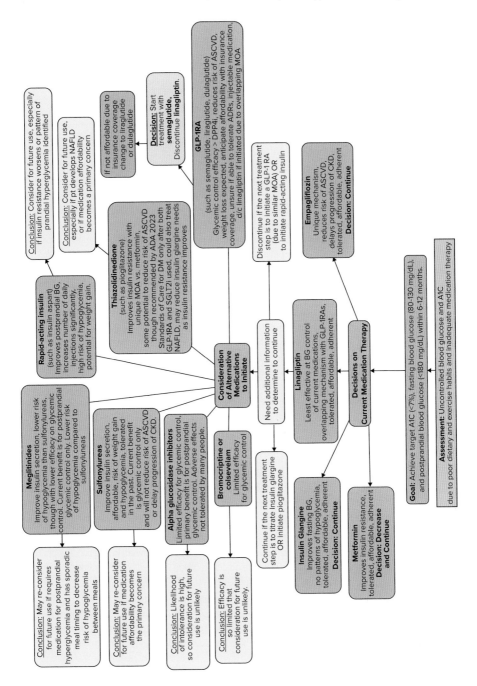

FIGURE 4-2. Decision tree for T2DM medication treatment options to improve glycemic control for continue, discontinue, and/or initiate. ADA, American Diabetes Association; ASCVD, atherosclerotic cardiovascular disease; BG, blood glucose; CKD, chronic kidney disease; DPP4i, dipeptidyl peptidase 4 inhibitor; GLP-1RAs, glucagon-like peptide 1 receptor agonists; MOA, mechanism of action; NAFLD, nonalcoholic fatty liver disease; SGLT2i, sodium-glucose cotransporter 2 inhibitor.

Plan: HTN/CKD	

Goals:
1. Reduce the blood pressure to <130/80 mm Hg within the next 3 months.
2. Delay progression in kidney function decline for as long as possible.

Conclusions	Rationale: Information or Premise to Support the Conclusion
Initiate chlorthalidone 25 mg by mouth once daily	Management of HTN requires either increasing the current antihypertensives or adding additional agents. Upon review of the current medications, lisinopril and empagliflozin are lowering the blood pressure and are at their maximum recommended doses. Metoprolol succinate can be increased to a higher dose for blood pressure control; however, his heart rate is 64 bpm and increasing this medication could cause him to be bradycardic. With the concomitant diagnoses of T2DM and CKD, recommended treatment options include an ACEi, ARB, calcium channel blocker (CCB), and thiazide-like diuretics.[21] continue, discontinue, and/or initiate is currently on an ACEi (lisinopril) and therefore another medication from this class should not be added due to compounding adverse effects with duplication of therapy. An ARB should also not be added as it has been shown that in patients with T2DM and nephropathy, acute kidney injury occurs significantly more frequently among patients receiving both ACEi/ARB therapy compared to ARB monotherapy.[42] This combination is also associated with an increased incidence of hypotension, serum creatinine elevation, hyperkalemia, and adverse events.[43] That leaves the decision between starting a CCB or a thiazide-like diuretic. CCBs could be a good option as they are inexpensive, well-tolerated, and have been shown to reduce stroke risk. However, this reduction is comparable to diuretics.[44] Diuretics are also inexpensive, well tolerated, and have been shown to prevent future cardiovascular events.[45] Diuretic options include hydrochlorothiazide or chlorthalidone and the decision then becomes which one to select. Both agents have demonstrated equivalent cardiovascular benefits, with chlorthalidone having a slightly greater risk of renal and electrolyte abnormalities.[45] However, the landmark trials that proved diuretic reduction of cardiovascular events primarily used chlorthalidone, leading clinicians to selecting this agent.[46–48] Nevertheless, either CCBs or diuretics are the most appropriate classes of medications to consider at this time and would involve a discussion with CP to decide.
Continue lisinopril, metoprolol succinate, and empagliflozin for blood pressure control	As CP is tolerating these medications and they are having a positive effect on his blood pressure, it is recommended that they be continued. In addition, lisinopril and metoprolol succinate are guideline-driven therapies recommended post-MI and empagliflozin reduces the risk of future ASCVD events.[39,49] Patients with T2DM in the presence of albuminuria and/or HTN should be treated with the highest tolerated dose of either ACEi or ARB therapy.[17] These medication classes have been shown to have renal protective effects by reducing urinary protein excretion, improving blood pressure, and slowing the progression of CKD.[50,51]

 KEY POINT

When intensifying treatment for hypertension, the mechanism of action of each agent should be unique and complementary to the other medications included in the treatment plan.

Critical Thinking Checks for Carlos P.'s HTN/CKD

Pharmacists need to be **objective** when selecting optimal therapy by practicing evidence-based medicine. This requires analyzing available literature for supporting evidence that is most closely aligned with your patient to provide positive benefits and health outcomes. In pursuit of the most **logical** and optimal therapy for the patient, it also requires **breadth** and **depth** of thought when deliberating on the many medication therapy options for controlling blood pressure and when considering the complexity of these options in terms of their potential impacts, positive or negative, on the patient's other conditions.

- For CP, adding an antihypertensive medication will not only reduce blood pressure, but can also affect laboratory values, organ systems, and increase risk of possible adverse effects. Using pharmacological agents that target the renin-angiotensin-aldosterone system is appropriate for patients with albuminuria, like CP, as these agents have proven benefit in reducing urinary protein and progression of CKD and should be used in all patients with albuminuria in absence of contraindications.

PLAN: Cardiovascular Disease Risk

Goals:

1. Secondary prevention of ASCVD events for as long as possible.
2. Reduce LDL by at least 50% from baseline (before drug therapy was initiated).

Conclusions	Rationale: Information or Premise to Support the Conclusion
Increase atorvastatin to 40 mg by mouth once daily	CP is currently taking atorvastatin 20 mg by mouth once daily, which is classified as moderate-intensity statin therapy. Since he is less than 75 years of age with established clinical ASCVD (MI), he is indicated for high-intensity statin therapy.[34] High-intensity statin therapy consists of rosuvastatin 20 to 40 mg/day and atorvastatin 40 to 80 mg/day. As he is currently tolerating atorvastatin without any reported adverse effects or barriers to therapy, this favors titrating his current medication rather than switching to rosuvastatin. Both the 40 mg and 80 mg dose of atorvastatin have the same effect on cholesterol levels; however, higher doses may have an increased risk of adverse effects, such as myalgias.[52] Either dose would be considered a viable option and would require a discussion with CP to determine the appropriate course of therapy.
Continue medications with cardiovascular disease risk reduction	CP is currently taking medications that have proven benefit in cardiovascular risk reduction such as empagliflozin, aspirin, and antihypertensive therapies.[39,49] As he denies any adverse events from these medications or barriers to therapy, they should be continued for their cardiovascular benefits and comorbid disease state control.

KEY POINT

The dosing of statins should be based on the intensity categorization determined by the indication for use.

Critical Thinking Checks for Carlos P.'s Cardiovascular Disease Risk

From a patient perspective, a statin dosage increase would mean better control of lipid levels; however, this would also mean increasing the chance of side effects. There should be **clarity** when explaining to CP that his cholesterol medication is being increased to a dose that was not only studied to have a greater reduction in cholesterol, but also shown to have a greater impact on cardiovascular risk reduction.[34] The **significance** of this increase needs to be explained so that he can assess the risk of possible side effects at an increased dose vs the cardiovascular benefits. However, the pharmacist having a **depth** of knowledge surrounding possible therapy options and adverse effects of statin therapy can discuss this with CP to reduce the risk of adverse effects or of statin tolerance with high-intensity statins.

PLAN: Hypothyroidism	
Goal: Maintain TSH 0.45 to 4.12 mIU/L without symptoms of hypo or hyperthyroidism	
Conclusions	Rationale: Information or Premise to Support the Conclusion
Continue levothyroxine at its current dose	As CP is asymptomatic with a TSH within goal range, no therapy adjustment is needed at this time

Critical Thinking Checks for Carlos P.'s Hypothyroidism

When considering thyroid disorders, there is a **depth** of understanding between the association of thyroid disorders and T2DM. Left untreated, thyroid disorders can impair metabolic control in people with diabetes.[28] If CP had issues with medication adherence, he could experience weight gain, fatigue, and muscle pains, which are common symptoms of hypothyroidism and could be a barrier in controlling other chronic disease states. There needs to be **clarity** when explaining the purpose of this medication to him as medication nonadherence is common for patients with chronic disease states.[53] He should be educated on the **significance** of consistently taking this medication appropriately and future drug interactions that may occur. For example, calcium in over-the-counter (OTC) agents can bind to levothyroxine, leading to reduced levothyroxine absorption, thus necessitating separate administration times.

 KEY POINT

There needs to be clarity when explaining the purpose of the medications to the patient, as medication nonadherence is common for patients with chronic disease states, and therefore the patient should be educated on the significance of consistently taking medications appropriately.

IMPLEMENT/MONITOR: Type 2 Diabetes—Glycemic Control	
Conclusions	Rationale: Information or Premise to Support the Conclusion
Implement: Write a new prescription for metformin with reduced dose (500 mg BID) and educate CP on the updated dosing.	*Implement:* A new prescription needs to be sent to the pharmacy. CP needs to be educated to expect a change when he receives the next fill of the medication. The prescription will be signed by an authorized prescriber (eg, MD, DO, APRN, PA).
Monitor: 1. eGFR via results of the basic metabolic panel (BMP) every 3 to 6 months. 2. Vitamin B12 concentration annually.	*Monitor:* 1. Decline in kidney function occurs in patients with T2DM. The rate of decline can vary between patients. Due to the risk of lactic acidosis when using metformin and the current stage of CKD for CP, eGFR should be monitored at least every 3 to 6 months to ensure continued safe use of metformin.[50] If the eGFR declines below 30 mL/min/m^2 then metformin will need to be discontinued. 2. Long-term use of metformin can cause a decrease in vitamin B12 concentrations. Low vitamin B12 can result in a macrocytic anemia that can also present with neurologic symptoms that is difficult to differentiate from diabetic peripheral neuropathy. Therefore, annual monitoring of vitamin B12 should be conducted to quickly identify and correct vitamin B12 deficiencies.[50]
Implement: 1. Initiate semaglutide 0.25 mg SC once weekly. Increase semaglutide to 0.5 mg SC once weekly after 4 weeks. 2. Educate on proper steps of administration and storage based on product labeling. 3. Educate on nausea/vomiting as an adverse reaction. 4. Educate on what to do if a dose is missed.	*Implement:* 1. The starting dose of 0.25 mg SC once weekly for semaglutide is used to reduce frequency/severity of nausea/vomiting when the dose is subsequently titrated to 0.5 mg weekly. It is expected that glycemic control will improve when CP has used 0.5 mg SC once weekly for 4 weeks. If glycemic control is not achieved at this dose, it can be titrated to 1 mg SC weekly after 4 weeks, with a maximum dose of 2 mg weekly.[54] 2. The manufacturer provides detailed guidelines for proper administration and storage of subcutaneous semaglutide, including needle attachment, removal, and discarding; dosing, skin swabbing, injecting, and storage conditions to maintain sterility and stability.[54] 3. Semaglutide decreases the gastric emptying rate, which results in food remaining in the stomach longer and can result in nausea/vomiting. Therefore, the more slowly you consume food, the more likely you will be to recognize you are full, which will prevent you from overeating. Severe nausea/vomiting may also be a sign of pancreatitis, so it is important for CP to notify healthcare providers in the event this occurs. 4. The manufacture provides directions on what to do if a dose is missed in consideration of how long it has been since the dose was missed.[54]

Monitor: 1. Adverse effects such as nausea, vomiting, injection site reaction/pain 2. Body weight 3. Symptoms of pancreatitis	*Monitor:* 1. Semaglutide can cause nausea and vomiting due to delays in gastric emptying rate. Therefore, CP should be educated on what to expect and to monitor the frequency of these adverse effects with instructions on when to notify a healthcare provider. 2. Semaglutide can also contribute to weight loss, which is beneficial for CP because he is obese (class I). Reducing weight by 5% to 10% can significantly improve insulin resistance and improve glycemic control.[33] Therefore, weight monitoring will be needed to help him identify potential benefits of this treatment option beyond glycemic control itself. Weight can be monitored at home by CP and during each office visit. 3. Pancreatitis can occur in patients while taking semaglutide.[54] CP should be educated on symptoms of pancreatitis (upper abdominal pain, abdominal pain may radiate to the back, nausea, vomiting, fever, tachycardia). If these symptoms are present, use of semaglutide should be discontinued and not reinitiated if pancreatitis is confirmed.
Implement: Educate patient on strategies, such as earlier medication administration and using daily reminders to improve his medication adherence with a focus on evening medication administration.	*Implement:* CP is exhibiting situational nonadherence, where medications are missed because he falls asleep in the evening. One strategy to avoid this in the future is to adjust medication administration timing to earlier in the day, such as with the evening meal or just prior to watching television in the evening. Another strategy may be to set automatic daily reminders on his cell phone. The finalized strategy will need to be discussed with CP to identify the best approach that will work best for him.
Implement: Goal weight loss of 5% to 10% total body weight. The approach to achieve this goal will be to implement sustainable strategies. For example, to decrease caloric intake, CP can employ the "plate method" and replace sugar-sweetened beverages with beverages without sugar. He can also gradually work toward increasing his physical activity to eventually meet a target of 150 minutes weekly of moderate-intensity activity. *Monitor:* Body weight, enjoyment of food	*Implement:* To help CP achieve his weight loss goals, he needs to be educated on actions to take that will be sustainable for the long term. One such approach is to use the plate method, which divides a 9-inch plate into sections (½ plate of nonstarchy vegetables, ¼ plate of carbohydrates (whole grains preferred), ¼ plate of lean protein (limit intake of saturated fats and avoid trans fats). This method can be adapted to a variety of cultures to ensure CP continues to consume the foods he enjoys. Another approach is to discontinue consumption of sugar-sweetened beverages. These beverages provide no nutritional value and include a significant amount of carbohydrates and calories. Instead, encourage him to consume water (preferred) or change to diet versions of his favorite beverages. Physical activity should begin at the level he is capable of and comfortable starting with, regarding type, intensity, and duration of activity. Encourage continued increase in intensity and duration to eventually meet a target of 150 minutes weekly of moderate-intensity activity or 75 minutes weekly of high-intensity activity. He should be educated to avoid spans longer than 2 days of inactivity. Physical activity plans should also include strength and balance training at a frequency of every 2 to 3 days on nonconsecutive days.[55]

Implement:	*Implement:*
Educate on signs, symptoms, and management of hypoglycemia using the "rule of 15".	The "rule of 15" specifies to administer 15 g of simple carbohydrates (eg, glucose, honey, table sugar, fruit juice) when the blood glucose is below 70 mg/dL. If the blood glucose is below 50 mg/dL, he should administer 30 g of simple carbohydrates instead of 15 g. Then wait 15 minutes and recheck the blood glucose. If at that time the blood glucose remains below 50 mg/dL or 70 mg/dL, then ingest an additional 30 g or 15 g of simple carbohydrates, respectively. Once blood glucose is ≥70 mg/dL, CP should consume a meal consisting of carbohydrates and protein to stabilize blood glucose.[13]
Monitor:	*Monitor:*
Blood glucose (fasting, preprandial, bedtime, and as needed for hypoglycemic episodes), A1C every 3 months.	Measuring the blood glucose allows CP to become familiar with behavior patterns (medication adherence, food choices, physical activity) that influence changes in blood glucose. It also provides additional information for healthcare providers on patterns observed regarding control and frequency/severity of hypo- and hyperglycemia, both of which contribute to making informed decisions on medication and lifestyle modifications needed in the future. Timing of blood glucose testing is a balance between how the measured information will be used to direct treatment decisions, convenience for him, and cost. Having CP check blood glucose four times a day will provide information needed to determine if treatment escalations are needed so patterns of hyperglycemia can be identified. For example, a pattern of preprandial hyperglycemia may signal that the current treatment plan needs adjusted to improve postprandial blood glucose elevations, whereas fasting hyperglycemia may signal a different approach to medication adjustments. Also, of note, it is important to consider patterns of hypoglycemia to identify either medication causes, or behavior patterns that are leading to these events. Changes in blood glucose occur faster than changes in A1C allowing healthcare providers to optimize medications prior to when the next A1C is due. However, the A1C is also important, as it is viewed as a measure of long-term glycemic control compared to the blood glucose alone. The A1C can be reassessed every 3 months for patients who have not yet achieved a target A1C.

 KEY POINT

To help patients maintain positivity throughout the duration of their treatment for diabetes, pharmacists must also be positive and set achievable goals with the patient, and encourage the patient to implement small changes that will collectively help achieve the goals.

KEY POINT

The approach to achieving a weight loss goal will be different for each person. The most important factors to consider when creating a plan are to identify what the patient enjoys doing and is able to fit into their lifestyle. These interventions are more likely to be successful for the long term.

KEY POINT

Frequency of blood glucose monitoring will be determined based on risk of hypoglycemia, medication adjustments based on glucose values, identified patterns of glucose control throughout the day, patient ability/access, and cost. It is essential to have a specific reason for the blood glucose to be measured by the patient at each timepoint to prevent unnecessarily inconveniencing the patient and wasting resources.

IMPLEMENT/MONITOR: Type 2 Diabetes—Microvascular Complications	
Conclusions	**Rationale: Information or Premise to Support the Conclusion**
Implement: Refer to ophthalmologist for dilated retinal exam and physician for comprehensive foot exam. *Monitor:* Dilated retinal exam Comprehensive foot exam	*Implement/Monitor:* Microvascular complications do not always present in a similar time frame, so while Carlos already had nephropathy, it is important to continue to also monitor for other microvascular complications such as retinopathy and neuropathy. Screening for retinopathy via dilated retinal exam and for peripheral neuropathy via comprehensive foot exam that includes sensory exam and visual inspection should be conducted at least annually.[8]

IMPLEMENT/MONITOR: HTN/CKD	
Conclusions	**Rationale: Information or Premise to Support the Conclusion**
Implement: 1. Write a new prescription for chlorthalidone 25 mg daily 2. Educate on chlorthalidone's indication, common adverse effects, and when to anticipate a change in blood pressure *Monitor:* BMP every 3 months, blood pressure, heart rate	*Implement/Monitor:* 1. A new prescription needs to be sent to the pharmacy. CP needs to be educated that this will be a new prescription that he will be receiving. The prescription will be signed by an authorized prescriber (eg, MD, DO, APRN, PA). 2. Educate CP that chlorthalidone is being used to treat hypertension, which also will decrease risk of future atherosclerotic cardiovascular events. Explain to him that the medication has historically been used as a diuretic, so to expect that initially he will experience increased urination. Because of this, it is recommended to take this medication in the morning to avoid waking up at night to urinate. Also explain that while taking chlorthalidone, his healthcare providers will monitor his blood pressure, heart rate, and electrolytes in the blood and that he can expect his blood pressure to improve within 1 to 2 months of starting this medication. Also tell him that 1 to 2 months after initiating chlorthalidone, we can check the blood electrolytes with a simple blood test.

Monitor:	*Monitor:*
BMP with eGFR every 3 months, albumin-to-creatinine ratio annually.	CP has Stage 3b CKD and albuminuria. It is necessary to continue to monitor his kidney function using eGFR (that can be obtained from ordering a basic metabolic panel) and urine albumin-to-creatinine ratio. These measures will help to identify if interventions being made are assisting to slow the decline in kidney function. eGFR is also important to follow as a safety measure to identify if and when medication dosing adjustments are needed. At this stage of CKD, it is advised to reassess the eGFR every 3 to 6 months and the urine albumin-to-creatinine ratio once annually.[17,50]
Implement: Educate CP on therapeutic lifestyle changes to minimize risk of future atherosclerotic cardiovascular disease, including reducing his sodium intake to less than 2300 mg/day, with an ideal goal of less than 1500 mg/day. *Monitor:* Sodium intake to a goal less than 2300 mg/day, and ideally less than 1500 mg/day.	*Implement/Monitor:* Consuming a diet that is low in sodium has been shown to improve blood pressure control, reduce risk of future cardiovascular disease events, and stroke.[56] The current recommendation from the AHA is to restrict sodium consumption to less than 2300 mg/day, with an ideal goal of less than 1500 mg/day.[57]

IMPLEMENT/MONITOR: Cardiovascular Disease Risk	
Conclusions	**Rationale: Information or Premise to Support the Conclusion**
Implement: 1. Write new prescription for atorvastatin 40 mg daily 2. Educated on side effects of statins, including myalgia. *Monitor:* Fasting lipid panel within 4 to 12 weeks of beginning atorvastatin 40 mg.	*Implement:* 1. A new prescription needs to be sent to the pharmacy. CP needs to be educated to expect a change when he receives the next fill of the medication. The prescription will be signed by an authorized prescriber (eg, MD, DO, APRN, PA). 2. The most commonly reported adverse effect of high-intensity statins is myalgia. When myalgia presents with elevations in creatinine kinase, this is referred to as statin-induced myopathy. Rarely, this can escalate to the most severe form of myopathy, rhabdomyolysis (myalgia with creatinine kinase 40 times greater than the upper limit of normal).[58] *Monitor:* Fasting lipid panels can be obtained 4 to 12 weeks following the change in atorvastatin dose. The results of this test will indicate if the expected decrease in LDL has been achieved. In the event CP experiences muscle pain, he should contact the provider as a creatinine kinase level can be considered to rule out rhabdomyolysis.

Implement:	Implement:
Educate CP on therapeutic lifestyle changes, including reducing consumption of food high in saturated and trans fats, to minimize risk of future atherosclerotic cardiovascular disease.	Consuming a diet low in saturated and trans-fat (and instead replacing these fats with polyunsaturated fat) can result in a reduction in cardiovascular disease by as much as 30%.[59] Trans fats should be avoided as they can increase the risk of cardiovascular disease.
Monitor:	Monitor:
Blood pressure, heart rate, BMP every 3 months, signs, and symptoms of bleeding	A comprehensive monitoring approach for cardiovascular disease risk will include blood pressure, heart rate, basic metabolic panel, and signs and symptoms of bleeding. Antihypertensive medications and empagliflozin directly impact blood pressure, so this should be monitored every visit with a healthcare provider. In addition, consideration could be given to monitoring blood pressure and heart rate periodically at home until target blood pressure is achieved. Heart rate will also be documented at the time of blood pressure measurement, due to the impact of metoprolol on the heart rate via beta-blocking activity. The basic metabolic panel should be monitored to assess the impact of ACEi and chlorthalidone on electrolytes and to measure kidney function (as previously stated). Signs and symptoms of bleeding will need to be monitored by CP regularly due to concurrent use of aspirin to assist with reducing risk of bleeding, which can vary from minor to major bleeding events.

IMPLEMENT/MONITOR: Hypothyroidism	
Conclusions	**Rationale: Information or Premise to Support the Conclusion**
Implement:	Implement:
Educate on proper administration of levothyroxine with regard to time of day and potential drug interactions.	Levothyroxine has many drug interactions, including interactions with medications/supplements/foods with di- and trivalent cations (eg, aluminum, calcium, iron). This medication is typically administered 30 minutes prior to the first meal of the day and with at least 4 hours of separation from administration with these cations to avoid erratic absorption.
Monitor:	Monitor:
TSH annually	The TSH is currently controlled, so annual monitoring is appropriate. However, if CP presents with worsening symptoms of hypothyroidism, then a TSH would be warranted at the time of symptom onset.

Critical Thinking Checks for Carlos P.'s Implementation and Monitoring Plan

The final step of the PPCP is to implement and monitor the treatment plan. When considering implementation, there needs to be **clarity** in the plan to ensure CP has a firm understanding of how to achieve his disease state goals. In the setting of T2DM management, much of the implementation is providing individualized education to patients. This requires the engagement of CP with decision-making in a **fair-minded** manner free of bias or judgment, and with an empathetic understanding that he can become overwhelmed with the amount of information that is conveyed to him. During this step in the process, the pharmacist also needs to serve as a patient advocate to assist with gaining access to necessary medications and monitoring supplies. It is also important that the pharmacist confirms patients are knowledgeable of the steps of their treatment plans, as they are responsible for implementing the plan with sufficient **accuracy** and **precision** to help assure achievement of therapeutic goals. During the Monitoring step of the PPCP, the cycle of critical thinking repeats. With the collection of new information provided by various sources, the pharmacist is required to revisit previous conclusions and reassess their **accuracy** in the setting of newly acquired information. There should also be a systematic approach in place to consistently reassess the **depth** and **breadth** of the comprehensive care plan for patients with T2DM. The **breadth** of the plan needs to extend beyond glycemic control and be inclusive of microvascular and macrovascular complications to detect and assess their presence and future risk.

 KEY POINT

To help assure successful implementation of the plan, there needs to be clarity to assure the patient has a firm understanding of the actions needed to achieve disease state goals. It should be conveyed to the patient in a fair-minded manner with an empathetic understanding that patients can become overwhelmed with the amount of information they are receiving.

CONCLUSION

The management of T2DM requires patient-centered care through treatment individualization, as there is no set standard for treatment progression. An interprofessional team should be used to provide the highest quality of care for patients with T2DM. For a pharmacist to achieve this personalized level of high-quality care, the PPCP must be applied with critical thinking and sound clinical reasoning at each step (Collect, Assess, Plan, Implement/Monitor) to create and implement an optimal course of action for achieving treatment goals in a manner that best meets the patient's needs, values, and beliefs. Critical thinking and clinical reasoning skills are not stagnant and will continue to grow through experience in chronic disease management and overcoming patient barriers to therapy.

Summary Points

- T2DM is a multifactorial disease state that requires a team approach to care. An interprofessional team is desirable to provide support needed by the patient, while keeping in mind that the patient is at the center of this team, not simply a receiver of information and treatment.
- In the Collect step, the accuracy of information collected is critical to decision-making for patients with T2DM. To help assure accuracy of collected information

from the patient, the pharmacist can engage the patient with a fair-minded approach that builds an empathetic, trusting relationship that shows fairness toward the information divulged, free from any biasing assumptions or attitudes. This approach can provide a rapport that encourages openness, objectivity, and honesty in the patient.

- When working with people who have T2DM and comorbid conditions, pharmacists must think deeply and broadly to assess and develop an understanding of how these disease states affect each other, as they cannot be assessed in isolation. This depth and breadth of thought is also needed for determining appropriate therapy for the patient, as this requires the consideration of the many different treatment choices for T2DM and complexities to consider, including the complexity and dynamics of the relationships between the patient's medications and disease states.

- In the Plan step, treatment considerations for glycemic control need to be individualized for the patient based on clinical guidelines and patient-specific factors, including the efficacy and safety of the patient's current medications, comorbid conditions, glycemic patterns, treatment goals, and patient preferences. While following the most current guidelines is a starting point for considering potential treatment options, those options then need to be critically reviewed to identify those that will be most appropriate for the patient. Arguments for and against alternative treatment strategies are developed, culminating in the selection of strategies that have strong supporting rationale.

- To help assure successful implementation of the plan, there needs to be clarity to assure the patient has a firm understanding of the actions needed to achieve disease state goals. When explaining the purpose of the medications to the patient, the patient should be educated on the significance of consistently taking medications appropriately as medication nonadherence is common in patients with chronic disease states, such as TD2M and commonly occurring comorbid conditions. Communication to the patient should occur in a fair-minded manner, with an empathetic understanding that patients can become overwhelmed with the amount of information they are receiving.

Abbreviations

ACC	American College of Cardiology
ACEi	Angiotensin-Converting Enzyme Inhibitor
ADA	American Diabetes Association
ADR	Adverse Drug Reaction
AHA	American Heart Association
APRN	Advanced Practice Registered Nurse
ARB	Angiotensin Receptor Blocker
ASCVD	Atherosclerotic Cardiovascular Disease
A1C	Glycated Hemoglobin
BG	Blood Glucose
BGM	Blood Glucose Monitoring
BMI	Body Mass Index
BMP	Basic Metabolic Profile
BP	Blood Pressure

CCB	Calcium Channel Blocker
CGM	Continuous Glucose Monitoring
CKD	Chronic Kidney Disease
CMP	Comprehensive Metabolic Panel
CVD	Cardiovascular Disease
DPP4i	Dipeptidyl Peptidase 4 Inhibitor
DM	Diabetes Mellitus
DO	Doctor of Osteopathic Medicine
eGFR	estimated Glomerular Filtration Rate
EHR	Electronic Health Record
GOP-1	Glucagon-like Peptide-1
GLP-1 RA	Glucagon-like Peptide Receptor Agonists
HDL	High-density Lipoprotein
HS	At Bedtime
HTN	Hypertension
IU	International Units
KDIGO	Kidney Disease Improving Global Outcomes
LDL	Low-density Lipoprotein
MD	Doctor of Medicine
MI	Myocardial Infarction
MOA	Mechanism of Action
NAFLD	Non-alcoholic Fatty Liver Disease
NVS	Newest Vital Sign
PA	Physician Assistant
PPCP	Pharmacists Patient Care Process
REALM	Rapid Estimate of Adult Literacy in Medicine
SC	Subcutaneously
SCr	Serum Creatinine
SGLT2i	Sodium/Glucose Cotransporter-2 Inhibitor
TC	Total Cholesterol
TG	Triglyceride
TOFHLA	Test of Functional Health Literacy in Adults
TSH	Thyroid Stimulating Hormone
T2DM	Type 2 Diabetes Mellitus
US	United States
WNL	Within Normal Limits

References

1. World Health Organization. *Diabetes.* Available at https://www.who.int/news-room/fact-sheets/detail/diabetes. Accessed April 28, 2022.

2. American Diabetes Association Professional Practice Committee. 2. Classification and diagnosis of diabetes: Standards of Care in Diabetes—2023. *Diabetes Care.* 2023;46(Suppl. 1): S19-S40.

3. American Diabetes Association Professional Practice Committee. 1. Improving care and promoting health in populations: Standards of Care in Diabetes—2023. *Diabetes Care.* 2023;46(Suppl. 1):S10-S18.

4. American Diabetes Association Professional Practice Committee. 4. Comprehensive medical evaluation and assessment of comorbidities: Standards of Care in Diabetes—2023. *Diabetes Care.* 2023;46(Suppl. 1):S49-S67.

5. Weiss BD, Mays MZ, Martz W, Castro KM, DeWalt DA, Pignone MP, Mockbee J, Hale FA. Quick assessment of literacy in primary care: the newest vital sign. *Ann Fam Med.* 2005;3(6):514-522.

6. Duell P, Wright D, Renzaho AM, Bhattacharya D. Optimal health literacy measurement for the clinical setting: a systematic review. *Patient Educ Couns.* 2015;98(11):1295-1307.

7. Wallace L; North American Primary Care Research Group. Patients' health literacy skills: the missing demographic variable in primary care research. *Ann Fam Med.* 2006;4(1):85-86.

8. American Diabetes Association Professional Practice Committee. 12. Retinopathy, neuropathy, and foot care: Standards of Care in Diabetes—2023. *Diabetes Care.* 2023;46(Suppl. 1): S203-S215.

9. Berbudi A, Rahmadika N, Tjahjadi AI, Ruslami R. Type 2 diabetes and its impact on the immune system. *Curr Diabetes Rev.* 2020;16(5):442-449.

10. Centers for Disease Control and Prevention. Adult immunization schedule by medical condition and other indication: recommendations for ages 19 years or older, United States, 2022.

11. U.S. Department of Agriculture and U.S. Department of Health and Human Services. Dietary guidelines for Americans, 2020-2025. 9th Edition. December 2020. Available at https://www.dietaryguidelines.gov/.

12. Prochaska JO, Velicer WF. The transtheoretical model of health behavior change. *Am J Health Promot.* 1997;12(1):38-48.

13. American Diabetes Association Professional Practice Committee. 6. Glycemic targets: Standards of Care in Diabetes—2023. *Diabetes Care.* 2023;46(Suppl. 1): S97-S110.

14. Inzucchi SE, Bergenstal RM, Buse JB, et al. Management of hyperglycemia in type 2 diabetes, 2015: a patient-centered approach: update to a position statement of the American Diabetes Association and the European Association for the Study of Diabetes. *Diabetes Care.* 2015;38:140-149.

15. American Diabetes Association Professional Practice Committee. 9. Pharmacologic approaches to glycemic treatment: Standards of Care in Diabetes—2023. *Diabetes Care.* 2023;46(Suppl. 1): S140-S157.

16. American Diabetes Association Professional Practice Committee. 10. Cardiovascular disease and risk management: Standards of Care in Diabetes—2023. *Diabetes Care.* 2023;46(Suppl. 1):S158-S190.

17. American Diabetes Association Professional Practice Committee. 11. Chronic kidney disease and risk management: Standards of Care in Diabetes—2023. *Diabetes Care.* 2023;46(Suppl. 1):S191-S202.

18. Corbo JM, Breslin TM, Hill LG, Rindfuss SL, Nashelsky J. ACE inhibitors or ARBs to prevent CKD in patients with microalbuminuria. *American Family Physician.* 2016;94(8):652-653.

19. Chu CD, Powe NR, McCulloch CE, et al. Angiotensin-converting enzyme inhibitor or angiotensin receptor blocker use among hypertensive US adults with albuminuria. *Hypertension.* 2021;77(1):94-102.

20. Whelton PK, Carey RM, Aronow WS, et al. 2017 ACC/AHA/AAPA/ABC/ACPM/AGS/APhA/ASH/ASPC/NMA/PCNA guideline for the prevention, detection, evaluation, and management of high blood pressure in adults: a report of the American College of Cardiology/American Heart Association Task Force on Clinical Practice Guidelines. *J Am Coll Cardiol.* 2018;71:e127-e248.

21. Unger T, Borghi C, Charchar F, et al. 2020 International Society of Hypertension Global Hypertension Practice Guidelines. Hypertension. 2020;75(6):1334-1357.

22. Kidney Disease: Improving Global Outcomes (KDIGO) CKD Work Group. KDIGO 2012 Clinical practice guideline for the evaluation and management of chronic kidney disease. *Kidney Inter Suppl.* 2013;3:1-150.

23. Carey RM, Calhoun DA, Bakris GL, et al. Resistant hypertension: detection, evaluation, and management: a scientific statement from the American Heart Association. *Hypertension.* 2018;72:e53-e90.

24. Inzucchi SE, Lipska KJ, Mayo H, Bailey CJ, McGuire DK. Metformin in patients with type 2 diabetes and kidney disease: a systematic review. *JAMA.* 2014;312(24):2668-2675.

25. Jellinger PS, Handelsman Y, Rosenblit PD, et al. American Association of Clinical Endocrinologists and American College of Endocrinology guidelines for management of dyslipidemia and prevention of cardiovascular disease. *Endocr Pract.* 2017;23(Suppl 2):1-87.

26. Garber JR, Cobin RH, Gharib H, et al. Clinical practice guidelines for hypothyroidism in adults: cosponsored by the American Association of Clinical Endocrinologists and the American Thyroid Association. *Thyroid.* 2012;22(12):1200-1235.

27. Wang C. The Relationship between Type 2 Diabetes Mellitus and Related Thyroid Diseases. *J Diabetes Res.* 2013;2013:390534. doi:10.1155/2013/390534.

28. Biondi B, Kahaly GJ, Robertson RP. Thyroid dysfunction and diabetes mellitus: two closely associated disorders. *Endocr Rev.* 2019; 40:789-824.

29. Safeer RS, Keenan J. Health literacy: the gap between physicians and patients. *Am Fam Physician.* 2005;72(3):463-468

30. UKPDS 34: UK Prospective Diabetes Study (UKPDS) Group. Effect of intensive blood-glucose control with metformin on complications in overweight patients with type 2 diabetes (UKPDS 34). *Lancet.* 1998:352:854-865.

31. UKPDS 33: UK Prospective Diabetes Study (UKPDS) Group. Intensive blood-glucose control with sulphonylureas or insulin compared with conventional treatment and risk of complications in patients with type 2 diabetes (UKPDS 33). *Lancet.* 1998;352:837-853.

32. UKPDS 10-year f/u: Holman RR, Paul SK, Bethel MA, Matthews DR, Neil HAW. 10-year follow-up of intensive glucose control in type 2 diabetes. *N Engl J Med.* 2008;359:1577-1589.

33. Kong DX, Xiao YX, Zhang ZX, Liu YB. Study on the Correlation between metabolism, insulin sensitivity and progressive weight loss change in type-2 diabetes. *Pak J Med Sci.* 2020;36(7):1523-1528.

34. Grundy SM, Stone NJ, Bailey AL, et al. 2018 AHA/ACC/AACVPR/AAPA/ABC/ACPM/ADA/ AGS/APhA/ASPC/NLA/PCNA Guideline on the Management of Blood Cholesterol: A Report of the American College of Cardiology/American Heart Association Task Force on Clinical Practice Guidelines [published correction appears in Circulation. 2019;139(25): e1182-e1186]. *Circulation.* 2019;139(25):e1082-e1143.

35. de Jong M, van der Worp HB, van der Graaf Y, Visseren FLJ, Westerink J. Pioglitazone and the secondary prevention of cardiovascular disease. A meta-analysis of randomized-controlled trials. *Cardiovasc Diabetol.* 2017;16(1):1-11.

36. Marso SP, Bain SC, Consoli A, et al. Semaglutide and cardiovascular outcomes in patients with type 2 diabetes. *N Engl J Med.* 2016;375(19):1834-1844.

37. Gerstein HC, Colhoun HM, Dagenais GR, et al. Dulaglutide and cardiovascular outcomes in type 2 diabetes (REWIND): a double-blind, randomised placebo-controlled trial. *Lancet.* 2019;394(10193):121-130.

38. Marso SP, Daniels GH, Brown-Frandsen K, et al. Liraglutide and cardiovascular outcomes in type 2 diabetes. *N Engl J Med.* 2016;375(4):311-322.

39. Zinman B, Wanner C, Lachin JM, et al. Empagliflozin, cardiovascular outcomes, and mortality in type 2 diabetes. *N Engl J Med.* 2015;373(22):2117-2128.

40. Wanner C, Inzucchi SE, Lachin JM, et al. Empagliflozin and Progression of Kidney Disease in Type 2 Diabetes. *N Engl J Med.* 2016;375(4):323-334.

41. DeFronzo R, Flemming GA, Chen K, Bicsak TA. Metformin-associated lactic acidosis: current perspectives on causes and risk. *Metabolism.* 2016; 65:20-29.

42. Fried LF, Emanuele N, Zhang JH, et al. Combined angiotensin inhibition for the treatment of diabetic nephropathy. *N Engl J Med.* 2013;369(20):1892-1903.

43. McMurray JJV, Ostergren J, Swedberg K, et al. Effects of candesartan in patients with chronic heart failure and reduced left-ventricular systolic function taking angiotensin-converting-enzyme inhibitors: the CHARM-added trial. *Lancet.* 2003; 362:767-771.

44. Chen GJ, Yang MS. The effects of calcium channel blockers in the prevention of stroke in adults with hypertension: a meta-analysis of data from 273,543 participants in 31 randomized controlled trials. *PLoS One.* 2013;8(3): e57854.

45. Hripcsak G, Suchard MA, Shea S, et al. Comparison of cardiovascular and safety outcomes of chlorthalidone vs hydrochlorothiazide to treat hypertension. *JAMA Intern Med.* 2020;180(4):542-551. doi:10.1001/jamainternmed.2019.7454.

46. Carter BL, Ernst ME, Cohen JD. Hydrochlorothiazide versus chlorthalidone: evidence supporting their interchangeability. *Hypertension.* 2004;43(1):4-9.

47. The ALLHAT Officers and Coordinators for the ALLHAT Collaborative Research Group. Major outcomes in high-risk hypertensive patients randomized to angiotensin-converting enzyme inhibitor

or calcium channel blocker vs diuretic: the Antihypertensive and Lipid-Lowering Treatment to Prevent Heart Attack Trial (ALLHAT). *JAMA*. 2002;288(23):2981-2997.

48. Perry HM Jr, Davis BR, Price TR, et al. Effect of treating isolated systolic hypertension on the risk of developing various types and subtypes of stroke: the Systolic Hypertension in the Elderly Program (SHEP). *JAMA*. 2000;284(4):465-471.

49. Jneid H, Addison D, Bhatt DL, et al. 2017 AHA/ACC clinical performance and quality measures for adults with st-elevation and non-st-elevation myocardial infarction: a report of the American College of Cardiology/American Heart Association Task Force on Performance Measures. *Circ Cardiovasc Qual Outcomes*. 2017;10(10):e000032.

50. Kidney Disease: Improving Global Outcomes (KDIGO) Diabetes Work Group. KDIGO 2020 clinical practice guideline for diabetes management in chronic kidney disease. Kidney Int. 2020;98(4S): S1-S115.

51. Xu R, Sun S, Huo Y, et al. Effects of ACEIs versus ARBs on proteinuria or albuminuria in primary hypertension: a meta-analysis of randomized trials. *Medicine (Baltimore)*. 2015;94(39): e1560.

52. Agrawal D, Manchanda SC, Sawhney JPS, et al. To study the effect of high dose Atorvastatin 40 mg versus 80 mg in patients with dyslipidemia. *Indian Heart J*. 2018;70(Suppl 3):S8-S12.

53. Kleinsinger F. The unmet challenge of medication nonadherence. *Perm J*. 2018; 22:18-033.

54. Ozempic [package insert]. Plainsboro, NJ: Novo Nordisk. https://www.novo-pi.com/ozempic.pdf. Accessed June 16, 2022.

55. U.S. Department of Health and Human Services. Physical activity guidelines for Americans, 2nd edition. Washington, DC: U.S. Department of Health and Human Services; 2018.

56. Whelton PK, Appel LJ, Sacco RL, et al. Sodium, blood pressure, and cardiovascular disease: further evidence supporting the American Heart Association sodium reduction recommendations. *Circulation*. 2012;126:2880-2889.

57. Lloyd-Jones DM, Hong Y, Labarthe D, et al. Defining and setting national goals for cardiovascular health promotion and disease reduction. *Circulation*. 2020; 121:586-613.

58. Newman CB, Preiss D, Tobert JA, et al. Statin safety and associated adverse events: a scientific statement from the American Heart Association. *Arterioscler Thromb Vasc Biol*. 2019;39(2):e38-81.

59. Sacks FM, Lichtenstein AH, WU JHY, et al. Dietary fats and cardiovascular disease: a presidential advisory from the American Heart Association. *Circulation*. 2017;136:e1-e23.

5

Ambulatory Care— Warfarin Management Clinic

Lihui Yuan

CHAPTER AIMS

The aims of this chapter are to:
- Discuss the roles of clinical reasoning and critical thinking skills in each step of the Pharmacists' Patient Care Process (PPCP) to assess and resolve warfarin management-related problems.

- Describe elements of clinical reasoning and critical thinking applied to the PPCP-guided care of a patient being provided warfarin management in an outpatient warfarin management clinic.

KEY WORDS
- Pharmacists' Patient Care Process • critical thinking • problem solving • anticoagulation
- warfarin • international normalized ratio • drug interaction • diet • vitamin K

INTRODUCTION

Anticoagulation management serves an important role in preventing thromboembolic events that are related to stroke, heart attack, deep vein thrombosis/pulmonary embolism (DVT/PE), among others. According to the Centers for Disease Control (CDC), each year in the United States, as many as 795,000 people have a stroke and 900,000 people could be affected by DVT/PE. The vast number of patients who can benefit from anticoagulation medications warrants the participation of ambulatory pharmacy services to help manage the patient's anticoagulation therapy.

Among the different classes of anticoagulation medications are the vitamin K antagonist, warfarin, and the Novel Oral Anticoagulants (NOACs) that include direct thrombin inhibitors (dabigatran) and factor Xa inhibitors (apixaban, betrixaban, edoxaban, and rivaroxaban). NOACs have fewer drug–drug interactions than warfarin, and unlike warfarin, they do not require routine laboratory monitoring. These are among the reasons that NOACs are supplanting the use of warfarin for anticoagulation therapy.[1] However, warfarin is favored under some circumstances, and currently there are 20 million Americans taking warfarin, with an additional 2 million who start taking the medication each year.[2]

Warfarin requires frequent drug therapy monitoring due to a variety of reasons, including optimizing the dosing to assure proper efficacy for thromboembolism prevention and to reduce the risk of bleeding. The unique drug properties associated with warfarin, such as slow onset of action and long half-life, complicated pharmacokinetics, pharmacogenomic variance,[3] drug–drug and drug–food interactions[4] warrant the need for warfarin drug therapy management by the ambulatory care pharmacist.

OUR PRACTICE—AN OUTPATIENT PHARMACIST MANAGED WARFARIN CLINIC

Our practice is a pharmacist-managed outpatient clinic overseen by a hematologist. The patient population includes patients who have suffered from a thromboembolic event and were initiated warfarin during a recent hospital admission, patients referred by a primary care physician (PCP) for chronic anticoagulation management, and patients who are on a medical assistance program who are not currently under the care of a PCP. Currently in our clinic, the patient population ranges in age from the 20s to 90s, with most of the patients being over 50 years of age.

The pharmacist's responsibilities are to initiate and optimize warfarin therapy, monitor its therapeutic effects, assess drug–drug and drug–food interactions, and provide overall management of the patient's warfarin regimen. Due to the high patient volume in this clinic, non-warfarin-related health issues are directed to the patient's PCP or other healthcare professionals, unless the patient experiences an emergent medical situation, in which case the patient will be transported to the emergency room (ER) by a readily available transport team in the hospital.

UTILIZING CRITICAL THINKING SKILLS IN OUR PRACTICE

In our clinic, the pharmacist applies clinical reasoning and critical thinking skills to provide quality patient care throughout the PPCP process.[5,6] This includes applying these skills when collecting and assessing patient information, and when planning, implementing, and monitoring therapy. Applying standards for critical thinking can ensure important factors are considered and can optimize the quality of our reasoning, thereby optimizing the care we provide. The factors to consider are many and include the patient's socioeconomic support, medication adherence, lifestyle, and autonomy towards therapy, and the care provided by others within an interprofessional practice.[7-10] **Table 5-1** provides a list of sample intellectual standards-based questions that can be applied to ensure effective critical thinking when providing warfarin medication therapy management.

APPLICATION OF THE PPCP IN OUR PRACTICE

In our clinic, the patient care process starts with the patient visit. The first step is to collect information, which is done through reviewing the patient's medical chart, reviewing other healthcare professionals' notes, and reviewing notes from previous visits at our clinic. This is followed by a patient interview to continue to collect further information and confirm information obtained through the chart review. A thorough

TABLE 5-1	
Sample Standards-Based Questions That Can Be Applied to Assure That Intellectual Standards for Thinking Are Met as the Pharmacist Provides Warfarin Medication Therapy Management	
Clarity (explicit, unambiguous, intelligible, free from confusion or doubt)	• Did I communicate clearly when I was collecting information about the patient's warfarin dosing regimen, missed/repeated doses, lifestyle changes, medication changes, signs and symptoms of bleeding, and any previous medical procedures? • Did I document the collected information so it can be clearly understood by other healthcare professionals? • When needed, did I seek a clear understanding of the information I gathered for example, when reading information written by other healthcare professionals, calling pharmacies, or communicating with family members? • What questions can I ask to assess the patient's understanding of drug interactions with warfarin?
Relevance (pertinent, applicable, germane)	• What collected information is relevant for warfarin management? • Did I formulate a list of all the collected information to determine which information is most relevant? • Did I review and evaluate the relevant lab values?
Significance (important, nontrivial, necessary, critical, required, impactful)	• What collected information is most significant for warfarin management? • What drug therapy problems are most critical for this patient's warfarin management? • What recommendation can I suggest to the patient that will have a positive and significant impact on medication management?
Objectivity (fact-based, unbiased)	• Was I aware of the potential provider bias in the way I asked questions? For example, instead of asking: You did not miss any doses, did you? I could ask: How many doses did you miss within the last 7 days? • Was I objective when speaking with the patient about the therapeutic plan based on the guidelines and the patient's specific situation? • Did I review the lab values to ensure objectivity when assessing the patient?
Fairness (unbiased, equitable, impartial)	• Did I collect the information in an unbiased way? • Were there any barriers during the interview process that prevented me from gathering needed information? • Is the therapeutic plan fair for the patient?
Accuracy (verifiable, valid, true, credible, undistorted)	• What steps do I need to take to verify the accuracy of the information collected? • What information sources do I need to verify the collected information? • Did I communicate with the patient in a way to ensure that accurate information was collected?
Precision (exact, specific, detailed)	• What questions can I ask to obtain the exact medication dosing? • What level of detail do I need to document? • How do I advise the patient on specific instructions of properly taking medications, improving medication efficacy, and preventing side effects?

Depth (roots, fundamentals, complexities, interrelationships, cause/effect, implications)	• What factors are contributing to the complexity of the patient's warfarin management? • How do the patient's other conditions and medications, and lifestyle factors such as patterns of Vitamin K intake, tobacco-use, and alcohol-use impact my assessment and therapeutic planning? • What level of detail about the patient's vitamin K intake do I need to be able to explain its impact on the International Normalized Ratio (INR)?
Breadth (comprehensive, encompassing, alternative perspectives)	• Am I assessing the patient's medications thoroughly, taking into consideration of all the relevant information? • What references do I need to investigate to ensure that I considered most, if not all, of the factors that affect the warfarin therapy? • Did I review the notes from other healthcare professionals to ensure a complete assessment of the patient?
Logic (reasonable, rational, without contradiction, well-founded, sound)	• Is the medication management plan reasonable for the patient to implement? • Does the therapeutic plan correspond to the assessment details and the current goals of therapy? • Did I consider alternative dosing regimens for the patient to aid in adherence?

and comprehensive assessment is then completed from the collected information, which becomes the basis for developing or adjusting a therapeutic plan for warfarin management. A patient-specific plan is developed based on the patient's goals for therapy. The selected treatment plan is then effectively communicated to the patient to ensure the patient's clear understanding of the treatment plan. Our notes are included in the patient's medical chart, which improves the collaboration between the healthcare providers that can help assure an effective implementation of the treatment plan.

THE COLLECTION OF PATIENT INFORMATION IN OUR PRACTICE

As mentioned, the PPCP begins with the collection of patient information, which includes a chart review followed by a patient interview. **Table 5-2** lists common information needed to be collected from the patient chart review.

TABLE 5-2

Examples of Data That Can Be Collected During Chart Review in Preparation for a Patient Interview

Data to Collect During Chart Review	Rationale for Collecting Specific Data
Patient profile: age, weight, past medical history, relevant past and recent lab results (eg, INR, renal/hepatic function, basic metabolic panel, complete blood cell count).	Medication therapy is related to the overall patient profile. We can identify risk factors for side effects by obtaining the patient's age, weight, and medical history. The previous lab results, especially the INR, can help the pharmacist understand the effectiveness of warfarin pharmacotherapy.[11]
Diagnosis for warfarin indication	The specific diagnosis helps with determining the INR range and duration of warfarin therapy.[12]

Complete medication list	The pharmacist must have a complete understanding of all medications the patient is taking—including the name, dosage form, indication, frequency, and refill history—to better assess medication effectiveness, adherence, duplication of therapy, drug interactions, and potential side effects.
Patient lifestyle, including vitamin K consumption, and alcohol and tobacco use	Certain lifestyle factors, including the consumption of vitamin K-containing food, alcohol use, and tobacco use, can influence the effectiveness of warfarin through different mechanisms.
Recent ER visits	If a recent ER visit is related to thrombosis or bleeding, it is time for the pharmacist to assess the warfarin effectiveness or side effects to determine if a warfarin dose adjustment is warranted.
Insurance coverage	Collecting insurance information is important for evaluating the affordability of the medications and copays for the patient.

 KEY POINT

It is important to collect information about all of the patient's medications, including medications prescribed by healthcare providers that practice outside of the warfarin clinic.

 KEY POINT

For a patient who is on warfarin, the warfarin regimen sometimes changes during the hospital stay. For example, if a patient had a thromboembolism event, they will receive other anticoagulation therapy instead of warfarin. It is important to check that information.

The next step after the comprehensive chart review is the patient interview. During the patient interview, there are a variety of topics that must be explored. During the interview, the pharmacist should utilize open-ended questions to verify adherence to all medications and their regimens, screen for any possible signs or symptoms of bleeding or thromboembolisms, and use this opportunity to educate the patient on the common signs and symptoms of bleeding seen with warfarin management. The information typically collected during the interview is listed in **Table 5-3**.

TABLE 5-3

Patient Interview: Examples of Data That Can Be Collected During the Patient Interview

- Indication of warfarin therapy
- Length of therapy
- Warfarin tablet strength, color, and dosing regimen
- Medication adherence (eg, number of missed doses in the past week)
- Vitamin K intake (especially green leafy vegetables on a weekly basis)

- Alcohol use
- Tobacco use
- Bleeding signs/symptoms (eg, easy bruising, bleeding gums, nose bleeds, dark-colored urine, and tarry stools, etc.)
- Thromboembolic signs/symptoms (eg, palpitations, chest pain, dizziness, fainting, memory lapse, vision loss, etc.)
- Specific dates and reasons for ER visits. Determine if the visits were related to warfarin therapy
- Adjustments or additions to the medication profile
- Future medical procedures or surgery. Determine if planned procedures or surgery will lead to increased bleeding risks
- Refills needed
- Availability for a follow-up visit
- Transportation concerns

 KEY POINT

When discussing the warfarin dosing with the patient, make sure to focus on the color of the tablet since each dose has a specific assigned color.

 KEY POINT

Make sure patient has refills before they come for the next appointment, as lack of refills can cause medication adherence issues.

We will utilize a fictitious patient case to illustrate how our clinic is managed and how critical thinking, clinical reasoning, and the PPCP can integrate to provide optimal care for our patients.

The Case of Robert S.: Overview

Robert S. (RS) is a 66-year-old male (body weight 86 kg) who presents to the clinic for INR management. RS had two unprovoked pulmonary embolism events from January 2017 and February 2020 and was referred by his PCP to the warfarin clinic in January 2021. RS presents to clinic today (May 20, 2021) reporting that he continues to take his warfarin as prescribed but does admit to missing doses periodically due to forgetfulness. He uses a shoe box to manage his medications and organizes his medications by moving vials from one side of the shoe box to the other after he takes the medication for the day. However, he struggles to remember if he moved the vials to the correct side of the box on certain days. He reports he was also seen by his PCP today and was prescribed Bactrim DS for a complicated urinary tract infection (UTI).

He is planning to start taking Bactrim DS today after clinic this afternoon.

The following information was collected from the patient's medical chart review:

Past medical history:

1. Pulmonary embolism: Diagnosed in 2017 and 2020

2. Unspecified chest pain: Diagnosed in 2020

3. Hyperlipidemia: Diagnosed in 2008

4. Hypertension: Diagnosed in 2016

Indications for warfarin therapy:
- Warfarin indications: Pulmonary embolism in 2017 and 2020.

Factors affecting INR: information collected from the previous visit (4/16)
- Missed warfarin doses: one dose on Wednesday in the week previous to this visit
- Diet (Vitamin K): RS usually consumes three to four servings of vegetables weekly, although intake is not consistent
- Alcohol use: RS reports consistent alcohol intake averaging one to two beers a day, along with intermittent heavy drinking with friends (average one time per month)
- Tobacco use: cigarettes—0.5 pack/day for 20 years

 KEY POINT

Dietary vitamin K intake is assessed on a weekly basis rather than on a daily basis.

Review of Systems (ROS): information collected from the previous visit (4/16)
- CV: No chest pain, shortness of breath, or palpitations
- Hematologic: No bruising or bleeding
- Extremities: No abnormal leg pain or swelling
- Neuro: No abnormal dizziness, lightheadedness, or vision changes. History of vertigo.

CLINICAL REASONING, CRITICAL THINKING, AND THE PPCP FOR THE CARE OF ROBERT S.

The following series of tables illustrate the application of the PPCP in the care of Robert S., from the initial Collect step to the last step of Monitoring in the PPCP cycle. The conclusions column in the tables lists the data to be collected, and the rationale column describes the clinical reasoning for collecting the specific data.

Collect

The Collect step is the process of gathering subjective and objective data from both the chart review and the patient interview, with the information collected from the chart confirmed during the patient interview. This includes but is not limited to medications, medical conditions, allergies, labs, social history, lifestyle, thrombosis/bleeding symptoms, and treatment history.

Although it is important to collect the patient's vital signs, it is not routinely done at our clinic due to their indirect relationship with warfarin therapy and the large number of patients and the limited number of staff members. The electronic medical record (EMR) contains previous vital signs from other clinics, so review of vital sign trends can be conducted during our visit if needed. If the patient has a nonemergent health condition, a referral will be placed to the primary care provider for evaluation. If the patient has an emergent health condition, a request for hospital transportation will be done so the patient can be assessed in the ER.

COLLECT: Current Medications	
Conclusions	Rationale: Information or premise to support the conclusion
Conduct a complete medication history review from the medical record and from the medication review with the patient during the interview. *(Collected during the chart review and the interview.)* • Verify the indication of each medication, dosing regimen, effectiveness, side effects, and medication adherence.	It is important for the pharmacist to collect a completed list of past and current medications for the following purposes: • To confirm the indication for each medication and identify any medication that does not have a corresponding disease state. • To ensure the effectiveness of the medication • To prevent duplicate therapy • To identify and prevent drug-drug interactions • To prevent or minimize drug side effects • To identify drug adherence issues

Critical Thinking Checks for the Collect Plan for This Patient's Current Medications

One of the important tasks for a pharmacist is to **objectively** review/collect the patient's medication list with the **accuracy** and **precision** necessary for evaluating the medication effectiveness, drug interaction, side effects and adherence. **Clear** and open communication with the patient is crucial to ensure that information gathered and conveyed is clearly understood by both the patient and the pharmacist.

• Although our clinic focuses on warfarin management, completing a full and detailed medication review, which includes all prescription and nonprescription medications, is very important. During my interview with RS, it was discovered that a new prescription for Bactrim DS for a UTI had been prescribed during his primary care appointment earlier today (5/21). This is a prescription written by a physician outside of our healthcare system, which was not listed in the EMR. Bactrim DS can increase the INR and bleeding risk.[13] Evaluating the potential impact of the patient's Bactrim DS therapy will be vital to prevent or decrease adverse drug effects.

Collected Current Medication Information Entered into Health Record

Current medication regimen:
Warfarin 10 mg po daily except 5 mg on Tuesday and Thursday, occasionally missed doses, no reported signs/symptoms of bleeding or thrombosis

Nitroglycerin 0.4 mg SL as needed for chest pain, the patient takes as needed, was not having chest pain during the interview

Atorvastatin 80 mg po daily for hyperlipidemia, the patient takes daily with occasional missed doses, no adverse drug reactions reported

Amlodipine 10 mg po daily for hypertension, the patient takes daily with occasional missed doses

Lisinopril 10 mg po daily for hypertension, the patient takes daily with occasional missed doses

Bactrim DS one tablet po every 12 hours for 7 days for complicated UTI, the patient will start taking this medication the day of the warfarin clinic on 5/21

COLLECT: Allergies and Labs	
Conclusions	**Rationale: Information or Premise to Support the Conclusion**
Collect/verify patient's allergies. Report specific symptoms the patient experienced. *(Collected during the chart review and the interview.)*	• Collecting all information surrounding any history of allergic reactions is important to ensure medication safety and to help assess if the reactions to a drug indicate a true allergy or a drug intolerance.
Collect the patient's previous and current pertinent labs, including those related to liver and kidney function and the most recent comprehensive metabolic panel (CMP). *(Collected during the chart review.)*	• Results from a CMP can help identify if the patient is experiencing any hepatic or renal impairment that could result in the need for dose adjustments for a variety of medications. There are no specific dosing adjustments for warfarin in renal impairment.[12] Patients with hepatic impairment could have a pronounced response to warfarin, resulting in higher INR levels and increased bleeding risk.
Collect the INR results, including those from the previous 6 months or longer. *(Collected during the chart review.)*	• The INR can fluctuate due to a variety of reasons, so it is recommended to monitor the INR closely. The INR will be collected at each visit for warfarin monitoring and dose adjustments are completed when the INR is out of range. • Up to 6 months of INR results aid in identifying trends and outliers to aid in identifying changes in the patient's adherence to drug therapy, diet consistency, or other factors that can impact the overall INR. • When the INR is within therapeutic range, warfarin is effective in preventing stroke and thrombosis. When the INR is lower than the therapeutic range (subtherapeutic), the patient is at increased risk for thromboembolic events. When the INR is higher than the therapeutic range (supratherapeutic), the patient is at increased risk for bleeding.

  KEY POINT

It is important to maintain the INR in the therapeutic range for the prevention of thromboembolic and bleeding events.

Critical Thinking Checks for the Collect Plan for This Patient's Allergies and Labs

It is critical to **accurately** collect the patient's allergic responses. This will ensure the patient's safety by avoiding allergens. Meanwhile, pharmacists need to conduct an **objective, in-depth** assessment on the allergic responses to **logically** determine if the responses are related to allergy or to adverse drug responses.

The INR value is one of the most **significant** lab values for the pharmacist to collect for patients taking warfarin. It is collected during each warfarin clinic visit since it serves as a therapeutic indicator and aids in identifying and evaluating the **broad** range of factors that can affect INR and that may need to be considered for developing or maintaining a **logical** therapy plan. A **detailed** list of the patient's INR values for the previous 6 months enables the determination of trends, outliers, and changes in factors that can affect the INR.

• For RS, I was able to record approximately 4 months of data going back to his first INR obtained shortly after he began taking warfarin.

Collected Allergy and Lab Information from the Health Record

Allergies: Lovastatin: Pt reports severe itching. Of note: patient is able to tolerate atorvastatin without similar reactions.

Labs: CMP: Within Normal Limits (WNL)

Current and past INR results with warfarin dosing: (RTC = Return To Clinic)

Date	INR	Old Dose	Weekly Dose	RS Reported Warfarin Use Pattern
05/21 (today's visit)	3.7	10 mg po daily except 5 mg Tue/Thurs	60 mg	No missed doses last week, decreased vitamin K intake, increased alcohol intake
04/16	1.7	10 mg po daily except 5mg Tue/Thurs	60 mg	Missed two doses last week, plan: no change in dosing, RTC 2 weeks
03/26	1.9	10 mg po daily except 5 mg Tue/Thurs	60 mg	Missed a dose last week, plan: no change in dose, RTC 2 weeks
03/12	2.3	10 mg po daily except 5 mg Tue/Thurs	60 mg	No change in dosing, RTC 2 weeks
02/26	3.6	10 mg po daily except 5 mg Mon/Thurs	60 mg	Hold one dose on 2/27 and continue current regimen, RTC in 2 weeks
01/29	2.8	10 mg po daily except 5 mg Mon/Thurs	60 mg	No change in dosing; RTC in 4 weeks

Collect: Past Medical History

Conclusions	Rationale: Information or Premise to Support the Conclusion
Complete a full medical history on the patient. *(Collected during the chart review.)*	The past medical history can help the pharmacist to evaluate the overall health condition of the patient and indications of the medications the patient takes. It also helps to understand the complexity of the treatment.

Critical Thinking Checks for the Collect Plan: This Patient's Past Medical History

It is important to adopt a **broad** perspective when collecting information about all of the patient's conditions, as it can be critical to assess their potential impact on his warfarin therapy and, conversely, the potential impact of warfarin therapy on the patient's other conditions.

- For RS, I have listed information about all of his conditions, including his previous history of two pulmonary embolisms (PE), which were the basis for his need for anticoagulation therapy.

Collected Past Medical History Entered into Health Record

Past medical history:
- Pulmonary embolism: Diagnosed in 2017 and 2020
- Unspecified chest pain: Diagnosed in 2020
- Hyperlipidemia: Diagnosed in 2008
- Hypertension: Diagnosed in 2016

Collect: Social history

Conclusions	Rationale: Information or Premise to Support the Conclusion
Collect the social history of the patient during interview, including information about socioeconomic status, living conditions, family support, and alcohol and tobacco use. *(Collected during the interview.)*	• The patient's social history is an important part of the patient care process. The socioeconomic status, living conditions, family support, and lifestyle can all affect the patient's health status and healthcare plan. For example, the patient's financial status is important in determining the affordability of medications for the patient. • The use of alcohol can impact warfarin therapy. For example, acute alcohol intoxication can inhibit warfarin metabolism, thereby increasing INR and bleeding risk. Chronic alcoholism can induce warfarin metabolism, thereby decreasing INR. • Smoking can affect warfarin clearance, so information about changes in smoking status should be collected.[14]
Collect information about the patient's occupation. *(Collected during the chart review and the interview.)*	Information about occupation is relevant for assessing potential risks related to warfarin therapy. For example, if a patient's occupation involves work that easily causes cuts on the skin, it will be very important to educate the patient on the potential bleeding risk associated with warfarin therapy.
Collect information on the patient's diet, particularly vitamin-K-containing food. *(Collected during the interview.)*	Given that warfarin is a vitamin K antagonist, a patient's intake of vitamin K from food can have a significant effect on their INR and can be very influential in warfarin therapy management. Thus, it is important to collect diet information during the interview.

Critical Thinking Checks for the Collect Plan: This Patient's Social History

The interview process should be **clear** and free of confusion, and I should therefore ask questions as needed to clarify what the patient is communicating to me.

Information collected during the interview about the patient's social history should be **broad** to fully assess its potential relationships with warfarin therapy.

- For example, it was important to gather information from RS about his alcohol and tobacco use, his occupation, and his vitamin K intake, as all of these can impact or be impacted by his warfarin therapy. The interview questions should be **specific**, including ascertaining the details of the type, frequency, and consistency of vitamin K food consumption.

The interview process should be unbiased to obtain an **in-depth** and **broad** understanding of the social history. The pharmacist should not ask questions that express the pharmacist's own opinion that creates biases. Instead of asking: "What vegetables do you eat since they are good for you?" The pharmacist can ask: "What type of vegetables do you eat?"

Collected Social History Entered into Health Record

Social history:

- Currently working part-time as a chef at a restaurant
- Lives with wife who requires aid with activities of daily livings (ADL). He has three adult children living in other states
- Tobacco use: Smokes 0.5 pack/day, no changes in use pattern, and no intention to quit at this moment
- Alcohol use: Reports heavy drinking one time a month, consistent use of one to two beers per day. However, the patient has been drinking six to seven beers per day for the last 2 days, prior to presenting for follow-up today
- Illicit drug use: Denies current or past use
- Current Dietary Habits: Reports three to four servings of vegetables weekly although intake is not consistent. Typical vegetables he eats include cucumber, lettuce, and collard greens.

 KEY POINT

When assessing alcohol use, it is important to ask open-ended questions to identify the frequency, type, and amount of alcohol a patient consumes in a given time period.

Collect: Warfarin Therapy Adverse Effects

Conclusions	Rationale: Information or Premise to Support the Conclusion
Investigate signs and symptoms of supratherapeutic warfarin levels, such as signs of bruising or bleeding, and subtherapeutic levels such as new thromboembolic events (eg, DVTs). *(Collected during the interview.)*	Identifying any new bruising or signs or symptoms of bruising or signs of bleeding in the gums, blood in the urine or stool can alert the pharmacist to supratherapeutic warfarin levels. Conversely, if the patient is reporting pain or swelling in the calf, this can be a possible DVT, which could be a sign of subtherapeutic warfarin levels, which would increase the risk of a clot development.

Critical Thinking Checks for This Patient's Warfarin Therapy Adverse Effects

When collecting the signs/symptoms of potential adverse effects, the pharmacist needs to obtain **accurate** and **precise** descriptions of signs and symptoms from the patient to be able to determine if they are related to his medication therapy. For RS, we were focused on collecting information about signs and symptoms potentially related to subtherapeutic or supratherapeutic warfarin levels.

Collected Warfarin Therapy Adverse Effects Entered into Health Record

RS did not report signs/symptoms of thromboembolism or evidence of new bruising or bleeding.

Example Collect Statement for Robert S.

RS is a 66-year-old male who reports to the clinic today for INR management. He experienced separate incidences of pulmonary embolisms, the first episode occurred in 2017 and the second episode occurred in 2020. It was determined by his cardiologist that he would continue warfarin therapy indefinitely to reduce the risk of a repeat PE. His current warfarin regimen is 10 mg po daily except 5 mg on Tuesday and Thursday. Over the last 6 months, his INR values have not consistently been within the appropriate range of 2-3, with two instances where it was below two, two instances where it was between two and three, and two instances where it was above three, including today's level of 3.7. He does not report signs/symptoms of thromboembolism or evidence of new bruising or bleeding. RS admits to missing warfarin doses: He is not currently using a pill box and recognizes his current system of using a shoe box is resulting in confusion regarding his medications. He has voiced interest in using a pill box to help improve his adherence to his current medications. RS also continues to have an inconsistent diet of Vitamin K: His favorite vegetables include lettuce, cucumbers, and collard greens, which are consumed approximately three times a week, but he does vary on consistency and frequency of consumption of these vegetables. He drinks one to two beers every day consistently and admits to heavy drinking once a month: Over the last 2 days, he drank six to seven beers per day. He continues to smoke ½ pack of cigarettes per day and has been consistent on his tobacco use for many years. RS is a part-time chef in a restaurant and has limited exercise but does perform yard work periodically. During the visit today, RS reports that he was seen by his primary care provider earlier this morning and was prescribed Bactrim DS for 7 days to treat a complicated UTI. He has not started taking this antibiotic but plans to start this evening.

 KEY POINT

Tobacco can affect the metabolism of warfarin and the INR. The interaction between tobacco and warfarin is consistent when the patient uses the same amount of tobacco, but a dose adjustment may be needed if patient decides to quit smoking.

Assessment of Collected Information

During the Assess step of the PPCP, it is important to thoroughly evaluate the collected information to determine the patient's medication-related clinical status and to identify and prioritize drug therapy problems. This will enable the development of an appropriate therapeutic plan. It is essential to utilize critical thinking skills when evaluating the collected information to identify and explain the factors that can be critical for the patient's pharmacotherapy. The full medication list needs to be reviewed to assess the indications, dosing regimen, effectiveness, and potential drug side effects and interactions. It is also important to evaluate the factors that can affect the medication affordability and accessibility. The drug-taking behaviors of the patient, such as adherence will also need to be considered.

ASSESS: Supratherapeutic INR	
Conclusions	**Rationale: Information or Premise to Support the Conclusion**
Supratherapeutic INR of 3.7 (INR range 2-3)	The patient's indication for warfarin is pulmonary embolism. His therapeutic range of INR should be 2-3, his INR on the clinic day was 3.7, which is supratherapeutic.[15]
Multiple factors can contribute to the patient's increased INR including decreased vitamin K intake, heavy drinking of alcohol 2 days before the clinic appointment, and inappropriate adherence to his warfarin therapy.	The patient reported that he did not consistently consume vitamin-K-containing food the prior week. Vitamin K is involved in the synthesis of coagulation factors II, VII, IX, and X and anticoagulant proteins C and S. Decreased vitamin K intake will decrease the synthesis of the coagulation factors II, VII, IX, and X and result in an increase of INR.[16] During the last two previous visits, the INR was subtherapeutic and one contributing factor identified was missed doses of warfarin. During this current visit, RS reported that he did not miss any doses for the past 7 days. Due to consistent daily dosing of warfarin, the INR is now supratherapeutic at 3.7. The patient reported that he was drinking alcohol heavily the past 2 days before coming to the clinic. Binge drinking of alcohol can result in a reduced rate of metabolism of warfarin resulting in an increase in INR.[17]

KEY POINT

The INR value is highly related to warfarin adherence. If a patient is having nontherapeutic INR values due to inappropriate adherence, the pharmacist must address the adherence issue and work with the patient to help improve adherence.

Critical Thinking Checks for Assessing This Patient's Supratherapeutic INR

Given that there were multiple factors affecting this patient's INR, a great **depth** of thought was needed to determine the **relevance**, **significance**, and **complexity** of the factors to fully explain their impact on his INR and his warfarin management.

- For example, factors to consider include the more significant factors of RS's inconsistent warfarin adherence, vitamin K intake, and his recent binge alcohol drinking. Less significant contributing factors also should be considered such as his current use of a shoe box to organize medications which has resulted in incidences of confusion surrounding his medication use. All contributing factors will be considered when designing RS's therapeutic plan.

Note: The following drug interaction is from a report focusing on interactions of warfarin with recently-added or recently-discontinued drugs. If an interaction exists between warfarin and a routine drug, the effect of the interaction is likely to remain stable and will not cause clinically significant adverse events.

ASSESS: Drug Therapy Problem	
Conclusions	**Rationale: Information or Premise to Support the Conclusion**
Adverse drug reaction: Drug interaction between warfarin and Bactrim DS	The patient has been prescribed Bactrim DS for 7 days for treatment of a complicated UTI. Bactrim can decrease the metabolism of warfarin and therefore will likely increase INR with increased risks of bleeding.[18]

Critical Thinking Checks for Assessing This Patient's Drug Therapy Problem

This patient takes multiple medications and presents with multiple drug interaction issues, which may affect pharmacotherapy and cause adverse effects. **Deep** thinking is required to identify the most **relevant** and **important** drug interactions.

Our clinic focuses on warfarin management; thus, the drug interaction with warfarin is more relevant for this clinic. It is important to use **accurate** and **precise** medication information to generate the drug interaction report.

The drug interaction report needs to be analyzed considering the **complexity** and necessity of the warfarin regimen. Intervention may be needed for some drug interactions but not for others. For example, for a routine chronic medication such as atorvastatin, even though there is a drug interaction, RS takes it consistently and no dose changes have occurred. In this case, it is not necessary to modify his regimen.

 KEY POINT

When analyzing drug interactions, it is important to pay attention to the medications that are newly added or discontinued. For the medications the patient takes routinely, the interaction should be stable and less likely to cause impactful events.

Multiple factors can influence this patient's anticoagulation therapy, including medications, lifestyle, and potential drug interactions. It can be beneficial to create a concept map to visualize the interrelationships among these factors and develop an enhanced understanding of how each factor can affect the therapeutic outcome (see **Figure 5-1**).

Example Assess Statement for Robert S.

RS is a 66-year-old male who visits the clinic for INR management. His medical record included a history of two pulmonary embolism events and he was prescribed warfarin for indefinite anticoagulation.

Supratherapeutic INR

The patient's INR is 3.7 (INR range 2-3). Multiple factors may be contributing to his increased INR, including inappropriate adherence to his warfarin therapy, decreased vitamin K intake, and heavy drinking of alcohol 2 days before the clinic.

His current warfarin regimen is 10 mg po daily except 5 mg on Tuesday and Thursday, but he reports he misses an average of one dose per week. RS struggles to organize all of his medications effectively. He is currently not using a pill box, but he is open to suggestions on how to improve his current process, including the addition of a pill box, which could positively impact his overall adherence to all medications.

RS's weekly vitamin K intake is not consistent in frequency or quantity. Fluctuations in vitamin K intake can lead to inconsistent INR levels, resulting in subtherapeutic levels when intake of vitamin K is high, and supratherapeutic levels when intake of vitamin K is low. Improvement in consistency of intake in quantity and frequency is needed to reach a more stable INR.

RS drinks alcohol heavily once per month. He admits to drinking six to seven beers per day 2 days in a row before his appointment. Large increases in alcohol consumption can decrease the metabolism of warfarin, resulting in an increase in INR. Continued education on alcohol's interaction with warfarin is warranted at this time.

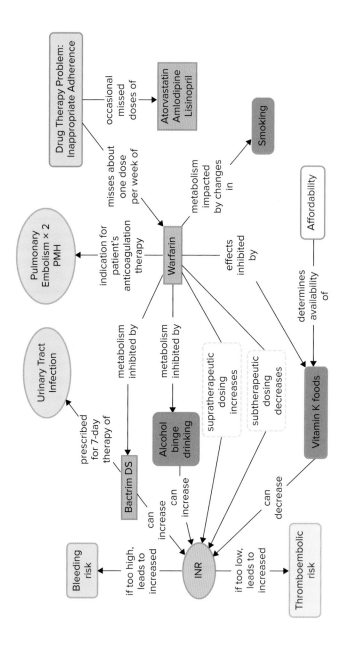

FIGURE 5-1. Concept map illustrating the interrelationships of RS's medications, lifestyle, and conditions.

RS continues to smoke ½ pack of cigarettes daily on a consistent basis and is not interested in smoking cessation at this time. Tobacco has the potential to increase metabolism of warfarin, thereby decreasing the INR.[19] Since RS uses tobacco consistently on a regular basis, his consistent tobacco use pattern will not cause INR fluctuations.

RS was prescribed Bactrim DS for 7 days for the treatment of a complicated UTI. He has not started this antibiotic at this time but will start it this evening after picking up the prescription from the pharmacy. Bactrim DS, specifically the sulfamethoxazole component, inhibits warfarin metabolism, thereby increasing INR. Given that RS already has a supratherapeutic INR, the initiation of Bactrim DS therapy can significantly increase his bleeding risk and therefore must be accounted for in therapeutic planning, which will include an appropriate adjustment of warfarin dosing.

Drug therapy problems include the following:

- *Inappropriate adherence*: Warfarin, average of one dose missed per week
- *Adverse drug reaction*: Drug interaction between warfarin and Bactrim DS

Plan, Implement, and Monitor

PLAN: Goals	
Conclusions	Rationale: Information or Premise to Support the Conclusion
Goals include: 1. Reach a therapeutic INR range of 2-3 within 1 to 2 weeks and maintain the therapeutic INR 2. Improve medication adherence to avoid missing more than one warfarin dose per month instead of one dose per week 3. Ensure the patient's understanding of lifestyle factors impacting the INR levels and risk associated with subtherapeutic and supratherapeutic levels.	1. The therapeutic range of INR for RS is 2-3, the current INR is 3.7, and the INR value needs to stay in the therapeutic range for the prevention of thrombotic and bleeding events. This goal can be achieved within 1 to 2 weeks with appropriate dosing adjustments, proper adherence, and adjustment in contributing lifestyle factors. 2. The patient struggles with adherence to his warfarin therapy. Strategies for improving adherence should enable him to achieve a goal of no more than one missed dose per month or better. 3. The patient has lifestyle factors that contributed to his supratherapeutic INR, including reduced vitamin K intake and acute elevated alcohol intake. The influence of these nonpharmacological factors on warfarin therapy needs to be discussed with RS.

Critical Thinking Checks for Developing This Patient's Goals

The SMART goals were developed based on a **clear** and **thorough** understanding of the patient's disease state and pharmacotherapeutic plan.

The SMART goals were developed with **objective** consideration of the available data and of the **complexity** of the disease state.

The SMART goals were developed with **logical**, **deep**, and **broad** thinking. For example, the pharmacist worked with RS to set a goal to improve the patient's medication adherence by reducing missed doses to no more than one time per month. Setting this goal to allow for one missed dose in a month compared to missing no doses is **logical** and **fair minded**, since it accommodates the patient's busy schedule and will decrease the stress of perfection. The SMART goals were communicated **clearly** to the patient in terms of expected outcomes.

PLAN: Supratherapeutic INR—Nonpharmacological	
Goals:	
• Improve medication adherence to avoid missing more than one warfarin dose per month instead of one dose per week • Ensure the patient's understanding of lifestyle factors that affect warfarin therapy	
Conclusions	**Rationale: Information or Premise to Support the Conclusion**
Educate the patient on the importance of medication adherence. Advise him to set up alarms for medications and use a pill box to manage his multiple medications.	RS misses warfarin doses periodically due to forgetfulness. He currently utilizes a shoe box to organize his medication, which has resulted in confusion. Adopting the use of a pill box and utilizing an alarm on his phone to remind him to take medications is a good strategy to improve medication adherence.
Educate the patient on lifestyle effects on warfarin therapy, including diet, alcohol, and tobacco. An education brochure on these topics is provided to the patient to serve as the resource.	RS lacks understanding of the effects of vitamin K intake, alcohol, and tobacco use on warfarin therapy. The pharmacist needs to work with him to develop a plan outlining a plan for a consistent diet of vitamin-K-containing foods. Motivational interviewing techniques can be utilized to approach the discussion of alcohol abstinence and tobacco cessation and their potential implications for his thromboembolic and bleeding risks and for his warfarin therapy. Included in his education will be a discussion of his increased bleeding risk associated with his occupation as a chef.
Educate the patient on the importance of adhering to all therapies and attending all follow-up appointments.	RS is already supratherapeutic and will now begin to take Bactrim DS, which can result in an increase in the INR due to the drug's interaction with warfarin. He should be educated on the importance of following all warfarin dosing instructions very carefully and follow-up as scheduled for INR monitoring. Close monitoring of the INR is indicated.

Critical Thinking Checks for This Patient's Nonpharmacological Plan for Supratherapeutic INR Management

The development of the nonpharmacological plan was based on **accurately** collecting and thoroughly assessing the **objective** data, combined with **deep** and **broad** consideration of patient-specific factors in warfarin therapy, such as adherence, lifestyle, and understanding of medications. It is important to **clearly** convey the plan to the patient with **logical** consideration of the feasibility of the plan.

• For example, RS sometimes misses his warfarin doses due to forgetfulness and ineffective process of managing his medications. Recommending the use of a pill box and a phone alarm could be effective strategies.

PLAN: Supratherapeutic INR and Antibiotic Therapy for Complicated UTI—Pharmacological Plan
Goal:
• Reach a therapeutic INR range of 2-3 within 1 to 2 weeks and maintain the therapeutic INR.

Conclusions	Rationale: Information or Premise to Support the Conclusion
Hold one dose of warfarin on the day of the clinic and then decrease warfarin dose to 5 mg daily except 10 mg on Tuesday and Thursday (total weekly dose (TWD) of 45 mg, 25% decrease).	The patient's INR is 3.7, which is supratherapeutic since the INR goal is two to three. The patient will start Bactrim DS today, which can decrease the metabolism of warfarin leading to an increased INR. A dose reduction is warranted for the patient to decrease the risk of further supratherapeutic INRs. The patient will hold one dose today and then reduce the TWD by 25% to obtain and maintain an INR within a therapeutic range of two to three.[20] The patient was on 10 mg daily except 5 mg on Tuesday and Thursday with TWD of 60 mg. A 25% decrease in TWD is 15 mg. The new regimen is 5 mg daily except 10 mg on Tuesday and Thursday with a new TWD of 45 mg.[21]
Take the Bactrim DS for 7 days for complicated UTI.	RS needs to finish the antibiotic regimen to resolve his complicated UTI. It is important to educate the patient on drug interactions, in this case, Bactrim DS with warfarin.
Schedule follow-up visit in 1 week for INR measurement and evaluation to determine if further warfarin dosing adjustment is warranted.	RS needs to be monitored closely to prevent adverse events with his warfarin dosing change while taking Bactrim DS. Warfarin has a long half-life, so it takes about 4 to 5 days to reflect the dosing change. Therefore, an appropriate time to evaluate the INR after dose adjustment is one week, at the conclusion of the Bactrim DS regimen.

Critical Thinking Checks for This Patient's Pharmacological Plan for Supratherapeutic INR Management

The pharmacological plan was developed with a complete assessment of the patient's disease states, and addressed the **significance** and **complexity** of drug interaction issues. The plan considered the factors affecting drug therapy to ensure it was **logical** and feasible.

• For example, there are a list of factors that affect the patient's warfarin therapy, including alcohol use, tobacco use, Bactrim DS, and diet. The pharmacist considered all the factors to perform a **complete** assessment, and focused on addressing the drug interaction, vitamin K intake, and alcohol consumption, to develop a **logical** and **feasible** plan.

IMPLEMENT/MONITOR: Nonpharmacological Plan for Supratherapeutic INR Management	
Conclusions	Rationale: Information or Premise to Support the Conclusion
Implement: Implement the patient education outlined in the plan: 1. Educate the patient on the importance of medication adherence. • Advise the patient to develop strategies to remind himself to take medications, such as setting alarms on the phone and utilizing a pill box.	*Implement:* 1. The main reason for the patient's nonadherence is forgetfulness. Thus, it is reasonable to utilize pill boxes and to create reminders on his cell phone, which he carries with him all the time. 2. Given the amount and complexity of information that the patient will be given related to lifestyle factors, providing a brochure that the patient can read and repeatedly refer to can be a valuable tool to empower the patient to self-manage his anticoagulation care.

2. Educate the patient on lifestyle effects of warfarin therapy, including diet, alcohol, and tobacco.
   - An education brochure on these topics is provided to the patient to serve as the resource.
3. Educate the patient on the importance of adherence to all therapies and attending all follow-up appointments.

Monitor:

1. INR monitoring
2. Patient self-report of:
   - The specific strategies he implemented to improve his medication adherence and their success
   - Intake of vitamin K, alcohol, and tobacco

3. Adherence to all of his therapies will be critical to the quality of his healthcare, as will attending follow-up appointments where his care can be evaluated and adjusted as needed to optimize the safety and efficacy of his care.

Monitor:

1. Warfarin adherence can be reflected in the INR values. As INR values can be affected by the lifestyle factors, monitoring INR is a quantitative way of assessing the effects of the lifestyle factors.
2. Having the patient self-report can be valuable to engage him in his own care. This includes a self-report of his adherence strategies and their success. His self-reported intake of vitamin K, alcohol, and tobacco can help him establish the relationship between INR values and the lifestyle factors for a better understanding.

IMPLEMENT/MONITOR: Pharmacological Plan for Supratherapeutic INR Management and Antibiotic Therapy for Complicated UTI	
Conclusions	Rationale: Information or Premise to Support the Conclusion
Implement: Hold one dose of warfarin and then decrease dose to 5 mg daily except 10 mg on Tuesday and Thursday with TWD of 45 mg. *Monitor:* Monitor the INR at next visit after a week.	*Implement:* Holding one dose of warfarin and then decreasing the dose is an appropriate strategy to decrease the INR to the therapeutic range. The patient presented with an INR of 3.7. There is a risk of further increase in INR due to the drug interaction with the Bactrim DS. *Monitor:* Warfarin has a long half-life and INR changes occur approximately 4 to 5 days after a warfarin dosage adjustment. The Bactrim DS is prescribed for 7 days. A repeat INR and reassessment to evaluate for signs and symptoms of bleeding should be scheduled in 1 week to determine if warfarin dosing adjustments are needed.
Implement: Educate the patient to take Bactrim DS for 7 days for the treatment of complicated UTI and educate the patient on the effects of Bactrim DS on his INR and bleeding risk. *Monitor:* INR, thromboembolic events, bleeding events, and signs and symptoms of a complicated UTI.	*Implement:* Treatment length of 7 days is appropriate for treating this patient's complicated UTI. It is important to explain to the patient the drug interaction between warfarin and Bactrim DS, so that he understands the reason for the warfarin dosing adjustment. *Monitor:* A higher INR is associated with bruises and bleeding events. The bleeding risk increases further with open wounds. Symptoms associated with a complicated UTI should be monitored to assure the effectiveness of Bactrim DS.

Implement:	*Implement:*
Educate the patient on the side effects of warfarin, includes bruising, bleeding, headache, dizziness, leg pain, respiration, etc. *Monitor:* Patient self-report of bruises and bleeding, such as nose bleeding, gum bleeding, blood in the urine and/or tarry stool, or signs and symptoms of thromboembolism.	Bruising and bleeding are common adverse effects related to warfarin therapy. *Monitor:* Patient self-reported nose-bleeding, gum-bleeding, blood in the urine, and/or tarry stool can be used to assess the bleeding symptoms. Thromboembolism symptoms such as headache and dizziness will also need to be monitored. If there are concerning symptoms associated with warfarin therapy that are addressed but do not improve within a reasonable time period, the patient will be directed to seek medication attention.
Follow-up plan: Set follow-up times: 1. The immediate follow-up time is 1 week from today (ie, 5/28) at the clinic. The INR value will be measured at that visit. 2. The next follow-up depends on the patient assessment from the appointment on 5/28. During follow-ups: 3. Assess warfarin efficacy, side effects, and adherence. 4. Assess factors that can affect the therapeutic plan of warfarin, such as diet, alcohol, tobacco intake, and drug interactions	*Follow-up plan:* 1. Scheduling a 1-week follow up appointment on 5/28 is appropriate since the dose adjustment was initiated during clinic. The patient also is starting Bactrim DS today to treat the complicated UTI. Average changes in INR occur in 4 to 5 days so a repeat INR in 7 days should reflect the changes made. 2. The second follow-up appointment will be determined based on the INR results and information obtained during the patient assessment on 5/28. Once the INR is stable over time and no signs of adverse effects are detected, follow-up visits can be extended based on provider comfort level. 3. Assessing warfarin efficacy, safety, and adherence at each follow-up are standards of the care we provide to our patients. Assess warfarin efficacy by monitoring INR. Assess the side effects by evaluating bleeding risk and signs and symptoms of bleeding and thrombosis. 4. To provide optimal care, continuous monitoring of contributing factors associated with fluctuations in INR are reviewed with patient, including consistency and amount of vitamin K containing food, alcohol intake, tobacco use, and addition or removal of any medications.

 KEY POINT

The earliest follow-up on INR monitoring after warfarin dosing adjustment is about 1 week due to the pharmacokinetic features of warfarin.

 KEY POINT

The follow-up time on INR monitoring varies based on a list of factors, including the INR value, disease states, surgeries, new medications, etc. If a patient presents with a stable therapeutic INR with no complications, the follow-up time can be extended accordingly.

Critical Thinking Checks for This Patient's Implementation and Monitoring Plan

The implementation of the plan has been developed **fairly**, in full consideration that the patient can become overwhelmed with the actions needed for successful implementation and adoption into his daily life. The instructions in the plan should be **accurate**, **precise**, and **specific**, and communicated to the patient in a **clear** and understandable way. It is important for the pharmacist to avoid using jargon and difficult terms to achieve an unequivocal understanding by the patient, and communicate in a manner that assures that RS is empowered to self-manage his health.

- For example, I clearly instructed RS on how to take his warfarin: Hold one dose tomorrow and then take one tablet (5 mg) daily except take two tablets (10 mg) on Tuesday and Thursday. Additionally, I provided RS a brochure to serve as a resource on the effects of diet, alcohol, and tobacco on his warfarin therapy, and clearly educated him on the importance of adherence to all therapies, on attending all follow-up appointments, and on specific signs and symptoms to be on alert for with regard to warfarin's adverse effects.

CONCLUSION

Warfarin therapy is important in the prevention of thromboembolic events in patients. Overall, there are a broad range of factors affecting the warfarin therapy, including dosing, patient adherence, drug interactions, diet, lifestyle, etc. The warfarin therapy plan needs to be individualized considering the different individual factors of each patient. When engaging in clinical problem-solving through application of the PPCP, it is important for the pharmacist to utilize effective critical thinking and clinical reasoning skills in each step to provide optimal individualized patient care.

Summary Points

- Warfarin management involves the broad and deep consideration of many different factors that contribute to the complexity of the patient's condition. The pharmacist needs to collect all relevant information to have a complete and thorough understanding of all the associated contributing factors to accurately assess the disease state, medication effectiveness, and adverse drug effects.
- Goals of therapy for the warfarin therapeutic and monitoring plan need to be developed with a fair-minded consideration of patient-specific factors and are based on an assessment of collected data that is thorough, subjective, and unbiased.
- When caring for patients on warfarin therapy, it is important to broadly analyze all current disease states to identify any drug-related problems to aid in developing an optimal plan for warfarin therapy and monitoring.
- The therapy and monitoring plans need to be clear and concise, and communicated to the patient at a proper level and with appropriate details to ensure the patient has a full understanding of dosing, monitoring, and proper follow-up.

Abbreviations

ADL	Activities of Daily Living
CDC	Centers for Disease Control
CMP	Comprehensive Metabolic Panel
DVT	Deep Vein Thrombosis
EMR	Electronic Medical Record
ER	Emergency Room

INR	International Normalized Ratio
NOAC	Novel Oral Anticoagulant
PCP	Primary Care Physician
PPCP	Pharmacists' Patient Care Process
PE	Pulmonary Embolism
RTC	Return to Clinic
TWD	Total Weekly Dose
UTI	Urinary Tract Infection
WNL	Within Normal Limits

References

1. Cardoso R, Ternes CMP, Justino GB, et al. Non-vitamin k antagonists versus warfarin in patients with atrial fibrillation and bioprosthetic valves: a systematic review and meta-analysis. *Am J Med.* 2022;135(2):228.e1-234.e1.

2. Carlson B. Declaring war on warfarin misdosing. *Biotechnol Healthc.* 2008;5(2):54-55.

3. Sanderson S, Emery J, Higgins J. CYP2C9 gene variants, drug dose, and bleeding risk in warfarin-treated patients: a HuGEnet systematic review and meta-analysis. *Genet Med.* 2005;7(2):97-104.

4. Holbrook AM, Pereira JA, Labiris R, et al. Systematic overview of warfarin and its drug and food interactions. *Arch Intern Med.* 2005;165(10):1095-1106.

5. Persky AM, Medina MS, Castleberry AN. Developing critical thinking skills in pharmacy students. *Am J Pharm Educ.* 2019;83(2):7033.

6. Joint Commission of Pharmacy Practitioners. *Pharmacist' Patient Care Process.* Available at https://jcpp.net/wp-content/uploads/2016/03/PatientCareProcess-with-supporting-organizations.pdf. Accessed April 28, 2022.

7. Mohammed E, McDonald WG, Ezike AC. Teamwork in health care services delivery in Nigeria: a mixed methods assessment of perceptions and lived experiences of pharmacists in a tertiary hospital. *Integr Pharm Res Pract.* 2022;11:33-45.

8. Collins JL, Thomas LJ. The influence of social determinants of health among young adults after they have left foster care in the US. *J Clin Nurs.* 2018;27(9-10):2022-2030.

9. Deen R. Use of direct observed therapy to confirm compliance in a warfarin clinic. *J Patient Saf.* 2011;7(4):232-233.

10. Mwita JC, Damasceno A, Chillo P, et al. Vitamin K-dependent anticoagulant use and level of anticoagulation control in sub-Saharan Africa: protocol for a retrospective cohort study. *BMJ Open.* 2022;12(2):e057166.

11. Nordstrom BL, Evans MA, Murphy BR, Nutescu EA, Schein JR, Bookhart BK. Risk of recurrent venous thromboembolism among deep vein thrombosis and pulmonary embolism patients treated with warfarin. *Curr Med Res Opin.* 2015;31(3):439-447.

12. Kearon C, Akl EA, Comerota AJ, et al. Antithrombotic therapy for VTE disease: Antithrombotic Therapy and Prevention of Thrombosis, 9th ed: American College of Chest Physicians Evidence-Based Clinical Practice Guidelines [published correction appears in Chest. 2012 Dec;142(6):1698-1704]. *Chest.* 2012;141(2 Suppl):e419S-e496S. doi:10.1378/chest.11-2301.

13. Clinical Pharmacology [database on the Internet]. Tampa; FL: Elsevier; 2022. Available at https://www.clinicalkey.com/pharmacology/reports/interactions?gpcid=226&gpcid=1036&dt=true&type=p. Accessed April 18, 2022.

14. Nathisuwan S, Dilokthornsakul P, Chaiyakunapruk N, Morarai T, Yodting T, Piriyachananusorn N. Assessing evidence of interaction between smoking and warfarin: a systematic review and meta-analysis. *Chest.* 2011;139(5):1130-1139.

15. Goldhaber SZ, Elliott CG. Acute pulmonary embolism: part II: risk stratification, treatment, and prevention. *Circulation.* 2003;108(23):2834-2838.

16. Donaldson CJ, Harrington DJ. Therapeutic warfarin use and the extrahepatic functions of vitamin K-dependent proteins. *Br J Biomed Sci.* 2017;74(4):163-169.

17. Sellers EM, Holloway MR. Drug kinetics and alcohol ingestion. *Clin Pharmacokinet.* 1978;3(6):440-452.

18. Clinical Pharmacology [database on the Internet]. Tampa; FL: Elsevier; 2022. Available at https://www.clinicalkey.com/pharmacology/reports/interactions?gpcid=226&gpcid=1036&dt=true&type=p. Accessed April 20, 2022.

19. Tan CSS, Lee SWH. Warfarin and food, herbal or dietary supplement interactions: a systematic review. *Br J Clin Pharmacol.* 2021;87(2):352-374.

20. Powers A, Loesch EB, Weiland A, Fioravanti N, Lucius D. Preemptive warfarin dose reduction after initiation of sulfamethoxazole-trimethoprim or metronidazole. *J Thromb Thrombolysis.* 2017;44(1):88-93.

21. UW Medicine Pharmacy Services Anticoagulation Services. *Warfarin Maintenance Dosing Nomogram.* Available at https://depts.washington.edu/anticoag/home/content/warfarin-maintenance-dosing-nomogram. Accessed April 20, 2022.

6

Inpatient Critical Care— Diabetic Ketoacidosis

Carinda Feild

The aims of this chapter are to:
- Discuss the roles of a systematic patient care process, clinical reasoning, and critical thinking in assessing and resolving medication-related problems as part of a collaborative effort to provide patient-centered care in diabetic ketoacidosis (DKA).
- Illustrate common medication-related problems encountered in an example DKA case using clinical reasoning and critical thinking techniques through the utilization of the Pharmacists' Patient Care Process.

KEY WORDS

• Diabetic ketoacidosis • electrolyte disturbances • hypovolemia • clinical reasoning • clinical problem solving • medication-related problems • Pharmacists' Patient care Process • critical thinking • cognitive biases

INTRODUCTION

Pharmacy practice in critical care environments provides many opportunities for managing a variety of acute disease states and is a place where pharmacists can play an impactful role in treatment plan development and treatment safety and efficacy monitoring. Critical care pharmacists are deemed essential members of the multiprofessional critical care team and multiorganizational recommendations have been made regarding foundational responsibilities of a critical care pharmacist.[1] Responsibilities include assisting in discussions with patients and/or family members to help make informed decisions regarding pharmacotherapy options, collaborating with the healthcare team to prevent potentially inappropriate drug therapy, and providing clinical consultation for pharmacotherapeutic issues related to critical illness. Additional responsibilities include providing reviews of the medication history to determine which maintenance medications should be continued during the acute illness; providing medication reconciliation for ICU patients at the time of ICU admission, upon transfer from the ICU to the ward, or upon discharge to home or another facility; and educating patients and/or caregivers regarding medications used to treat patients during and after acute illness. A valuable element of the care that the critical care pharmacist provides is using the medical record as one means to communicate with other healthcare professionals, and/or to document specific pharmacotherapeutic recommendations or activities.[1]

In this chapter, the care provided for a fictitious patient with diabetic ketoacidosis (DKA) by a pharmacist applying critical thinking and clinical reasoning during the Pharmacists' Patient Care Process (PPCP) will be described. DKA is considered a hyperglycemic, endocrine emergency and is the most serious and life-threatening acute complication of diabetes.[2,3] Patients can present severely ill with hemodynamic instability due to severe dehydration, electrolyte abnormalities, acidosis, nausea, vomiting, and significantly altered mental status. The mortality rate can be over 7%. Rapid diagnosis and treatment are key to minimizing poor outcomes. Pharmacist involvement in the management of DKA has been shown to decrease the incidence of hypoglycemia and helps with protocol interpretation and compliance.[4]

 KEY POINT

Using the PPCP and critical thinking, pharmacists can minimize adverse effects associated with DKA treatment.

MY PRACTICE—A MEDICAL/SURGICAL INTENSIVE CARE UNIT AT A COMMUNITY-BASED TEACHING HOSPITAL

My practice site is in intensive care units (ICUs) that care for surgical, trauma, and medical patients who require critical care. The care for some patients is delivered by a critical care team that has primary responsibility for the patient. For other patients, a critical care consult team provides recommendations to the primary care providers. Pharmacists participate in daily patient care rounds with both teams. At my institution, pharmacists cover the ICU 24 hours a day, 7 days a week. They evaluate the patient's medication therapy prior to rounds and make recommendations regarding treatment to the team during rounds and throughout their shift as data indicates. If possible, the pharmacist will communicate directly with patients to obtain or clarify information. Often, patients are not able to communicate or are an unreliable source of information due to the severity of their illness. In these cases, the pharmacist may speak with a surrogate, such as a family or household member. If this is not possible, pharmacists may utilize other resources, such as information already stored in the health record from prior visits, companion databases accessed through the health record, or outside sources such as local pharmacies or a Prescription Drug Monitoring Program (PDMP). During their shift, pharmacists may also evaluate and process medication orders for patients in the ICUs. They monitor medication therapy and are also available to answer medication-related questions and consult on challenging cases.

Patients may come to the ICU from a variety of places, including the emergency department (ED) or operating room (OR), which can be other critical care environments. Communication between pharmacists is important for continuity and smooth transitions of care as patients move from one critical setting to another or transfer between a critical and a noncritical setting. It has been reported that almost half of patients experience a medication error when going from an ICU to a non-ICU setting.[5] Based on a systemic review, Bethishou and colleagues concluded that pharmacists play a crucial role by promoting medication adherence and providing effective medication reconciliation.[6] The pharmacist's important role in transitions of care has been outlined in two American College of Clinical Pharmacy (ACCP) white papers.[7,8]

UTILIZING CRITICAL THINKING SKILLS IN OUR PRACTICE

In this practice, critical thinking must be utilized continually throughout patient care process. For example, the pharmacist will need to constantly question and reflect on all information gathered to determine if it is factual and reliable.[1] As a treatment plan is considered, pharmacists must reflect to verify that decisions are evidence-based and that cognitive biases have been identified and addressed.[1] This chapter will use the hyperglycemic emergency of DKA to explore critical thinking skills needed for the care of critically ill and injured patients. **Table 6-1** provides a list of sample standards-based questions that can be applied to assure that intellectual standards for critical thinking are met as the pharmacist facilitates DKA medication therapy management. Proper application of these standards will enable the pharmacist to gain a clear comprehensive understanding of the patient's clinical status and healthcare needs and develop the best strategy for optimal treatment while limiting potential side effects.

TABLE 6-1

Sample Standards-Based Questions That Can Be Applied To Assure That Intellectual Standards for Thinking Are Met as the Pharmacist Provides DKA Medication Therapy Management

Clarity (explicit, unambiguous, intelligible, free from confusion or doubt)	• Has all information been collected from the patient (or surrogate), or obtained from pharmacy records to ensure clarity regarding prior diabetes therapy and history of present illness? • Have I reconciled conflicting information? • Have I documented the information I have obtained in a clear format so others may clearly understand? • Have I utilized approved protocols or algorithms for determining treatments or adjusting doses?
Relevance (pertinent, applicable, germane)	• What collected information during the evaluation/record review is relevant to DKA? • As I work through the process, is it clear I am following applicable standards of care and DKA management guidelines?
Significance (important, nontrivial, necessary, critical, required, impactful)	• What information that have I gathered from the patient, caregivers, and other providers' notes is most significant? • Have I evaluated all potential information to determine what is clinically most significant, and then can I apply it to develop an effective treatment plan?

Objectivity (fact-based, unbiased)	• Are there biases that could affect my judgment? (eg, race, socioeconomic status, sexual gender, religious or political beliefs) • Have I worked to identify any biases and worked to verify my objectivity? • Have I identified when emotion could possibly impact my objectivity? When this occurs, do I identify this is occurring and work to focus on the objective facts rather than the emotions?
Fairness (unbiased, equitable, impartial)	• What perspectives do I need to consider? The patient, the caregivers, the family, the providers? • How do I ensure I am considering all of these viewpoints in a fair-minded way and utilize proper empathy when considering these perspectives? • Have I avoided biases such as confirmation, anchoring, and availability bias as I search for and evaluate information regarding the patient?
Accuracy (verifiable, valid, true, credible, undistorted)	• Have I verified that laboratory values are accurate (eg, sample not hemolyzed, chemistry and arterial blood gas drawn at the same time) for use in assessing the patient's condition and response to therapy?
Precision (exact, specific, detailed)	• What are some proper questions that can be asked during the patient interview to obtain specific details regarding events leading up to admission, compliance with diet, and medication regimens • While educating the patient (family, caregivers), what level of detail should be provided to the patient (family, caregivers)? • What format of education is appropriate for this particular patient? (eg, handout, teach-back method)?
Depth (roots, fundamentals, complexities, interrelationships, cause/effect, implications)	• When developing the treatment plan, it is important to deeply consider the disease pathology relationships. For example, how will administering insulin and correcting glucose affect other clinical parameters so that changes can be anticipated and proactively addressed? • When considering treatment recommendations, what medical complexities must be considered when choosing proper therapy and dosing? • When planning transition therapy and discharge, it is important to consider the etiology of the DKA and diabetes control confounders to develop the most appropriate home regimen.
Breadth (comprehensive, encompassing, alternative perspectives)	• Who are the stakeholders aside from the patient? Family members, caregivers? • What providers are involved in this patient's care? How might their perspectives differ? What impact can different perspectives have on recommendations and changes to medication therapy or diet/lifestyle? • How do I navigate interdisciplinary conflicts or differences in perspective?
Logic (reasonable, rational, without contradiction, well-founded, sound)	• How do I evaluate the logicalness of my hypotheses? • Have I worked to identify assumptions and addressed them accordingly? • What are the steps I need to take to evaluate my alternative explanations for the problems I am focusing on?

APPLICATION OF THE PPCP IN OUR PRACTICE

In the application of the PPCP for providing care to patients with DKA, the pharmacist begins by collecting information about the patient who is usually presenting to the ED. From this collected information, a comprehensive patient assessment is completed in the Assess step. This comprehensive assessment serves as the basis for validating or eliminating hypotheses related to etiology and diagnosis. This is key to developing an accurate prioritized medication problem list and development of a comprehensive treatment strategy in the Plan step. Treatment strategies can be based on institutional protocols. Protocols are treatment algorithms developed in a multidisciplinary fashion by experts at the institution, are based on well-agreed-upon literature, and can be helpful in diseases with complex treatment plans. In the ensuing Implementation step, the treatment and monitoring plan, determined by the protocol, is often effectively communicated to the inpatient caregivers through use of order sets, which operationalize the elements of the protocol. Order sets can be paper orders or can be built into the electronic medical record (EMR). The required treatment elements are automatically ordered when the order set is activated to help ensure critical steps are not missed. They also contain all the necessary prompts to select the appropriate therapy in cases where treatment needs to be tailored to the patient. This ensures all the steps in complex treatments are addressed. The use of protocols and order sets has been shown to increase adherence to guidelines and decrease time to DKA resolution, time to DKA treatment outcomes, and incidence of hypokalemia.[9,10]

 KEY POINT

The use of institutional protocols and order sets facilitates the critical thinking and clinical reasoning by providing prompts to ensure all critical elements of treatment are considered.

In addition to ensure that protocols and order sets are properly implemented, pharmacists perform efficacy and toxicity monitoring. They will communicate recommendations to the team directly or through charting notes, which will be the same medium for communication with other members of the pharmacy team to ensure continuity of care from shift to shift.

As mentioned, the process of patient care facilitated by pharmacists begins with the gathering of information about the patient. For deeper understanding of this Collect step, details are provided below. This will be followed by a patient case review in which all PPCP steps will be elaborated on with the clinical reasoning and critical thinking that can be employed by an ICU pharmacist care provider who engages in a systematic and deliberate clinical problem-solving process.

THE COLLECTION OF PATIENT INFORMATION IN OUR PRACTICE

Typically, data collection begins with a record review (**Table 6-2**). This can include the hospital medical record and internal and external electronic resources, which provide information on prescription and admission history. This can be followed by a patient/surrogate interview (**Table 6-3**). Often patients in this setting are not able to provide a history due to their illness severity, and in these cases, the pharmacist must rely on those close to the patient (family, friends, household members) to provide information. There are times when these other individuals may not be present or may be inaccurate with the information they provide, and therefore the pharmacist may be called upon to make initial therapy recommendations with limited or suboptimal information. If the patient is able or if a surrogate is available, the interview will include obtaining a medication history and the history of present illness. Obtaining information from multiple sources allows for data confirmation. This can be important when historian reliability is questionable.

 KEY POINT

There are times when the pharmacist may need to employ their critical thinking and clinical reasoning with absent or incomplete data as the patient's severity of illness requires prompt intervention. This is when it is particularly important to employ critical thinking and clinical reasoning to develop the most appropriate plan given the limited available data.

TABLE 6-2

Examples of Data That Can Be Collected During Chart Review in Preparation for a Patient Interview

Data to Collect During Chart Review	Rationale for Collecting Specific Data
History of present illness	To better understand events that may have led to the episode of DKA.
Past medical/social history	To determine what therapy was needed to control the patient's diabetes prior to admission. To determine if there are contributing or interacting medications, psychosocial factors, or disease states.
Laboratory values (chemistry, complete blood count, arterial blood gas, urine, and serum ketones)	To assess glucose (degree of hyperglycemia), measured osmolality (impact of hyperglycemia), sodium (to assess impact of hyperosmolar state on dilution of sodium and help make decisions about the most appropriate initial fluid therapy), bicarbonate (to assess acid-base status), potassium (to assess impact of disease on potassium levels and to determine if insulin can be administered and if potassium needs to be added to the IV fluid), urine and serum ketones (eg, beta-hydroxybutyrate [BHT]), (to verify diagnosis of DKA), white blood cell count (to determine if infection might be part of the etiology of the DKA), arterial blood gas (to assess acid-base status)

TABLE 6-3

Patient/Caregiver Interview: Examples of Data That Can Be Collected During the Patient/Surrogate Interview

- Medication history with details on antidiabetic regimen
- Adherence with prescribed medications
- Concomitant diseases
- Family disease history
- History of present illness
- Social history such as hobbies or habits that might impact current illness and treatment
- Insurance

This background knowledge of DKA and our practice is applied below with an in-depth analysis of a fictitious case of a patient presenting with DKA. This analysis will illustrate the reasoning that occurs during each PPCP step and demonstrate how critical thinking can be applied to optimize the reasoning process in each step, thereby optimizing patient-centered care.

The Case of Monroe P.: Overview

Monroe P. (MP) is a 27-year-old male presenting to the ED with his girlfriend via ambulance, secondary to a sharp decline in mental status, nausea and vomiting, and worsening diffuse abdominal pain. Of note, MP's girlfriend reports he has been complaining of 6/10 abdominal pain over the past 3 days after attending a local buffet with his friends.

> **Insurance:** Blue Cross Blue Shield
> **Family history:** Sister and mother have Type 1 (insulin-dependent) Diabetes
> **Inpatient course to date:** Patient with nausea, vomiting, increased abdominal pain, and altered mental status. The girlfriend suspects he ate something spoiled and noted that he has not been eating well nor taking his insulin × 72 hours.

With some background knowledge on the management of DKA and the intensive care environment, we will explore clinical reasoning, critical thinking, and the PPCP for the care of Monroe P.

CLINICAL REASONING, CRITICAL THINKING, AND THE PHARMACISTS' PATIENT CARE PROCESS FOR THE CARE OF MONROE P.

The following series of tables delineates the PPCP as it is applied for the provision of pharmacy care to MP. For each step, from Collect to Monitor, there is a description of the pharmacist's clinical reasoning along with examples of how the critical thinking standards can be applied to optimize the pharmacist's clinical reasoning. Clinical reasoning is described in terms of the conclusions drawn along with case information or premises on which the conclusions are based. Critical thinking intellectual standards are expressed in the form of past-tense statements, instead of the question format introduced in Chapter 1. This is because the case analysis was performed in *reflection* upon the clinical encounter. An exception to this past-tense format of critical thinking statements is with the Collect step, where the future-tense is used to illustrate how the standards can be applied in *preparation* for the clinical encounter. As a reminder, the critical thinking standards are embodied in the mnemonic "Clear ROAD for Logic". They are clarity, relevance, significance, objectivity, fairness, accuracy, precision, depth, breadth, and logic. (See Chapter 1.)

Collect

In the Collect step, the pharmacist collects the subjective and objective information about the patient in order to understand the relevant medical and medication history and clinical status of the patient. Information may be obtained by the pharmacist from the electronic health record and supplemental databases in preparation for a patient/surrogate interview and verified with the patient/surrogate, if possible, during the interview.

COLLECT: History and Medications	
Conclusions	Rationale: Information or Premise to Support the Conclusion
Perform a full and complete medication review from the chart and electronic health records and confirm with the patient/surrogate during the initial interview, if possible. Match each medication with its indication. Evaluate efficacy and any current side effects and drug interactions. Verify adherence to each medication.	• Though the focus will be on DKA management during the intensive care portion of the visit, it is vital the pharmacist has a good understanding of the complete medication regimen as this may help guide therapy beyond the ICU. • Confirming the indication with each medication can help identify any medications that might not be indicated while the patient is critically ill or can identify possible duplications of therapy. • Identifying possible drug–drug interactions or possible side effects is a fundamental role of pharmacists, as are determining adherence patterns and any barriers to adherence. • A thorough medication review can also help uncover any other relevant drug therapy problems such as adherence issues. • It is important to note that while a holistic view of the patient is important, DKA is an endocrine emergency. Thus, emphasis and focus are placed on the aspects of medicine therapy most directly related to this event. Assessment of medications not impacting the acute event may be deferred until the patient is not critically ill.
If possible and appropriate, during the medication review, for each medication, reinforce with the patient the indication and purpose, proper dosing and use, and possible side effects that can occur. If unable to communicate with the patient, and a family member, surrogate, or household member is available, assess their understanding of the medication's indication and purpose, proper dosing and use, and possible side effects that can occur if appropriate.	• Reinforcing medication purpose and use with the patient, or with the family, surrogate, or household member if unable to communicate with patient, can be valuable for improving overall adherence and the patient's understanding of the entire treatment regimen. The reported medication use can give the provider insight into what may have contributed to the development of DKA and may help prevent episodes in the future. While this reinforcement is important, the implementation may be deferred until the patient is not critically ill and is able to participate in the process. This step may be conducted by a non-ICU member of the pharmacy team later in the hospital stay.

Critical Thinking Checks for the Collect Plan for This Patient's History and Medications

In the medication review for this patient, it will be important to collect information with sufficient **accuracy** and **precision** to enable me to draw **sound** conclusions on medication effectiveness, safety, adherence, and any barriers negatively impacting the patient's medication use experience.

• This information may be challenging to obtain from critically ill patients and family/surrogates and may not be immediately available. Because DKA is a medical emergency I may have to proceed with the next steps in the PPCP with limited information.

As optimizing medication use is an essential part of my practice, it will be critical in our discussion of medications that I **clearly** understand the patient/surrogate and that they clearly understand me.

- There are times when confirming for **clarity** needs to be deferred as information may not be available at the moment or may not be able to be confirmed with the patient, surrogate, or via other records and treatment cannot wait until this is completed.

Given that the patient has a complex medical condition, it will be important for me to think **deeply** as we discuss medication usage and events leading up to the admission, so that I can gather the information needed for me to grasp the complexity of his medication experience.

Collected Current Medication Information and History Entered into Health Record

Current home medication regimen:
- Insulin glargine 22 units subcutaneous nightly
- Insulin aspart 5 units subcutaneous three times daily with meals
- Correctional aspart insulin at meals glucose 121 to 160 mg/dL—1 unit, glucose 161 to 200 mg/dL—2 units, glucose 201 to 250 mg/dL—3 units, glucose 251 to 300 mg/dL—4 units, glucose 301 to 350 mg/dL—5 units, glucose 351 to 500 mg/dL—6 units, glucose >400 mg/dL—7 units

History of present illness:
Per MP's girlfriend, he has been complaining 6/10 abdominal pain over the past 3 days after attending a local buffet with his friends. He has been nauseous and vomiting. His girlfriend suspects he ate something that was spoiled and noted that he has not been eating well nor taking his insulin for the last 72 hours.

Note that in our case we were able to obtain medication information from the surrogate (girlfriend), but there will be times when this information is not available and initial assessments and decisions will need to be made with limited or unconfirmed information.

COLLECT: Family/Social History

Conclusions	Rationale: Information or Premise to Support the Conclusion
Complete a full family/social history of the patient.	• The information obtained from a full family history may provide information that is consistent with being at risk for developing DKA and supports a DKA diagnosis. • A full social history which includes behaviors and recent activities, may provide insight into the etiology of the presumptive DKA.

Critical Thinking Checks for the Collect Plan for This Patient's Family/Social History

Am I gathering information that is **relevant** to evaluating the presumptive diagnosis of DKA?
- Am I thinking of the causes of DKA and checking to see if they are present? Am I thinking about the criteria for diagnosing DKA and making sure that the relevant information is collected?

Am I gathering data with enough **precision** to **accurately** evaluate the **significance** of the information collected?

- This would include knowing the timing of the events in enough detail to determine if they could be contributing factors. For example, is the timing of eating at the buffet consistent with development of food poisoning?

Have I verified information to confirm **accuracy**, especially in situations where I gathered information from sources that have a risk of being incomplete or unreliable?

- Did I confirm the information regarding the medication regimen provided by the girlfriend with another source, such as the medication labels or confirmation with the pharmacy if possible?

Have I gone into enough **breadth** and **depth** with the information gathered from the social history to be able to identify all the potential social history contributing factors for DKA or similar illness in the patient?

Collected Current Medication Information Entered into Health Record

- Family history: Sister and mother have Type 1 (insulin-dependent) Diabetes
- Social history: −tobacco/+alcohol (social use)

COLLECT: Allergies, Vital Signs, Physical Findings, Laboratory Values

Conclusions	Rationale: Information or Premise to Support the Conclusion
Verify the patient's allergy status. When entering any allergies into the system, report specific effects that the patient experienced.	• Knowledge of a patient's allergies or intolerances will help the pharmacist avoid medications that may result in negative outcomes. Knowledge of the specific effects experienced will allow the pharmacist to weigh the risks and benefits of therapy.
Collect the patient's current physical findings, vital signs, and pertinent labs.	• Physical findings, vital signs, and pertinent laboratory findings will help the pharmacist confirm a diagnosis, determine disease severity, and provide information that inform choices among treatment options.

Critical Thinking Checks for the Collect Plan for This Patient's Allergies, Vital Signs, Physical Findings, Laboratory Values

Have I **clarified** that blood gas and basic metabolic panel (BMP) were drawn at the same time so that the values can be used in concert?

Have I reviewed all of the available information and identified what is **relevant** to this patient's disease process and determined the **significance** of those values? Relevant laboratory values would include glucose, sodium, potassium, bicarbonate, ketones, and blood gas. All of these values are abnormal and consistent with DKA.

Have I ensured that the blood pressures were obtained using a reliable tool and **accurately** reflects the patient's blood pressure? Note in some cases, if pressures were measured from an arterial line where the catheter is positional (measurement changes based on position), the values may be off.

Have I ensured that the laboratory values are **accurate** and the sample(s) were not hemolyzed?

Have I looked into the allergy in **depth** enough to distinguish an allergy from an intolerance and determined if the reaction prohibits particular medications to be used in this patient?

Collected Allergies, Vital Signs, Physical Findings, Laboratory Values Entered into Health Record

- Drug Allergies: None
- Vital Signs:
  - Temp 38.2°C, HR 121, RR 29, BP 100/43
  - Height 5'11", Weight 175 lb
- Physical Exam:
  - Neuro: AO×2, moans and localizes pain but does not speak coherently
  - Skin: cool, dry with decreased turgor
  - Card: RR, tachycardia, no M/R/G
  - Pulm: lungs clear bilaterally, increased respiratory rate with deep breaths, fruity smell to breath
  - GI/GU: bowel sounds diminished, abdominal pain
- Pertinent Initial Labs:
  - *BMP:*
    - Sodium 131 mEq/L, Chloride 99 mEq/L, Potassium 5.9 mEq/L, Bicarbonate 6 mEq/L, BUN 25 mg/dL, Serum Creatinine 1.2 mg/dL, Glucose 504 mg/dL
  - *CBC:*
    - WBC 15,700 cells/uL, hemoglobin and hematocrit levels within normal limits
  - *Urinalysis:*
    - Glucose >1000 mg/dL, ketones 40 mg/dL, specific gravity 1.017
  - *Arterial blood gas:*
    - pH 6.96, $PaCO_2$ 20 mm Hg, PaO_2 150 mm Hg, HCO_3 7 mmol/L
  - *Coagulation parameters:*
    - PT/INR 1.1, PTT 21
  - *Amylase/Lipase:*
    - 30 U/L / 20 U/L
  - *Urine drug screen*—pending
  - *Blood alcohol*—pending
  - *Serum beta-hydroxybutyrate (BHB)*—20 mmol/L

EXAMPLE COLLECT STATEMENT FOR MONROE P.

MP is a 27-year-old male who presents to the ED for sharp decline in mental status, diffuse abdominal pain, nausea, and vomiting. MP's girlfriend reports he has been complaining 6/10 abdominal pain over the past 3 days after attending a local buffet with his friends. MP localizes the pain, but does not speak coherently. His skin is cool and dry with decreased turgor. He is an otherwise healthy Type 1 (insulin-dependent) diabetic who normally manages his diabetes with insulin glargine 22 units subcutaneous nightly, insulin aspart 5 units three times daily with meals, and correctional aspart insulin at meals. The girlfriend notes that he has not been eating well nor taking his insulin × 72 hours. He is currently tachycardic at 121 bpm, tachypneic with a respiratory rate of 29 bpm, hypotensive with a MAP of 62 mm Hg, and febrile with a temp of 38.2°C. Lungs are clear, breath has a fruity smell, bowel sounds are diminished, localizes to pain in abdomen. BMP is significant for Na 131 mEq/L, chloride 99 mEq/L, potassium 5.9 mEq/L, bicarbonate 6 mEq/L, BUN 25 mg/dL, serum creatinine 1.2 mg/dL, glucose 504 mg/dL. WBC is elevated at 15,700 cells/uL. ABG is notable for pH 6.96, PaCO$_2$ 20 mm Hg, PaO$_2$ 150 mm Hg, HCO$_3$ 7 mmol/L. Urinalysis is significant for glucose >1000 mg/dL, positive ketones, and elevated specific gravity. Serum BHB level is 20 mmol/L. Ethanol level and drug screen pending. No known drug allergies, no tobacco use, positive social EtOH use. Sister and mother are type 1 (insulin-dependent) diabetics.

Assessment of Collected Information

During the Assess phase, the pharmacist reviews all subjective and objective information obtained during the Collect step to provide the best explanation of the patient's current health status. During this time, it is important to understand what type of conclusions you are working toward to recognize how the information collected is related to the disease process and its etiology. The various manifestations of DKA can be directly impacting each other and it is important to understand these dynamics when working to develop a proper treatment regimen for this patient. To achieve these steps, it is vital to use critical thinking standards during this process to ensure the most logical and complete assessment of the patient's clinical situation. (See Table 6-1 and Chapter 1.) When assessing each specific medical condition, it is important to consider the impact of other conditions or other aspects of the same condition, other medications, and related patient treatment goals. Additionally, completing a full medication review ensuring each medication listed is linked to a current health-related problem and making note of unnecessary (or unnecessary during critical illness) drug therapy is important. Each medication should be assessed for efficacy, the patient's adherence patterns, current side effects, and any concerns the patient might have regarding each medication. Some medication therapy assessment aspects will need to be prioritized over others based on MPs disease acuity. Addressing less critical aspects of therapy may be deferred until he is no longer critically ill or is out of the hospital. An example of a deferred assessment is exploring an insulin adherence issue. While it is important to identify nonadherence as part of the initial patient workup and as a potential DKA trigger, addressing the cause and possible solutions is best done when the patient is not critically ill and can better participate in the process. It is also not a critical aspect of therapy until the DKA has resolved and it is time to reinitiate subcutaneous (SQ) insulin in preparation for discharge. DKA is a complex disease. When assessing and creating a problem list, it is helpful to break down the complications of DKA and look at them as individual but related problems and prioritize them based on the patient impact severity. Prioritizing your problem list in a critically ill or injured patient is very important as you need to address the most life-threatening problems first.

 KEY POINT

In DKA, the disease process is complex and manifestations are interconnected. It is important to use clinical reasoning and critical thinking to understand these relationships and consider how they may impact treatment plans and monitoring.

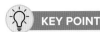 **KEY POINT**

Not all identified problems will be addressed at the same time. Problems need to be prioritized and plans that address life-threatening problems should be addressed first. Other problems may need to wait until the patient is stabilized and, in some cases, able to participate in care-plan decision-making.

ASSESS: Circulatory Status	
Conclusions	Rationale: Information or Premise to Support the Conclusion
Hypovolemia/Shock secondary to DKA	The patient has the following vital signs and laboratory findings that support the conclusion of volume loss and shock: • The patient's glucose is 504 mg/dL. The increased serum glucose increases serum osmolality and acts as an osmotic diuretic pulling fluid into the intravascular space and presenting a larger volume to the kidneys for excretion, which could be a cause of the hypovolemia. • The patient has been vomiting, which can contribute to fluid loss as well. • Patient is tachycardic (121 bpm), hypotensive (100/43 mm Hg = MAP 62 mm Hg), and has dry skin with poor turgor. These are all signs of hypovolemia. • The patient is presenting with altered mental status, which can be a manifestation of shock.

Critical Thinking Checks for Assessing This Patient's Hypovolemia/Shock Secondary to DKA

To evaluate this patient's volume status properly, all **relevant** and **significant** information needed to be gathered and fully considered.

• This included his blood pressure, urine output, skin turgor, etc., and other findings related to hypovolemia and shock.

It was also necessary to assure that the **accuracy** and **precision** of this information was sufficient to support accurate reasoning.

Given the interconnectedness of DKA manifestations and how they can impact volume and oxygen delivery, a **breadth** of information was considered, and great **depth** of thought was needed to determine their **relevance**, **significance**, and the interrelationships to fully explain their impact on the patient's shock state.

• This includes the relationships between hyperglycemia, serum osmolality, diuresis, vomiting, heart rate, blood pressure, skin turgor, and altered mental status.

To be **objective and avoid confirmation or availability bias**, it was important to be aware of other potential causes for the physical findings and see if there is data to support or refute the other causes before finalizing the assessment.

• An example is that the change in mental status could be due to shock, or it could be due to medication toxicity. This will need to be evaluated.

ASSESS: Glycemic/Osmolar State	
Conclusions	Rationale: Information or Premise to Support the Conclusion
Hyperglycemia/ Hyperosmolar state	The patient has the following laboratory values and history to support this conclusion: • The patient has an elevated serum glucose of 504 mg/dL (normal nonfasting, as we do not know when this patient last ate, is <140 mg/dL) and has a urine glucose level of >1000 mg/dL (greater than 250 mg/dL is considered abnormal). • The calculated serum osmolality is 298.5 mOsm/kg which is elevated (normal range 282 to 295 mOsm/kg). • Per the girlfriend, the patient has not been taking his insulin consistently for the past 72 hours. She also has a reported concern of history of a recent potential gastrointestinal infection from eating bad food at a buffet several days prior. Infection and nonadherence are two of the most common reasons for presenting with hyperglycemia (DKA).

Critical Thinking Checks for Assessing This Patient's Hyperglycemia/Hyperosmolar State

The collected data needed to be evaluated for accuracy.

• It is possible that if the labs were drawn through an infusion set with a dextrose-containing solution, the serum glucose results could be inaccurate. The other results supporting the finding give confidence in the accuracy of the serum glucose value.

It is important to be objective in assessing provided information. The history is from the girlfriend, who may have bias that we need to consider.

• She thinks MP has a gastrointestinal infection from the food he ate, but there could be other causes of the patient's complaints that do not readily come to her mind during the interview. To explore other potential causes of the patient's complaint, it is incumbent upon the pharmacist to ask appropriate follow-up questions to uncover any other potential factors or assumptions, in order to reach the most accurate and logical conclusions. An example would be probing in depth about medication history to see if the patient has taken medication that could cause gastrointestinal issues. We may need to look at other sources of information including labs, such as the white blood cell count, to see if the results support an infection diagnosis.

ASSESS: Serum Potassium Status	
Conclusions	Rationale: Information or Premise to Support the Conclusion
Hyperkalemia	The patient has the following laboratory findings and physiological processes to support this conclusion: • The patient had a serum potassium level of 5.9 mEq/L (3.5 to 5.5 mEq/L). Patients with DKA may present with normal or elevated serum potassium levels while actually being total body depleted in potassium. Potassium depletion can result from increased urination and increased potassium excretion that arises from vomiting. Elevations in serum potassium can still be seen in DKA due to the following factors that are present in our patient: – The lack of insulin can lead to more potassium remaining in the serum, as insulin drives the sodium/potassium pump that moves potassium into the cell. – The acidosis caused by the presence of ketones formed as a result of using fatty acids rather than glucose as the body's fuel source, leads to a buffering attempt by the potassium/hydrogen pump, driving hydrogen into the cell and moving potassium out.

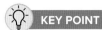

KEY POINT

Changes in serum potassium associated with DKA can be complex. It is important to be able to use critical thinking and clinical reasoning to evaluate all the ongoing processes that may impact serum potassium levels and anticipate how they may be affected by DKA treatment.

Critical Thinking Checks for Assessing This Patient's Changes in Serum Potassium

When a serum potassium level is reported as elevated, is it important to confirm the **accuracy** of the lab results.

- For example, falsely elevated potassium levels can be seen in hemolyzed specimens. The presence of hemolysis is typically reported with the lab result, so this would be important to check.

It is also important to consider the **significance** and **relevance** of the potassium level.

- For example, is the level high enough to warrant immediate intervention? Is the elevated level causing a problem such as cardiac rhythm changes that need to be addressed right away?

It is important to revisit the physical findings with enough **breadth** and **depth** to determine if there is **relevant** information to answer these questions.

ASSESS: Serum Sodium Status

Conclusions	Rationale: Information or Premise to Support the Conclusion
Relative hyponatremia	The patient has the following laboratory finding to support this conclusion: • The patient has a serum sodium of 131 mEq/L (normal range 135 to 145 mEq/L). The conclusion of relative hyponatremia is consistent with the pathophysiology of hyperglycemia. The serum sodium can be diluted due to fluid being pulled into the intravascular space as a result of the osmotic effects of the hyperglycemia.

Critical Thinking Checks for Assessing This Patient's Serum Sodium

It is important to determine the **accuracy** of the assessment of dilutional hyponatremia. One step is to calculate a corrected sodium, which would consider the effects of dilution.

This step will also help determine **relevance** and **significance** of the laboratory finding. The corrected sodium being normal or elevated versus still being low will impact treatment plans regarding fluid resuscitation.

ASSESS: Acid-Base Status/Ketones

Conclusions	Rationale: Information or Premise to Support the Conclusion
DKA	The patient has the following laboratory and physical findings to support the assessment of DKA: • The patient has an arterial pH of 6.96 (normal 7.35 to 7.45) indicating acidosis, a $PaCO_2$ 20 mm Hg (normal 35 to 45 mm Hg), and a calculated HCO_3^- 7 mmol/L (normal 22 to 26 mmol/L) from the arterial blood gas indicating metabolic acidosis. • The anion GAP is 26 indicating an elevated anion gap metabolic acidosis. • Serum BHB 20 mmol/L and urine ketones 40 mg/dL. These are elevated, suggesting ketones as the source of the gap and thus ketoacidosis.

- Ketoacidosis is a diagnosis consistent with a type 1 (insulin-dependent) diabetic, like our patient, who has not been compliant with his insulin regimen and who may have a gastrointestinal infection. The stress response to infection can lead to increased glucose production, and unless the insulin dose is modified to compensate, there is inadequate insulin to facilitate the use of glucose as a fuel source, leading to use of fatty acids as a fuel source. This is augmented by the increase in counter-regulatory hormones such as glucagon. The by-product of fatty acid metabolism is ketones resulting in ketoacidosis.
- The patient is tachypneic (29 bpm) and has a low $PaCO_2$ which is consistent with a respiratory alkalosis to compensate for the metabolic acidosis. His breath has a fruity smell which is consistent with the presence of ketones.
- The patient presented with nausea, vomiting, worsening abdominal pain, and altered mental status. The nausea and vomiting may be associated with food poisoning but is also associated with DKA. The fact that the abdominal pain is worsening after 3 days is further suggestive of DKA as the abdominal pain is associated with ketones and would worsen as ketones rise.[11,12] This is in contrast to food poisoning, which should be resolving by this timeline. The altered mental status is also seen in DKA patients.

Critical Thinking Checks for Assessing This Patient's Acid-Base Status/Ketones

It is important to have **clarity** and **precision** on the timing of laboratory specimens.

- If the BMP and arterial blood gas are not obtained at the same time, the results cannot be used together as they represent different points in the disease process. Using them together could lead to an inaccurate diagnosis. Note: In this case the bicarbonate from the BMP was 6 mmol/L and from the arterial blood gas it was 7 mmol/L. The values should be within 1 to 2 mmol/L of each other if the samples were obtained at the same time, such as in our case. Either value can be used in the calculations.

It is important to review the laboratory and physical findings and history with enough **breadth** and **depth** to determine **relevance** to and ensure the **accuracy** of the diagnosis.

- There can be non-DKA reasons for having ketones present, such as in starvation diets or with alcohol use disorders. There can be nongap forms of acidosis resulting from excessive chloride intake, for example. There can be nonketone causes of gap metabolic acidosis such as toxic ingestions and elevated lactic acid. One needs to review all of the elements together to ensure accuracy.

ASSESS: Medication Adherence

Conclusions	Rationale: Information or Premise to Support the Conclusion
Drug therapy problem: Inappropriate adherence to insulin	According to MP's girlfriend, he has not been taking his insulin as prescribed for 3 days. Not taking insulin is one of the most common etiologies for DKA.

Critical Thinking Checks for Assessing This Patient's Medication Adherence

It is important to ensure the **accuracy** and **precision** of the patient's medication usage to discover, evaluate, and explain problems with medication adherence.

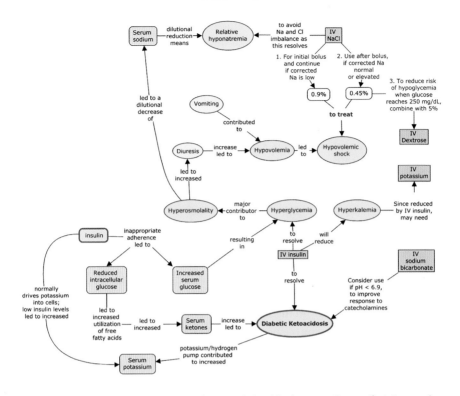

FIGURE 6-1. Concept map illustrating the interrelationships between the manifestations and treatment of DKA.

DKA is a multifaceted disease encompassing multiple physiological changes requiring multiple and interrelated therapies that will require frequent monitoring and adjustments before ultimate goals are met. Given the complexity of this patient's disease and presentation, and potential therapeutic strategies, it can be useful to create a concept map to help grasp some of the interrelationships that contribute to the complexity. (See **Figure 6-1.**) Understanding these interrelationships can be useful in the creation of this patient's comprehensive assessment, which is expressed in the Assess statement below.

 KEY POINT

A visualization of the interacting processes associated with DKA may help the clinician appreciate the disease and treatment complexities.

Example Assess Statement for Monroe P.

MP is a 27-year-old male presenting to the ED with hypovolemic shock secondary to DKA-associated volume loss.

(1) Hypovolemia/Shock secondary to DKA and vomiting

The patient is tachycardic at 121 bpm, hypotensive with a MAP of 63 mm Hg, and has dry skin with poor turgor. These are all signs of hypovolemia.[2] Patients with

DKA can lose in the range of 6 to 9 L of fluid due to excessive urination.[13] The patient is also presenting with signs of shock and impaired oxygen delivery, such as altered mental status.[14,15]

(2) Hyperglycemia/Hyperosmolality

The serum glucose is 504 mg/dL and the urine glucose is >1000 mg/dL. This glucose level is consistent with DKA but is approaching levels seen in hyperosmolar hyperglycemic state (HHS).[13] The calculated serum osmolality is 298.5 mmol/kg. This is elevated consistent with DKA. It would be expected to be higher in the setting of HHS. Per the girlfriend, the patient is an insulin-dependent diabetic and has not been using his insulin consistently for the past 72 hours. He also has a history of potential gastrointestinal infection. Infection and nonadherence are two of the most common reasons for presenting with hyperglycemia (DKA).[13]

(3) Electrolyte abnormalities—Hyperkalemia

The serum potassium is 5.9 mEq/L. Elevations in serum potassium can be seen in DKA due to the following:

1. As insulin drives the sodium/potassium pump that moves potassium into the cell, inadequate insulin due to problems with adherence leads to more potassium remaining in the serum
2. The acidosis caused by the presence of ketones formed as a result of using fatty acids rather than glucose as the body's fuel source. The resulting ketoacidemia leads to a buffering attempt by the potassium/hydrogen pump driving hydrogen into the cell and moving potassium out.[2] If the patient has developed renal damage due to the hypoperfusion/shock, potassium levels may be further elevated.[16] Conversely, the polyuria can lead to potassium losses, complicating the initial presentation picture.

(4) Electrolyte abnormalities—Hyponatremia

The serum sodium is 131 mEq/L. The serum sodium can be diluted due to the fluid being pulled into the intravascular space because of the osmotic effects of hyperglycemia This does not reflect a sodium deficit. A corrected sodium should be calculated to determine sodium status. Corrected sodium = measured sodium − [1.6 × (measured glucose − 100)/100].[2]

(5) Acid-Base Disorder—DKA

The patient has an arterial pH of 6.96, a $PaCO_2$ 20 mm Hg, and a calculated HCO_3^- 7 mmol/L. The patient is acidemic based on the pH with a metabolic acidosis based on the HCO_3^-, and a respiratory alkalosis based on the $PaCO_2$. Because the patient is acidemic, the primary disorder is the metabolic acidosis. The patient is tachypneic with a respiratory rate of 29 bpm and has a low $PaCO_2$ which is consistent with a respiratory alkalosis to compensate for the primary metabolic acidosis.[17] The anion GAP is 26, calculated using the formula: anion Gap = Na^+ − (Cl^- + HCO_3^-) = 131 − (99 + 6) = 26, indicating an elevated anion gap metabolic acidosis. The serum BHB is 20 mmol/L and urine ketones 40 mg/dL. These are elevated suggesting ketones as the etiology of the acidosis and thus a ketoacidosis. This is further supported by the patient's fruity smelling breath.[18,19] Ketoacidosis is a diagnosis consistent with a type 1 (insulin-dependent) diabetic who has not been compliant with their insulin regimen and/or who has an infection and a counter regulatory hormone-driven increase in glucose production and inadequate insulin, unless the insulin dose is modified. The inability to utilize glucose and the presence of counter regulatory hormones such as glucagon lead to the use of fatty acids as a fuel source. The byproduct of fatty acid metabolism is elevated ketone levels, resulting in ketoacidosis.[20] The degree of acidosis, in this case, may impair responsiveness to endogenous catecholamines and may further complicate the response to hypovolemia.[21]

(6) Medication Adherence—Nonadherence with insulin

Per the girlfriend, the patient had not been adherent with his insulin regimen for 3 days. Nonadherence with the insulin regimen is one of the most common reasons for the development of DKA. It is logical that the patient may have decided to not take his insulin if he was not eating.

Drug therapy problems include the following:

- *Needs additional medication therapy:* pharmacological treatment indicated for hypovolemia, hyperglycemia, hyperkalemia, and acidosis.
- *Inappropriate adherence:* nonadherence with insulin

These conclusions drawn in the Assess step serve as the basis for the therapeutic decision-making that will occur in the Plan step.

Plan, Implement, and Monitor

Because of interconnected relationships between the various disease manifestations in DKA, the treatment goals and plan are presented together in the tables below. The critical thinking checks that went into developing the goals are discussed later on in the text, and the critical thinking checks used for each plan element are provided after the Goal/Plan table.

PLAN: Goals	
Conclusions	**Rationale: Information or Premise to Support the Conclusion**
Goal 1: Resolve shock as soon as possible, but within 1 to 2 hours, and restore volume loss within 24 to 36 hours with half restored in the first 8 to 12 hours. Resolve excessive urinary losses.	Current MAP of 63 mm Hg and evidence of impaired oxygen delivery with altered mental status indicates shock. Immediate goal is to elevate MAP to greater than 65 mm Hg and see resolution of altered mental status. This is a medical emergency and should be accomplished immediately through bolus IV fluid.
	The subsequent goal is to restore volume loss due to excessive urination and possibly vomiting. Typical fluid loss in DKA is 6 to 9 L. Restoring the remaining volume over 24 to 36 hours minimizes side effects associated with rapid fluid treatment, such as cerebral edema.[20] The treatment used to replace volume may also impact serum sodium and needs to be considered as part of Goal 3. Decreasing the blood glucose will diminish the hyperglycemia related volume loss. Correcting glucose over 5 to 8 hours in this case will resolve the hyperglycemia in a timely manner, while avoiding cerebral edema associated with the rapid drop in serum osmolality resulting from a rapid decrease in serum glucose.[20]
	Insulin administration (see Goal 2) will lower plasma glucose, reduce serum osmolality, and resolve excessive urinary losses.

Goal 2: Decrease blood glucose and serum osmolality to normal range over 5 to 8 hours and avoid hypoglycemia.	The goal is to decrease plasma glucose level by 50 to 75 mg/dL/h. This approach would take approximately 4 to 6 hours to reach a goal of less than 200 mg/dL. Another target that is supported in the literature is a reduction of 10% over the first hour.[13,22] Serum glucose/osmolality should not be reduced too quickly due to risk of cerebral edema resulting from an imbalance between intracellular and extracellular osmolality. To avoid overcorrection and hypoglycemia, dextrose should be added to the IV fluid once the glucose level decreases to 250 mg/dL.[2] Another recommendation is that serum osmolality should, ideally, concurrently decrease by no more than 3 mOsm/kg/h.[23]
Goal 3: Maintain corrected serum sodium within the normal range over the course of volume resuscitation and glucose normalization.	The serum sodium is diluted by the intravascular volume shifts associated with hyperglycemic/hyperosmolar states. A corrected sodium should be used to make decisions regarding electrolyte therapy. As the glucose is normalized the corrected serum sodium and actual serum sodium will come into line, and then actual serum sodium can be used. It is also important that serum sodium not be corrected too quickly as the abrupt change in sodium concentration and thus osmolality can lead to pontine myelinolysis, a rare but devastating adverse effect.[24,25]
Goal 4: Maintain potassium between 3.3 and 5.2 mEq/L with a goal of 4 to 5 mEq/L during insulin infusion for glucose normalization and DKA resolution.	It is important to maintain proper potassium levels with the understanding of the multiple processes affecting serum potassium levels during DKA and its resolution. Patients have total body potassium depletion but may present with normal or elevated potassium levels due to: 1. Insulin, a driver of the sodium potassium pump, drives potassium into the cell. The absence of this driver leads to an increase in serum potassium. 2. The acidosis, which resulted from the formation of ketones formed from fatty acid metabolism as the body was unable to utilize glucose in the absence of insulin, results in a shift of potassium out of the cell and hydrogen ions (protons) into the cell to offset the acidosis. The result is an increase in serum potassium. 3. The osmotic diuresis caused by hyperglycemia can lead to potassium losses which would result in a decrease in serum potassium. 4. In the event of renal damage due to the hypovolemic shock that can occur, serum potassium is likely to be increased.[26]
Goal 5: Correct DKA within 12 hours and keep pH above 6.9 while DKA resolution is ongoing.	The goal for correcting DKA over 12 hours is not a fixed number, but the following factors were taken into consideration. 1. The goal minimum reduction rate is 50 mg/dL/h from Goal 2. This would result in it taking 6 to 7 hours to decrease to less than 200 mg/dL our target for DKA resolution (see below). 2. It is possible that the initial rate of reduction may be lower, and the dose of insulin would need to be adjusted, thus increasing the time to goal. 3. It is also possible that the potassium may drop below 3.3. If this happens, the insulin infusion needs to be held until the potassium is replaced. A potassium "bolus" is typically administered at 20 mEq/h. This could further delay resolution.

	Given these factors, achieving resolution within 12 hours is a reasonable goal. A slightly shorter or longer interval would also be reasonable.
	Resolution of DKA is defined as glucose <200 *and* two of the following:
	1. Serum bicarbonate ≥15 mEq/L
	2. Venous pH >7.3
	3. Calculated anion gap ≤12 mEq/L*
	The goal of considering treatment of a pH less than 6.9 is based on several considerations:
	1. Data suggest that patients may be less responsive to catecholamines in the setting of severe acidosis.[27,28]
	2. Data indicates no value in treating a pH greater than 6.85 in DKA patients.[29]
	3. In the absence of data on the value of treating a pH less than 6.85 in a DKA patient who also has shock (such as in our case), based on shock pathophysiology, responsiveness to catecholamines may be important to improving shock and thus sodium bicarbonate may be beneficial.[30,31]
	*These three elements are all indicators of acidosis. If the majority are resolved, the acidosis is considered resolved. Note: Not all elements will be measured in every patient.[13]
Goal 6: Address nonadherence with the insulin regimen before hospital discharge.	Because nonadherence is a leading cause of DKA, it is very important that issues associated with nonadherence be addressed to avoid future DKA episodes.
	These issues should be addressed once the patient's acute issues have been resolved and they have the ability (mental status and energy) to be involved in creating an adherence plan. This would typically be after DKA has resolved but before hospital discharge.

 KEY POINT

The hypovolemia seen in DKA can be a medical emergency. The volume lost can lead to shock which can be life-threatening. Volume replacement is the initial treatment of DKA and should be addressed even before initiating insulin therapy to treat hyperglycemia.

Critical Thinking Checks for Developing This Patient's Goals

The SMART goals were developed with a **clear** understanding of the knowledge of DKA and its resolution.

The SMART goals set for this patient are **clearly** stated including their timeframe and expected outcomes.

The SMART goals were developed in consideration of the most **significant** factors affecting this patient's health and the most **significant** expected outcomes.

• The goals for MP are listed in order of priority, beginning with his most urgent needs to restore his health and ending with a goal to maintain his health upon its restoration.

The SMART goals were developed with the necessary **precision** and **breadth** of thought needed for resolving MP's condition with a full consideration of factors and implications.

• For example, the time-setting of goal achievement carefully considered the potential negative implications of too rapid of a correction of serum glucose levels and osmolarity.

The SMART goals were developed with **deep** consideration of the complexities that could be involved in this patient's care.

- There are numerous complexities to consider for MP when determining his goals of therapy. These include the interrelated effects of the different physiological processes in DKA and its resolution and the interrelationships between the different goals, such as goals 1 and 2 above.

The SMART goals make **logical** sense based on disease pathophysiology, a full assessment of the patient, clinical guidelines, potential therapeutic strategies, and what is realistically achievable for this patient.

PLAN: DKA-Related Hypovolemia/Shock

Goal 1: Resolve shock as soon as possible but within 1 to 2 hours and restore volume loss within 24 to 36 hours with half restored in the first 8 to 12 hours. Resolve excessive urinary losses.

Conclusions	Rationale: Information or Premise to Support the Conclusion
Administer 1000 mL 0.9% NaCl IV during first hour	A bolus of IV fluid should be administered given that the patient is in shock. Recommended dose is 15 to 20 mL/kg/h × 1 h or 1 to 1.5 L. Normal saline is recommended for the initial bolus.[2,32] While there is emerging data on the use of balanced crystalloids, normal saline currently remains the recommended initial bolus fluid.[2,32]
In this case, 0.45% NaCl IV at 350 mL/h × 10 h. Rate can then be decreased to 250 mL/h × 18 h	Guidelines indicate that 50% of the fluid deficits should be corrected within 8 to 12 hours and remaining deficits within 24 to 36 hours. As previously mentioned, typical fluid loss is in the range of 6 to 9 L. Given that the patient is presenting with severe DKA and in shock, I estimated the volume loss to be at the higher end and based my calculations, on a 9-L volume loss. Since 1 L will be given as bolus, there is a need to replace an additional 3500 mL in the first 8 to 12 hours to meet the 50% recommendation. With a rate of 350 mL/h, the 3500 mL will be replaced over 10 hours. With the rate then decreased to 250 mL/h, the remaining 4500 mL deficit will be replaced over the subsequent 18 hours and the total deficits being replaced over 29 hours.
	For post-bolus resuscitation, in general, 0.45% saline IV at 250 to 500 mL/h is recommended if corrected serum sodium is normal or elevated (0.9% NaCl if corrected serum sodium is low). Because of the sodium and chloride content in 0.9% saline (154 mEq/L), it is not recommended for resuscitation.[33] The larger volumes infused can lead to a hyperchloremic metabolic acidosis and hypernatremia. There is some literature looking at the use of balanced crystalloids such as lactated Ringers (130 mEq/L sodium and 109 mEq/L chloride).[34,35] Data is not conclusive, and 0.45% saline remains the fluid recommended in guidelines.[32,36]
	Note: Fluid type may need to be adjusted during therapy based on decreasing glucose, corrected serum sodium, and decreasing serum potassium.
	Correcting serum glucose through insulin (see Goal 2) will decrease serum osmolality and thus the dilution of serum sodium (see Goal 3).
	Providing insulin (see Goal 2) and thus allowing glucose to be used as the preferred calorie source will stop the production of ketones and lead to resolution of DKA. Provision of insulin and resolution of acidosis will both result in a shifting of potassium into the cell (see Goal 4).

When glucose reaches 250 mg/dL change to 5% dextrose/0.45% NaCl at 250 mL/h (assuming 0.45% NaCl is the proper solution at that time). Continue until DKA resolves.	Because IV insulin should be continued until DKA resolves, which may be after glucose normalizes, when serum glucose reaches 250 mg/dL, dextrose needs to be administered to prevent hypoglycemia. Note an appropriate range for IV fluid rate at this time is 150 to 250 mL/h.[32] Resolution of DKA is defined as glucose <200 *and* two of the following: 1. Serum bicarbonate ≥15 mEq/L 2. Venous pH >7.3 3. Calculated anion gap ≤12 mEq/L

 KEY POINT

DKA must be resolved before transitioning from IV to SQ insulin due to the risk of rebound DKA. It is important to confirm the criteria for DKA resolution are met prior to insulin conversion.

Critical Thinking Checks for This Patient's Hypovolemia/Shock

Fluid therapy recommendations were developed with a **broad** and **deep** consideration of all of the **significant** contributing factors and the complexity of this patient's health such as severity of volume loss and associated electrolyte abnormalities that may impact fluid choices.

- This included the consideration of alternative fluid options, such as 0.9% sodium chloride solution versus 0.45% in relationship to his serum glucose, sodium, and potassium levels, and the dynamics of changes in MP's status during his IV fluid therapy.

The fluid therapy strategies for achieving the goals make **logical** sense based on disease pathophysiology, a full assessment of the patient, clinical guidelines, and available therapeutic strategies.

- For example, in developing the recommendation for infusion volumes and times, I followed the guidelines indicating that 50% of the fluid deficits should be corrected within 8 to 12 hours and remaining deficits within 24 to 36 hours.

In reasoning about the fluid therapy options for this patient's hypovolemia/shock, I have the **accurate** and **clear** medication knowledge needed to make these recommendations.

PLAN: Hyperglycemia/Hyperosmolality

Goal 2: Decrease blood glucose and serum osmolality to normal range over 5 to 8 hours and avoid hypoglycemia.

Conclusions	Rationale: Information or Premise to Support the Conclusion
Since potassium is greater than 3.3, start insulin infusion using regular insulin with an 8-unit bolus then an 8-unit/h insulin infusion.	There are two equally accepted insulin infusion regimens. The 0.1 u/kg bolus then a 0.1 u/kg/h infusion, or a 0.14 u/kg/h infusion with no bolus. See Figure 6-2 for an example of an insulin therapy argument map describing how to determine which therapy to use. In addition to the arguments in the map, I selected the 0.1 u/kg bolus and then a 0.1 u/kg/h infusion regimen in part because it is the regimen used in my institution's protocol/order set. I used the patient's actual body weight (175 pounds/80 kg) to calculate his insulin infusion rate of 8 units/h. Guidelines and reviews do not specifically state which weight to use, but notably do not indicate anything other than actual weight. Following a standardized approach to care is important, and practitioners should follow local protocols and order sets for consistency in treatment.[9,10,13,20,27,32,36]

The administration of insulin helps glucose enter cells where it can be used as a fuel source. It also signals the liver to store glucose for later use. These actions result in a decrease in serum glucose.[20] Serum glucose is a major contributor to serum osmolality $(2[Na^+] + glucose$ (mg/dL)/18 + BUN (mg/dL)/2.8) and, as can be seen in the osmolality formula, a drop in serum glucose leads to a decrease in serum osmolality as well.

Note that the potassium has to be at least 3.3 mEq/L to initiate insulin therapy, as the addition of insulin will drive the sodium-potassium pump and move potassium into the cell, lowering serum potassium. Insulin infusion needs to be held if the serum potassium drops below 3.3 mEq/L.[20] (See Goal 4.)

 KEY POINT

Even though problems are prioritized, operationalizing the plan for the higher-priority problems may be impacted by problems with lower priority. Critical thinking and clinical reasoning play an important role in accounting for these relationships when developing treatment plans.

Critical Thinking Checks for This Patient's Hyperglycemia/Hyperosmolality

I have considered insulin dosing approaches with enough detail to make recommendations that are **precise** and **clear** such as specifying which weight to use in dosing.

I have considered the **relevance** and **significance** of laboratory values such as potassium to the insulin plan development such as need to discontinue insulin if potassium is too low.

I have considered various insulin treatment approaches in enough **breadth** and **depth** to develop a **logical** plan suited to this specific patient.

- For example, in determining which insulin infusion regimen to recommend from among the accepted choices, I followed my institution's protocol in consideration of his actual body weight and serum potassium levels.

PLAN: Electrolyte Abnormality—Changes in Sodium

Goal 3: Maintain corrected serum sodium within the normal range over the course of volume resuscitation and glucose normalization.

Conclusions	Rationale: Information or Premise to Support the Conclusion
Initially give 0.45% NaCl IV at 350 mL/h for post-bolus resuscitation.	Use 0.45% saline if corrected serum sodium is normal or elevated. Use 0.9% saline if corrected serum sodium is low.
	• Because corrected sodium is in the normal range, initiate remaining resuscitation with 0.45% saline.
	• May need to adjust resuscitation fluid based on subsequent corrected sodium values to maintain sodium in normal range over the course of glucose normalization.
	See rationale under the plan for DKA-related hypovolemia/shock for additional details.

Critical Thinking Checks for This Patient's Electrolyte Abnormality—Changes in Sodium

I have evaluated the serum sodium in a **logical** fashion, taking into consideration the impacts of the disease process on the measured laboratory value.

I have considered the **relevance** of sodium alterations and the **significance** of these values to the development of a treatment plan such as which resuscitation fluid to utilize.

I have reviewed fluid administration options and approaches in enough **breadth** and **depth** to consider their impact on the rate of change of serum sodium. I have also considered the interrelationships between the goal of correcting MP's serum sodium and the goal of correcting his DKA-related hypovolemia and shock.

PLAN: Electrolyte Abnormality—Changes in Potassium	
Goal 4: Maintain potassium between 3.3 and 5.2 mEq/L with a goal of 4 to 5 mEq/L during insulin infusion for glucose normalization and DKA resolution.	
Conclusions	Rationale: Information or Premise to Support the Conclusion
Initiate a sliding scale potassium order. • For serum K$^+$ <3.3 mEq/L: No insulin; give 40 mEq potassium as a bolus infusion over 2 h • Serum K$^+$ 3.3 to 4 mEq/L: Add potassium 40 mEq/L to IVF • Serum K$^+$ 4.1 to 5 mEq/L: Add potassium 20 mEq/L to IVF • Serum K$^+$ >5 mEq/L remove potassium from IVF (do not give potassium replacement)	The net effect of the following is usually an increase in serum potassium, but serum potassium can be variable: 1. Lack of insulin moving potassium into the cell via the sodium-potassium pump 2. Acidosis leading to a shift of hydrogen into the cell and potassium out of the cell via the hydrogen-potassium pump 3. Osmotic diuresis leading to loss of potassium 4. The variable effects of potential kidney injury resulting from hypovolemia and shock As the processes are addressed, the net effect is a reduction in serum potassium which can be significant.[20] Proactive anticipatory interventions need to be in place to maintain serum potassium in the normal range. General recommendations from the ADA are:[33] • Serum K$^+$ <3.3 mEq/L: Stop or do not initiate insulin; given 20 to 40 mEq/dL as a bolus infusion • Serum K$^+$ 3.3 to 5.2 mEq/L: Acceptable to initiate or continue insulin; given 20 to 30 mEq/L in IVF to keep potassium between 4 and 5. • Serum K$^+$ >5.2 mEq/L: Acceptable to initiate or continue insulin, check potassium every 2 hours but do not give potassium replacement The recommended intervention is an example order where the general recommended dosing range has been made more patient-specific. Typically, an institution will have a protocol and/or order set with specific orders. This example is from my institution's order set. The recommendations can vary slightly based on the literature source but are generally consistent.[20]

Critical Thinking Checks for This Patient's Electrolyte Abnormality—Changes in Potassium

I evaluated treatment options based on guidelines and local protocols and order sets to recommend an approach that can be **specifically** applied for this patient.

- A sliding scale potassium order allows for adjustments to MP's potassium therapy based on his serum potassium levels.

I confirmed the **accuracy** of the potassium levels obtained from the lab, making sure that sample was not hemolyzed, to ensure appropriate orders are implemented.

PLAN: Acid/Base Status—DKA

Goal 5: Correct DKA within 12 hours and keep pH above 6.9 while DKA resolution is ongoing.

Conclusions	Rationale: Information or Premise to Support the Conclusion
See recommendations regarding infusion of insulin found under Goal 2.	As insulin is administered, glucose is able to be used as a fuel source. The body no longer needs to utilize fatty acids for fuel with its associated production of ketones. The ketones will be cleared and with no new production, the acidosis will resolve. For most patients, this is all that is needed to resolve the acidosis.[20]
Consider administration of sodium bicarbonate 100 mEq IV if pH <6.9	Some patients may present with severe acidosis. The following should be considered when deciding if sodium bicarbonate administration would be appropriate. 1. Data suggests that patients may be less responsive to catecholamines in the setting of severe acidosis.[27,28] 2. Data indicates no value in treating a pH greater than 6.85 in DKA patients.[29] 3. There is a lack of data on the benefit of treating a pH less than 7.0 with sodium bicarbonate in DKA patients.[37] In the absence of data on the value of treating a pH less than 6.85 in a DKA patient who also has shock (such as in our case), based on shock pathophysiology, responsiveness to catecholamines may be important to improving shock and thus sodium bicarbonate may theoretically be beneficial.[31,32] In our case, the pH is currently 6.96, so sodium bicarbonate is not indicated, but if pH drops below 6.9, and the patient is not responding to treatment, sodium bicarbonate could be given. Note: There is some variability in the literature in the recommended pH cut-off for administering sodium bicarbonate.[29,37] I have used the cut value in the order set at my institution.

Critical Thinking Checks for This Patient's Acid/Base Status—DKA

I have considered treatment options in enough **breadth** and **depth** to factor in information from guidelines and from the primary literature when needed.

- For example, I have considered how the plan for MP's insulin therapy to decrease his blood glucose and serum osmolality (Goal 2) will also resolve his acidosis, and if needed, the IV administration of sodium bicarbonate may also be utilized to help mitigate if he develops severe acidosis.

I have used **logic** and critical thinking to select options in the absence of **clear** definitive data to guide treatment decisions.

PLAN: Insulin Nonadherence

Goal 6: Address nonadherence with insulin regimen before hospital discharge.

Conclusions	Rationale: Information or Premise to Support the Conclusion
Action on this medication-related problem will be deferred until the patient is able to participate in the decision-making process. When patient is able to participate, I need to confirm barriers to adherence so they can be addressed. Educate patient on the importance of being adherent to insulin therapy and the importance of adjusting therapy based on intake but not discontinuing treatment.	As previously mentioned, nonadherence is one of the most common reasons for developing DKA. Adherence is not relevant during the acute treatment of DKA as the clinician will be dictating therapy. In addition, this patient is not able to actively participate in decisions regarding care, so addressing this problem will be deferred until time to transition from insulin infusion and re-establish SQ insulin therapy. At this time, the mental status changes should be resolved, and the patient should be able to participate in decisions regarding care. To prevent DKA in the future, it is important that the patient be educated on the importance of adherence with insulin therapy and the consequences of therapy discontinuation.[22]

Critical Thinking Checks for This Patient's Insulin Nonadherence

In developing and providing **clear** education to the patient on improving his adherence, I will:

- Ensure that the plan is developed with a **fair-minded** consideration of the patient's wants, needs, abilities, and a fair consideration of the roles and responsibilities of family members and other stakeholders. For example, this will include MP's girlfriend, whose participation was very instrumental for his healthcare in this case.
- Ensure the plan is developed and communicated with an empathetic understanding of perspectives of the patient and other stakeholders and in a manner that assures the patient is empowered to self-manage his health and health behaviors
- Carefully consider potential ambiguities, jargon, poor grammar, or other potential causes of unclear understanding by the patient.

As discussed in Chapter 1, in therapeutic reasoning, based on the pharmacist's knowledge, experience, and evidence-based practice, they generate potential strategies, and develop arguments for and against them. Conclusions are drawn about the best strategies for the patient, which are those that have the best supporting argument for realistically meeting the treatment goals. One of the ways the logic of an argument can be represented is in the form of an argument map, which shows the premises supporting an argument. An example of a map for supporting the argument for a specific insulin regimen recommendation for this patient is shown in **Figure 6-2**. The map shows part of the hidden underlying structure of the argument, beginning with conclusions drawn to create the Assessment, which support conclusions drawn for the SMART goal, which underlies the premises—including one of the assumptions—that collectively help support the recommendation for the recommended regimen. Note that there are other ways of constructing argument maps.

Recommendation
Insulin 0.1 u/kg bolus followed by 0.1 u/kg/h infusion

Insulin will enable glucose to be used as a fuel source, decreasing serum glucose and stopping the production of ketones	The listed insulin regimen is one of two regimens recommended by ADA guidelines[32] (0.1 u/kg bolus followed by 0.1 u/kg/h or 0.14 u/kg/h)	The bolus dose regimen has been recommended in severe acidosis to quickly achieve therapeutic insulin levels but has also been seen to have higher rates of hypoglycemia. This may be more of an issue when the presenting glucose level is lower[38] Higher dosing may be more beneficial in those likely to have insulin resistance such as the obese or pregnant[39,40]	Data suggests that there is no difference in time to DKA resolution based on regimen[41,42]	Assumption to verify: Patient is not likely to be more insulin resistant. Can verify once regimen initiated and adjust dose if needed

SMART Goals
1. Decrease blood glucose to normal range over 5 to 8 hours 2. Correct DKA within 12 hours

Assessment
Severe DKA due to insulin nonadherence and possible infection. Drug therapy problem: Needs additional therapy

FIGURE 6-2. Argument map for insulin regimen selection

 KEY POINT

While many of the elements of DKA treatment are standard and supported by recommendations from multiple sources, there are some elements where there may be several acceptable options. The use of critical thinking and clinical reasoning is important to the clinician when evaluating available evidence and considering patient-specific factors to arrive at a treatment choice.

IMPLEMENT/MONITOR: DKA-Related Hypovolemia/Shock

Plan:

- Administer 1000 mL 0.9% NaCl IV during first hour
- Then, in this case, 0.45% NaCl IV at 350 mL/h × 10 hours
- Rate can then be decreased to 250 mL/h × 18 hours
- When glucose reaches 250 mg/dL change to 5% dextrose/0.45% NaCl at 250 mL/h (assuming 0.45% NaCl is the proper solution at that time)

Conclusions	Rationale: Information or Premise to Support the Conclusion
Implement: DKA treatment order set. Ensure that a 1-L bolus of 0.9% sodium chloride and an infusion using 0.45% sodium chloride solution are selected on order set if available. Confirm proper solution hanging for the patient. Confirm target rate of 350 mL/h selected or that predetermined rate from order set in the 250 to 500 mL/h range. *Monitor:* Monitor blood pressure every 15 minutes (or continuously if arterial line present) until target of 65 mm Hg, then hourly. Monitor mental status hourly for normalization of mental status. Track total IV fluid administration volume hourly.	*Implement:* Shock is a medical emergency and prompt treatment is key to quality outcomes and survival.[20] Based on corrected serum sodium, the fluid should be 0.45% saline and an acceptable rate is 250 to 500 mL/h. While the 350 mL/h is targeted for this patient, the range is acceptable, and the fluid order should be operationalized based on the site protocol or order set. That might be slightly different from what we have calculated in this example, and as long as it is within the recommended range, it would be acceptable. Given that the initial bolus fluid is different than the subsequent resuscitation fluid, it is important to confirm the solution was changed. *Monitor:* Based on goals, expect shock to resolve within 1 to 2 hours, so frequent monitoring is needed. This is the timeframe listed in my institution's order set. Half the estimated 9-L volume loss should be replaced over 8 to 12 hours. Continue to monitor the replacement rate carefully to reach goals in the target timeframe without overadministering fluid.

IMPLEMENT/MONITOR: Hyperglycemia/Hyperosmolality
Plan: Since potassium is greater than 3.3, start insulin infusion with 8-unit bolus then an 8-unit/h infusion.

Conclusions	Rationale: Information or Premise to Support the Conclusion
Implement: Confirm that insulin can be initiated based on serum potassium. Ensure that insulin infusion is selected on order set if available. Confirm weight-based dose calculation and that the pump is set to deliver the correct amount of insulin. *Monitor:* Check glucose hourly.	*Implement:* Based on serum potassium of 5.9, insulin can be initiated. Weight-based calculations can be a source of medication errors, so they are important to confirm.[43] Setting the infusion pump is also a source of medication errors and so it is important to confirm the rate has been properly determined and entered.[44] *Monitor:* Need to ensure glucose is decreasing in the target range of 50 to 75 mg/dL/h. May need to decrease dose if dropping too quickly (risk of side effects) or increase dose if dropping too slowly (prolonging disease process). The time frame is the one listed in my institution's order set.

IMPLEMENT/MONITOR: Electrolyte Abnormality—Hyponatremia	
Plan: **Initially give 0.45% NaCl IV at 350 mL/h**	
Conclusions	**Rationale: Information or Premise to Support the Conclusion**
Implement: Ensure that 0.45% sodium chloride solution selected on order set. Confirm target rate of 350 mL/h selected or that predetermined rate from order set in the 250 to 500 mL/h range. *Monitor:* Serum sodium every 2 hours. Calculate corrected serum sodium at each measurement.	*Implement:* Based on corrected serum sodium, the fluid should be 0.45% saline and an acceptable rate is 250 to 500 mL/h. While the 350 mL/h is targeted to this patient given the desired correction time, the range above is acceptable and should be operationalized based on the site protocol or order set. *Monitor:* Need to ensure that the proper fluid is being administered and so there is a need to frequently monitor how serum sodium, and more importantly, how corrected serum sodium changes, to avoid hyper or hyponatremia. The frequency listed is the one in my institution's order set.

IMPLEMENT/MONITOR: Electrolyte Abnormality—Hyperkalemia	
Plan: **Initiate a sliding scale potassium order. For** **Serum K$^+$ <3.3 mEq/L: No insulin; give 40 mEq as a bolus infusion over 2 hours** **Serum K$^+$ 3.3 to 4 mEq/L: Add potassium 40 mEq/L to IVF** **Serum K$^+$ 4.1 to 5 mEq/L: Add potassium 20 mEq/L to IVF** **Serum K$^+$ >5 mEq/L: Remove potassium from IVF (do not give potassium replacement)**	
Conclusions	**Rationale: Information or Premise to Support the Conclusion**
Implement: Ensure that potassium sliding scale is implemented via the order set if available. Confirm solution hanging for the patient does not have potassium. *Monitor:* Check potassium every 2 hours.	*Implement:* Based on corrected sliding scale and a serum potassium of 5.9, no potassium is needed in the IV fluid at this time. It is important to confirm that orders are correct, but also that the correct solution is administered to the patient. *Monitor:* Significant changes in potassium are expected with treatment of DKA. Potassium may need to be added to IV fluid to avoid hypokalemia and so frequent monitoring is important to facilitate avoiding the development of hypokalemia. The frequency listed is the one in my institution's order set.

IMPLEMENT/MONITOR: Acid-Base Disorder—DKA	
Plan: See recommendations regarding infusion of insulin Consider administration of sodium bicarbonate 100 mEq IV if pH <6.9	
Conclusions	Rationale: Information or Premise to Support the Conclusion
Implement: See implementation recommendations regarding insulin administration for hyperglycemia/hyperosmolality. Ensure blood gas is set to coincide with BMP if using both to make decisions. *Monitor:* See monitoring recommendations regarding insulin administration for hyperglycemia/hyperosmolality. BMP every 2 hours to assess bicarbonate. Arterial blood gas 2 hours after initial arterial blood gas.	*Implement:* See implementation rationale regarding insulin administration for hyperglycemia/hyperosmolality. It is important to note when the BMP was drawn if used in conjunction with the arterial blood gas. Patient condition can change over time and lab values drawn at different times may reflect different patient conditions. *Monitor:* See monitoring rationale regarding insulin administration for hyperglycemia/hyperosmolality As insulin is administered and glucose drops, so should ketones, leading to resolution in DKA. Tracking blood gas and metabolic panel will provide insight into DKA resolution and need for transition therapy. Interval chosen is based on my site's order set.
Implement: Evaluate whether order for bicarbonate should be checked on order set in the event of a pH less than 6.9. *Monitor:* Arterial blood gas 2 hours after initial	*Implement:* As mentioned, severe acidosis may impact ability to respond to endogenous catecholamines. If felt to be a concern in a given patient, it is important to make sure pH does not drop too low. *Monitor:* The interval chosen is based on my site's order set to ensure arterial pH does not drop too low and to facilitate recognition if treatment needed.

IMPLEMENT/MONITOR: Medication Adherence—Insulin Nonadherence	
Plan: Address insulin nonadherence once patient's DKA has resolved.	
Conclusions	Rationale: Information or Premise to Support the Conclusion
Implement: Make note in pharmacy system to ensure patient education takes place. Communicate with the non-ICU pharmacist if plan is not developed before ICU discharge.	*Implement:* As patients undergo transitions in care, it is important to communicate plans to new providers to ensure the plan is executed.[7]

Monitor:	*Monitor:*
Encourage patient to follow up with the primary care provider, endocrinologist, or other relevant provider(s) to ensure adherence to and efficacy of the insulin regimen prescribed upon discharge.	In most healthcare systems, the monitoring will be completed by another provider outside of the system and monitoring by the health system may not be feasible. Efforts should be made to communicate plans to outpatient providers.[7]

Critical Thinking Checks for This Patient's Implementation and Monitoring Plan

I have considered the disease state with enough **breadth** and **depth** to evaluate the interacting elements and ensure the implementation plan is **logical** and that the interacting elements are addressed for all **significant** aspects of the implementation plan.

The steps for implementing the strategies were outlined and provided with enough **clarity** and **accuracy** and were detailed enough to facilitate their implementation by the care team.

I have included steps to confirm **accurate** implementation of the plan by the care team.

To facilitate successful implementation of strategies that are complex and interrelated, I have outlined and conveyed the most **significant** actions for strategy implementation.

The plan monitoring for a patient with DKA is frequent and iterative. To illustrate this, **Table 6-4** presents monitoring frequency and results for MP at admission and at different times on Day 1. **Tables 6-5** and **Table 6-6** depict the assessment of selected Day 1 monitoring results 2 and 8 hours after insulin initiation, respectively, along with subsequent plans and monitoring based on therapeutic goals.

 KEY POINT

Patient condition can change rapidly with DKA treatment. Frequent monitoring and adjustments to therapy may be needed. Given that a therapy adjustment to address one change may impact other treatments or results, clinical reasoning and critical thinking are important processes in determining how best to manage a rapidly changing clinical situation.

TABLE 6-4

Key Follow-up Monitoring Laboratory Values and Physical Findings for Monroe P.

	Day 1	Day 1	Day 1	Day 1	Day 1
	07:15 (admission)	10:00 (2 hours after insulin started)	12:00	16:00 (8 hours after insulin started)	20:00
Sodium (mEq/L)	131	133	135	136	135
Potassium (mEq/L)	5.9	5.1	4.3	3.8	3.7
Chloride (mEq/L)	99	100	101	102	104

Bicarbonate (mEq/L)	6	9	11	13	20
Blood urea nitrogen (mg/dL)	25	22	21	20	20
Creatinine (mg/dL)	1.2	1.0	1.1	0.9	1.0
Glucose (mg/dL)	504	375	275	175	180
pH	6.96	7.1	7.2		7.33
$PaCO_2$ (mm Hg)	20	25	29		32
PaO_2 (mm Hg)	150	146	148		154
BHB (mmol/L)	20				
MAP	62	67	70	72	73

TABLE 6-5

Sequential Assess, Plan, Implement, and Monitoring—2 Hours After Insulin Initiated

Day 1, 10:00, 2 hours after Insulin initiated	Assess Goal Achieved? Rationale	Plan/Implement Recommendations	Monitoring
Goal			
Resolve shock as soon as possible but within 1 to 2 hours Restore volume loss within 24 to 36 hours with half restored in the first 8 to 12 hours	Shock resolved based on MAP >65 mm Hg Resuscitation volume administered 1000 mL bolus + (350 mL/h × 2 hours) = 1700 mL. Estimated volume loss approximately 9 L not resolved	Continue the same rate for IV fluids as treatment ongoing	Monitor blood pressure, can be adjusted to hourly if done via cuff since shock resolved Track total volume of fluid administered via assessment of hourly administration volume
Decrease blood glucose to normal range (<200 mg/dL) over 5 to 8 hours	Glucose 375, not at goal of normal range, rate of decrease of 64.5 mg/dL/h within desired range of 50 to 75 mg/dL/h	Treatment ongoing, no need to change rate	Check glucose every hour to ensure it is decreasing at recommended rate
Maintain corrected serum sodium within the normal range over the course of volume resuscitation and glucose normalization	Serum sodium 133 mEq/L, corrected sodium = 133 + [1.6 × (375 − 100/100)] = 137.4 at goal of maintaining sodium in the normal range	Treatment ongoing as glucose as not normalized, no need to change IV fluid	Monitor serum sodium every 2 hours and calculate corrected sodium using the glucose collected at the same time

Maintain potassium between 3.3 and 5.2 mEq/L with a goal of 4 to 5 mEq/L during insulin infusion for glucose normalization and DKA resolution	Potassium 5.1. Goal of between 3.3 and 5.2 met. Ultimate goal not met as glucose not yet normalized and thus DKA not resolved. Glucose less than 200 is one of the required parameters for resolution. Until resolved, steps need to be taken to maintain in goal range	As potassium is likely to continue to drop with ongoing insulin administration and continued DKA resolution, need to operationalize adding potassium 20 mEq/L to resuscitation IV fluid to maintain in this range per the original treatment plan	Monitor serum potassium every 2 hours
Resolve DKA within 12 hours. Keep pH above 6.9 while DKA resolution ongoing	Goal of DKA resolution ongoing has not yet been met. pH goal currently being met	Continue insulin therapy to reduce glucose, and assist in resolution of DKA	Monitor glucose hourly until glucose <200 mg/dL then every 2 hours Assess at least two of the following at that time: pH, bicarbonate, and anion GAP

TABLE 6-6

Sequential Assess, Plan, Implement, and Monitoring—8 Hours After Insulin Initiated

Day 1, 16:00, 8 hours after Insulin initiated	Assess Goal Achieved? Rationale	Plan/Implement Recommendations	Monitoring
Goal			
Restore volume loss within 24 to 36 hours with half restored in the first 8 to 12 hours	Resuscitation volume administered 1000 mL bolus + (350 mL/h × 8 hours) = 3800 mL. Estimated volume loss, approximately 9 liters, not resolved, but is on track for half the volume to be replaced within 12 hours	Continue IV fluids. As the glucose as dropped to within normal limits, can decrease IV fluid rate to 150 mL/h. This will still be on track for half the losses to be replaced in 12 hours	Track total volume of fluid administered via assessment of hourly administration volume
Decrease blood glucose to normal range (<200 mg/dL) over 5 to 8 hours	Glucose 175, at goal of normal range within 8 hours	As DKA not resolved (see goal below), continue insulin but decrease rate to 0.03 u/kg/h; add dextrose 5% to IV fluid	Check glucose every 2 hours to ensure glucose maintained in range less than 200 mg/dL and no hypoglycemia

Maintain corrected serum sodium within the normal range over the course of volume resuscitation and glucose normalization	Serum sodium 136 mEq/L, corrected sodium = 136 + [1.6 × (175 – 100/100)] = 137.2 at goal of maintaining sodium in the normal range	Glucose has normalized—no need to calculate corrected sodium	Monitor serum sodium every 4 hours
Maintain potassium between 3.3 and 5.2 mEq/L with a goal of 4 to 5 mEq/L during insulin infusion for glucose normalization and DKA resolution	Potassium 3.8. Goal of between 3.3 and 5.2 met. Ultimate goal not while glucose normalized, DKA not resolved (see goal below)	To maintain 4 to 5 mEq/L per the original treatment plan, increase potassium to 30 mEq/L, as potassium may continue to drop with ongoing insulin administration and continued DKA resolution, albeit perhaps more slowly	Monitor serum potassium every 4 hours
Resolve DKA within 12 hours Keep pH above 6.9 while DKA resolution ongoing	Patient met glucose goal of DKA resolution but has not met two of the three resolution criteria (anion gap, bicarbonate, pH)	Continue insulin therapy to assist in resolution of DKA	Monitor remaining criteria every 4 hours to assess if at least two of the following have normalized: pH, bicarbonate, and anion gap

Note that when identifying the goals at subsequent time points, those that were met (eg, resolution of shock) were dropped from the goal list on the subsequent table (Table 6-6).

CONCLUSION

Managing DKA in a critically ill patient is a complex process. Because DKA is considered a medical emergency, prioritizing problems and their corresponding treatment is key to successful management. Pharmacists can play a key role in determining and operationalizing successful treatment. With multiple and interconnected disease manifestations and a rapidly changing patient, critical thinking and clinical reasoning play vital roles in completing the PPCP steps of patient assessment, treatment development, and perhaps even more importantly monitoring, reassessment, and plan revision. These skills will develop and evolve as the critical care practitioner cares for complex patients with complex diseases.

Summary Points

- DKA is considered a medical emergency and management in a critically ill patient is a complex process. Using a systematic patient care process such as the PPCP in conjunction with clinical reasoning and critical thinking to identify and prioritize problems and their corresponding treatment is key to successful management.

As addressing the critical care patient's most urgent needs is paramount, the critical care pharmacist must often have to make decisions with information about the patient that is unclear or of questionable accuracy, as the patient may be unable to communicate, and family or caregivers may not be immediately available or may not provide sufficiently accurate information. Accordingly, adopting a broad critical thinking mindset, considering multiple information sources, can be valuable to help overcome this limitation. It is also important for the pharmacist to assure the accuracy of the lab values most significant for assessing the patient's clinical status and for the selection, implementation, and monitoring of the therapeutic strategy.

- With multiple and interconnected disease manifestations and a rapidly changing patient course, clinical reasoning and critical thinking play vital roles in treatment development, and perhaps even more importantly, in monitoring, reassessment, and plan revision. The critical care pharmacist must be able to think broadly and deeply to grasp and manage the complexity associated with interrelated and changing physiological processes that occur with the critical care patient in DKA.

- Pharmacists are key members of the critical care team and can play an important role in the care of complex patients with complex diseases by determining and operationalizing successful treatment through the use of institutional protocols and order sets. Their use of clinical reasoning and critical thinking when more than one option may be appropriate is also vital to the care process. For the patient in the physiologically complex state of DKA, the critical care pharmacist must apply deep thought in setting and prioritizing interdependent SMART goals of therapy, and for precise therapeutic decision-making within the parameters of the established institutional protocols and order sets.

Abbreviations

ABG	Arterial Blood Gas
ACCP	American College of Clinical Pharmacy
ADA	American Diabetes Association
BHB	Beta-Hydroxybutyrate
BMP	Basic Metabolic Panel
BP	Blood Pressure
BUN	Blood Urea Nitrogen
Cl	Chloride
DKA	Diabetic Ketoacidosis
ED	Emergency Department
GAP	Anion Gap
GI	Gastrointestinal
GU	Genitourinary
HCO$_3$	Bicarbonate
HR	Heart Rate
Ht	Height
ICU	Intensive Care Unit
INR	International Normalized Ratio
IV	Intravenous

IVF	Intravenous Fluids
Kg	Kilograms
MAP	Mean Arterial Pressure
Na	Sodium
NaCl	Sodium Chloride
OR	Operating Room
PaCO$_2$	Partial Pressure of Carbon Dioxide
PaO$_2$	Partial Pressure of Oxygen
PPCP	Pharmacists' Patient Care Process
PT	Prothrombin Time
Pulm	Pulmonology
Serum K+	Serum Potassium
SQ	Subcutaneous
U	Units
WBC	White Blood Cell
Wt	Weight

References

1. Lat I, Paciullo C, Daley MJ, et al. Position paper on critical care pharmacy services: 2020 update. *Crit Care Med.* 2020;48(9):e813-e834.

2. Long B, Willis GC, Lentz S, Koyfman A, Gottlieb M. Evaluation and management of the critically ill adult with diabetic ketoacidosis. *J Emerg Med.* 2020;59(3):371-383.

3. Brar PC, Tell S, Mehta S, Franklin B. Hyperosmolar diabetic ketoacidosis - review of literature and the shifting paradigm in evaluation and management. *Diabetes Metab Syndr.* 2021;15(6):102313.

4. Noll KM, Franck AJ, Hendrickson AL, Telford ED, Maltese Dietrich N. Integration of around-the-clock clinical pharmacy specialists into the critical care team can increase safety of hyperglycemic crisis management. *Clin Diabetes.* 2019;37(1):86-89.

5. Tully AP, Hammond DA, Li C, Jarrell AS, Kruer RM. Evaluation of medication errors at the transition of care from an ICU to non-ICU location. *Crit Care Med.* 2019;47(4):543-549.

6. Bethishou L, Herik K, Fang N, et.al. Evaluation of medication errors at the transition of care from an ICU to non-ICU location. *JAPhA.* 2020; 60(1):163-177.e2.

7. American College of Clinical Pharmacy, Hume AL, Kirwin J, et al. Improving care transitions: current practice and future opportunities for pharmacists. *Pharmacotherapy.* 2012;32(11):e326-e337.

8. Stranges P, Jackevicius C, Anderson S. ACCP White Paper Role of clinical pharmacists and pharmacy support personnel in transitions of care. *JACCP.* 2020;3(2):532-545.

9. Evans KJ, Thompson J, Spratt SE, Lien LF, Vorderstrasse A. The implementation and evaluation of an evidence-based protocol to treat diabetic ketoacidosis: a quality improvement study. *Adv Emerg Nurs J.* 2014;36(2):189-198.

10. Laliberte B, Yeung SYA, Gonzales JP. Impact of diabetic ketoacidosis management in the medical intensive care unit after order set implementation. *Int J Pharm Pract.* 2017;25(3):238-243.

11. Umpierrez G, Freire AX. Abdominal pain in patients with hyperglycemic crises. *J Crit Care.* 2002; 17(1):63-67.

12. Campbell IW, Duncan LJ, Innes JA, MacCuish AC, Munro JF. Abdominal pain in diabetic metabolic decompensation. Clinical significance. *JAMA.* 1975;233(2):166-168.

13. Nyenwe EA, Kitabchi AE. Evidence-based management of hyperglycemic emergencies in diabetes mellitus. *Diabetes Res Clin Pract.* 2011;94(3):340-351.

14. Bauer S, Maclaren R, Erstad B. Chapter e42 shock syndromes. In: DiPiro JT, ed. *Pharmacotherapy: A Pathophysiologic Approach.* 12th ed. New York, NY: McGraw Hill; 2021:417-439.

15. Marino P. Hemodynamic monitoring. In: Marino PL, ed. *The ICU Book.* 4th ed. Philadelphia, PA: Lippincott Williams & Wilkins; 2014:123-194.

16. Bellomo R, Kellum JA, Ronco C. Acute kidney injury. *Lancet.* 2012;380(9843):756-766.

17. Hamilton PK, Morgan NA, Connolly GM, Maxwell AP. Understanding acid-base disorders. *Ulster Med J.* 2017;86(3):161-166.

18. Bijland LR, Bomers MK, Smulders YM. Smelling the diagnosis: a review on the use of scent in diagnosing disease. *Neth J Med.* 2013;71(6):300-307.

19. Misra S, Oliver NS. Diabetic ketoacidosis in adults [published correction appears in BMJ. 2015;351:h5866]. *BMJ.* 2015;351:h5660.

20. Charfen MA, Fernández-Frackelton M. Diabetic ketoacidosis. *Emerg Med Clin North Am.* 2005; 23(3):609-vii.

21. Andersen MN, Border JR, Mouritzen CV. Acidosis, catecholamines and cardiovascular dynamics: when does acidosis require correction? *Ann Surg.* 1967;166(3):344-356.

22. Wilson JF. In clinic. Diabetic ketoacidosis. *Ann Intern Med.* 2010;152(1):ITC1-ITC16.

23. Trachtenbarg DE. Diabetic ketoacidosis. *Am Fam Physician.* 2005;71(9):1705-1714.

24. Danyalian A, Heller D. Central Pontine Myelinolysis. [Updated 2022 May 1]. In: StatPearls [Internet]. Treasure Island, FL: StatPearls Publishing; 2022 Jan. Available at https://www.ncbi.nlm.nih.gov/books/ NBK551697/. Accessed July 21, 2022.

25. Guerrero WR, Dababneh H, Nadeau SE. Hemiparesis, encephalopathy, and extrapontine osmotic myelinolysis in the setting of hyperosmolar hyperglycemia. *J Clin Neurosci.* 2013;20(6):894-896.

26. Bellomo R, Kellum JA, Ronco C. Acute kidney injury. *Lancet.* 2012;380(9843):756-766.

27. Kitabchi AE, Umpierrez GE, Miles JM, Fisher JN. Hyperglycemic crises in adult patients with diabetes. *Diabetes Care.* 2009;32(7):1335-1343.

28. From Intravenous fluid therapy in adults in hospital. NICE clinical guideline 174. Available at https://www.nice.org.uk/guidance/cg174/resources/composition-of-commonly-used-crystalloids-table-191662813. Accessed July 21, 2022.

29. Lactated Ringers Package insert. Available at https://www.accessdata.fda.gov/drugsatfda_docs/ label/2019/016682s117lbl.pdf. Accessed July 21, 2022.

30. Self WH, Evans CS, Jenkins CA, et al. Clinical effects of balanced crystalloids vs saline in adults with diabetic ketoacidosis: a subgroup analysis of cluster randomized clinical trials. *JAMA Netw Open.* 2020;3(11):e2024596.

31. Joint British Diabetes Societies for inpatient care (JBDS-IP). *The Management of Diabetic Ketoacidosis in Adults.* 2021. Available at https://diabetes-resources-production.s3.eu-west-1.amazonaws.com/ resources-s3/public/2021-06/JBDS%2002%20DKA%20Guideline%20amended%20v2.pdf. Accessed July 21, 2022;

32. Cardoso L, Vicente N, Rodrigues D, Gomes L, Carrilho F. Controversies in the management of hyperglycaemic emergencies in adults with diabetes. *Metabolism.* 2017;68:43-54.

33. Bauer SR, Sacha GL, Siuba MT, et al. Association of arterial ph with hemodynamic response to vasopressin in patients with septic shock: an observational cohort study. *Crit Care Explor.* 2022; 4(2):e0634.

34. Weil MH, Houle DB, Brown EB Jr, Campbell GS, Heath C. Vasopressor agents; influence of acidosis on cardiac and vascular responsiveness. *Calif Med.* 1958;88(6):437-440.

35. Chua HR, Schneider A, Bellomo R. Bicarbonate in diabetic ketoacidosis - a systematic review. *Ann Intensive Care.* 2011;1(1):23.

36. Duhon B, Attridge RL, Franco-Martinez AC, Maxwell PR, Hughes DW. Intravenous sodium bicarbonate therapy in severely acidotic diabetic ketoacidosis. *Ann Pharmacother.* 2013;47(7-8):970-975.

37. Kimmoun A, Novy E, Auchet T, Ducrocq N, Levy B. Hemodynamic consequences of severe lactic acidosis in shock states: from bench to bedside [published correction appears in Crit Care. 2017;21(1):40]. *Crit Care.* 2015;19(1):175.

38. Farkas J. Anatomy of a DKA resuscitation. *The Internet Book of Critical Care.* 2016. Available at https:// emcrit.org/ibcc/dka/. Accessed July 27, 2022.

39. Priya G, Kalra S. A review of insulin resistance in type 1 diabetes: is there a place for adjunctive metformin? *Diabetes Ther.* 2018;9(1):349-361.

40. Taylor R, Davison JM. Type 1 diabetes and pregnancy. *BMJ.* 2007;334(7596):742-745.

41. Kitabchi AE, Murphy MB, Spencer J, Matteri R, Karas J. Is a priming dose of insulin necessary in a low-dose insulin protocol for the treatment of diabetic ketoacidosis? *Diabetes Care.* 2008;31(11):2081-2085.

42. Tran TTT, Pease A, Wood AJ, et al. Review of evidence for adult diabetic ketoacidosis management protocols [published correction appears in front endocrinol (Lausanne). 2017;8:185]. *Front Endocrinol (Lausanne).* 2017;8:106.

43. Bokser S. Medication errors: significance of accurate patient weights a weighty mistake. *Pa Patient Saf Advis.* 2009;6(1):10-15. Available at https://psnet.ahrq.gov/web-mm/weighty-mistake.

44. Taylor M, Jones R. Risk of medication errors with infusion pumps a study of 1,004 events from 132 hospitals across Pennsylvania. *Patient Safety.* 2019;1(2):60-69. Available at https://doi.org/10.33940/biomed/2019.12.7.

7

Inpatient Psychiatry Care—Treatment-Resistant Schizophrenia

Ericka L. Crouse and Rebecca M. Reiss

CHAPTER AIMS

The aims of this chapter are to:

- Describe acute care pharmacy practice within an interprofessional inpatient psychiatric team.
- Discuss the Pharmacists' Patient Care Process (PPCP), critical thinking, and clinical reasoning in assessing and resolving medication-related problems as part of an interprofessional effort

to provide patient-centered care for schizophrenia or mental health.

- Illustrate the use of clinical reasoning, critical thinking, and the PPCP to address common medication-related problems, including adherence, encountered in an example case of a patient with schizophrenia and medical comorbidities.

KEY WORDS

- Nonadherence • clozapine • schizophrenia • critical thinking • clinical reasoning • PPCP

INTRODUCTION

Acute care pharmacy practice in an inpatient psychiatric unit provides ample opportunities for managing psychopharmacology, acutely decompensated mental health disease states, and comorbid medical conditions. Acute care psychiatry is a practice area where pharmacists can play a vital role in patient assessment, patient safety, treatment plan development, drug–drug interactions, pharmacotherapy and pharmacokinetic monitoring, patient education, and transitions of care.

 KEY POINT

The role of pharmacy on inpatient psychiatry is diverse and includes medication reconciliation, recognizing and managing drug therapy problems, input into pharmacotherapy plans, monitoring adverse effects, pharmacokinetic monitoring, and provider, patient, and caregiver education.

Patients receiving care in an acute care inpatient psychiatry unit may present with a variety of disease states, and many patients with the same diagnosis can have symptoms that vastly differ from one another, making it critical to individualize care. They often have comorbidities, both psychiatric and nonpsychiatric, that can increase the complexity of diagnosis and treatment. A survey of 334 psychiatric pharmacists found that 41.3% of respondents also treated nonpsychiatric disease states as part of their pharmacist care process.[1]

OUR PRACTICE—AN INPATIENT PSYCHIATRIC UNIT WHERE A CLINICAL PHARMACIST IS PART OF AN INTERPROFESSIONAL TEAM

Our practice is an acute care rotation at an adult inpatient psychiatric unit at an academic medical center with four care teams. Each team primarily focuses on one disorder (Medical Psychiatry, Geriatric Psychiatry, Mood Disorders, and Psychotic Disorders/Schizophrenia). We also have a separate child/adolescent inpatient psychiatry building/unit. This is specific to our hospital and may differ at other psychiatric inpatient units or institutions. Patients are admitted to the unit due to concerns that, as a result of a mental illness, they present a danger to themselves, a danger to others, or cannot meet their basic needs for survival (eg, finding food or shelter). Patients vary in their level of understanding or awareness of their symptoms (referred to as insight). Some patients have never before been diagnosed with a mental illness, while others have a history of multiple admissions with similar presentations. The average length of stay is 5 to 7 days.

Pharmacy is part of an interprofessional team comprised of an attending psychiatrist, a postgraduate year-one or-two (PGY1 or PGY2) medical psychiatric resident, a psychiatric nurse practitioner, licensed clinical social workers, nursing staff, occupational therapists, and many interprofessional learners (medical students, pharmacy residents/students, social work interns, nursing students, and psychiatric nurse practitioner students). Members of the interprofessional team work with patients individually or in group settings. The medical team conducts daily rounds where they discuss each patient including pertinent updates, information that needs to be gathered, and a tentative plan. They then walk the unit, meeting with patients individually to gather desired information and to discuss next steps. When not meeting with members of their treatment team, patients are encouraged to socialize, engage in activities, and attend group sessions (psychotherapy, recreational therapy, pharmacy education, etc.).

Other descriptions of the role of psychiatric pharmacy have been published, and the impact of a Mental Health First Aid course or a psychiatric clinical rotation on Doctor of Pharmacy Students' attitudes toward providing care to the mentally ill.[1-7] The reader is encouraged to review some of these to learn more about this aspect of pharmacy.

UTILIZING CRITICAL THINKING SKILLS IN OUR PRACTICE

The application of critical thinking skills is vital to assure optimal clinical reasoning in an acute care psychiatry practice setting, where pharmacists identify, assess, and manage multiple drug therapy problems and disease states, prioritizing those that have led to or are keeping the patient hospitalized. Many mental health conditions are chronic, and symptoms may not fully resolve. Therefore, it is important for the pharmacist to consider what goals are reasonable and practical while a person is inpatient versus what might be better suited for long-term management as an outpatient. Patient safety and patient-centered decision-making are therefore core components of an acute care psychiatric pharmacist's job.

Patients are admitted to acute psychiatry for many different reasons and mental health emergencies, including suicidal thinking, status postoverdose as a suicide attempt, acute manic episodes, or decompensation of their primary psychiatric illness due to a multitude of factors. This chapter will focus on the psychiatric pharmacist's involvement in care of a fictitious patient admitted for schizophrenia.

Lifetime prevalence of schizophrenia ranges from 0.3% to 0.7%.[8] With adequate treatment, patients can achieve symptomatic and functional improvement. However, nonadherence is very common in this patient population, secondary to lack of insight into the disease, and lack of motivation (which is a negative symptom of the disease), negative views of medication, or ongoing/concurrent substance use disorders.[9] Adherence may be overestimated by both patients and practitioners.[9] Schizophrenia is characterized by positive symptoms (most commonly auditory hallucinations [eg, hearing voices that are not there], delusions, and disorganized thinking), negative symptoms (characterized by lack of motivation, a blunted or flat affect, or lack of pleasure), and cognitive symptoms (eg, impaired executive function).[8,10] Medication treatment focuses primarily on reducing the positive symptoms of schizophrenia and prevention of relapse.[10]

 KEY POINT

Nonadherence is common in patients with schizophrenia due to lack of insight and negative views toward medication; thus, pharmacists can help identify barriers to adherence and work with patients to find a medication they are willing to continue.

Examples of where critical thinking standards can be valuable for optimizing reasoning is when interviewing a patient during an acute crisis, where consideration of the patient's thought process and ability to abstract should be taken into account. If a person is experiencing psychosis, we need to ask ourselves if their answer is based on reality, or if it is an overvalued idea or delusion. We need to confirm that the information is **accurate** and **undistorted**. If a patient has difficulty abstracting, we need to determine the relevance of the patient's answer. For example, if a patient has concrete thinking when asked: "When was the last time you took your risperidone?," they may respond: "The nurse gave it to me this morning," but might be unable to abstract to when they last took it prior to admission. The pharmacist must determine if the provided answer is **relevant** to the question. In persons who care for patients with mental illness, there is sometimes a stigma toward certain diagnoses. It is important to remain objective and make sure treatment decisions are unbiased. The value of critical thinking extends throughout the PPCP when caring for patients with schizophrenia. **Table 7-1** delineates some of the questions pharmacists in this practice can ask themselves to help assure effective critical thinking and clinical reasoning through the application of the intellectual standards of critical thinking: clarity, relevance, significance, objectivity, fairness, accuracy, precision, depth, breadth, and logic—embodied in the "Clear ROAD to Logic" mnemonic provided in Chapter 1.

TABLE 7-1

Sample Standards-Based Questions That Can Be Applied to Assure That Intellectual Standards for Thinking Are Met As the Pharmacist Provides Recommendations on the Pharmacologic Management of Treatment-Resistant Schizophrenia

Clarity (explicit, unambiguous, intelligible, free from confusion or doubt)	Have I confirmed with the patient that all information collected from their chart and pharmacy fill records is correct and reflective of their experience?
	Have I addressed any discrepancies?
	Have I spoken with past providers, family, friends, and others who may be able to verify or clarify information?
	Have I documented the collected information in a way that is clear to others?
	Did I ask questions in a way that the patient understood what information I was looking for?
Relevance (pertinent, applicable, germane)	Do I need to ask follow-up questions when gathering information to ensure I received all relevant information?
	Have I reviewed the PDMP (Prescription Drug Monitoring Program) and Medication Refill History?
	What information from the patient's history is relevant to medication management versus what information provides additional detail but does not impact medication management?
	When assessing past medication trials, did I gather information on timing, dose, concomitant treatments, positive effects, adverse effects, and reasons for discontinuation?
	What family and social history is relevant given the patient's presentation?
	Where will this patient live once discharged and what support or resources will be available to them?
	Did I gather information relevant to each drug therapy problem I have identified?
Significance (important, nontrivial, necessary, critical, required, impactful)	Have I considered what information is most significant to the treatment team and to the patient?
	Have I considered what information may guide me toward or away from certain treatment options?
	Of the information gathered, what will help me know if literature and guideline recommendations are applicable to this patient?
	What data will I need to gather to determine if a plan was appropriate or successful? When is the appropriate time to gather such information? Is there a plan in place to prospectively collect such data?
	What are the most pertinent problems? What is preventing the patient from being able to be discharged?
Objectivity (fact-based, unbiased)	Am I aware of my own implicit biases and how they may impact my feelings and decisions during this patient encounter? Have I taken steps to overcome these biases?
	Have I avoided assumptions on their willingness to take a medication or adherence?

	Have I maintained professional boundaries, addressed countertransference (pharmacist's personal reaction or feelings to the patient)? For example, "I like them, I really want to help them" or "They remind me of a patient who...which impacts my desire to help or not help them".
	Have I recognized any instances of staff-splitting that might have led me to a non-evidence-based decision? (An example of staff-splitting is when patients see certain staff or team members as "good" or "bad", which can impact team dynamics and decrease collaboration.)
	Have I made an unbiased and destigmatized recommendation?
	What objective information is available in the patient's chart that can be used to establish a baseline and then track progress after implementing a plan?
Fairness (unbiased, equitable, impartial)	Is this patient here voluntarily or against their will? Is the patient court-ordered to take certain medications?
	Have I avoided any gender, racial, or ethnic biases in the treatment plan of this patient?
	Have I asked the patient and their family about their willingness to try a medication and monitoring plan, or did we decide what was best without their input?
	Have I considered cultural norms and the patient's goals and when deciding if a symptom needs to be treated?
	What social determinants of health might be contributing to this patient's presentation and how have they been addressed when developing a treatment plan?
	Is the patient aware of nonpharmacologic treatment modalities with evidence for treating their illness and has the patient been offered the opportunity to include such modalities into their treatment plan?
	Have I avoided using my personal feelings, judgments, or values to make decisions?
Accuracy (verifiable, valid, true, credible, undistorted)	Did the patient understand my questions and actively participate in the discussion, or do I need to seek out additional sources of information?
	Have I sought input or collateral information from family and friends to determine if the information provided by the patient is factual or delusional?
	Have I identified and reconciled any discrepancies?
	If the treatment team has concerns for malingering, has the patient been appropriately assessed?
	Does the patient's mental status exam reveal any abnormalities in thought process, thought content, cognition, insight, or judgment that need to be accounted for when assessing the accuracy of information gathered?
	Have I used validated assessments or rating scales when available and appropriate?
	How will I measure if treatment goals are achieved?

Precision (exact, specific, detailed)	Have I collected all relevant lab values, vital signs, and test results?
	Do I have the details needed to understand a timeline of events?
	Have I collected enough detail to understand the scope and intensity of a symptom or adverse effect?
	When collecting a medication history, did I determine what dose the patient was taking, when was the last dose, how frequently a dose was missed, etc.?
	What medications are available based on the hospital's inpatient formulary? What medications are available as an outpatient based on the patient's insurance?
	Based on a patient's mental status and level of cognitive functioning, what approach and level of detail is appropriate when providing education?
Depth (roots, fundamentals, complexities, interrelationships, cause/effect, implications)	Have I assessed factors of nonadherence and patient's perception of more worrisome adverse effects?
	What role might stigma have in the patient's perception of their illness and willingness to participate in treatment?
	Does the patient have a support system? Does that support system encourage or inhibit the patient from achieving their health goals?
	Are there systemic factors, policies, or laws that might impact the patient's access to care or ability to participate in care?
	How might a patient's comorbidities impact their treatment?
	What factors may improve or worsen the patient's symptoms?
	Can a patient's response to a medication provide me information that will help guide what medication to choose or avoid next by comparing mechanisms of actions, side effect profiles, and pharmacokinetic parameters?
Breadth (comprehensive, encompassing, alternative perspectives)	Can bloodwork or other tests be done to verify the information collected?
	Will other providers be impacted by the treatment decisions made? Does anyone besides the patient need to be involved in the decision?
	Did I approach the drug therapy problems broadly enough to avoid "tunnel vision" when determining a path forward?
	What questions should I ask the patient to ensure we have developed a comprehensive plan?
	Have I looked at multiple treatment guidelines, review articles, and primary literature sources to ensure I am not missing relevant data?
Logic (reasonable, rational, without contradiction, well-founded, sound)	If I was unable to gather relevant information, are my assumptions logical?
	Is the information gathered from the patient logical, or is it possible that it is a symptom of their illness (eg, a delusion)?
	Can I clearly explain my reasoning to the patient and other members of the treatment team?
	Have I utilized guidelines and evidence-based medicine for my medication recommendations?
	Have I considered the patient's ability to access the medication and monitoring plan to ensure it is reasonable for the patient to follow?
	Have I considered pros/cons of long-acting injectable antipsychotics (LAIs) versus clozapine?

KEY POINT

Including the patient's input and perspective when choosing a medication may help improve adherence and long-term outcomes.

APPLICATION OF THE PPCP IN OUR PRACTICE

When utilizing the PPCP in providing care to inpatient psychiatric patients, the pharmacist often begins by collecting information about the patient from the electronic medical record. Input is also gathered from other disciplines during interprofessional team rounds, adding to the breadth of information available to the pharmacist. Additional details are then obtained from the patient interview and assessment, which may be done as part of the team or on a one-to-one basis, if appropriate. The patient interview includes clarification of any gaps or discrepancies noted while collecting information, discussion of bothersome symptoms and desired outcomes, assessment of adherence to their most recently prescribed medication regimen, exploration of beliefs about their illness and medications, conversations regarding side effects of concern (current or potential), and overview of past treatments. As necessary, the pharmacist may collect collateral information by reaching out to other providers, pharmacies, or people who are close to the patient in an effort to verify or clarify information. The pharmacist then comprehensively considers what information is reasonable and most relevant for determining and assessing drug therapy problems and for developing a medication therapy plan based on this assessment.

Following the assessment, SMART goals will be developed with the patient and/or interprofessional team, prioritizing the most distressing symptoms and concerns that are preventing the patient from being discharged. In fairness to the patient, it is important that the pharmacist ensure the plan is not only evidence-based and free of bias, but also practical given the patient's specific circumstances. While the focus is on creating a plan that addresses the patient's acute inpatient needs, it is also imperative that the pharmacist ensures that the plan sets patients up to be successfully transitioned to an outpatient setting upon discharge.

After presenting recommendations to the treatment team and patient, it is time to implement the plan. The pharmacist's role is often to ensure orders are entered accurately, timing is correct for new or changing medications, and both patients and staff are clearly educated on relevant details of the plans. Pharmacists then monitor the changes, looking for objective and subjective signs of improvement or worsening of symptoms that would trigger them to restart the PPCP. If during the follow-up phase treatment goals are reached, the patient will likely be evaluated for discharge and the pharmacist will assist in creating a smooth transition from one care setting to the next.

In an acute care setting, pharmacists may be completing PPCP steps for multiple medications or disease states simultaneously. Although it is a fast-paced environment, it is important to remain detail-oriented and organized during each phase of the process. The following sections of the chapter will review each step in greater detail and include a patient case that will help to illustrate these steps in practice.

> **KEY POINT**
>
> Each stage of the PPCP offers opportunities to identify and complete education on important topics during the patient interview.

THE COLLECTION OF PATIENT INFORMATION IN OUR PRACTICE

Data collection in acute psychiatry begins with reviewing the medical record as to why the patient was admitted and what symptoms the patient was experiencing before presenting to the hospital. Further information can be obtained through patient interview and, with the patient's consent, collateral information from family or friends. Contacting the patient's outpatient pharmacy can help gain further insight into their current medication regimen and adherence. In situations where patients present with a treatment-resistant illness or express they have tried many medications in the past, it is important to gather as much detail as possible on past medication trials. A list of medications used for the disease state can be helpful in sparking a person's memory and creating a table can help organize the information. This can help the pharmacist determine if they received an "adequate" trial of a medication at a therapeutic dose for a reasonable duration. See **Figure 7-1** for an example of a medication history chart.

> **KEY POINT**
>
> Collection of information should include a review of the medical record, reaching out to outpatient pharmacies, and discussions with the patient and caregivers.

During the patient's admission, it is important for the pharmacist to collect information on a daily basis. This should start with a review of current medication orders for scheduled, one-time, and as-needed (PRN) orders. Reviewing previously administered medications can help the pharmacist understand what changes have been made, including what has been added, discontinued, titrated, or tapered. Adherence to medications and use of PRN medications (PRNs) are important to assess before making medication changes or solidifying a diagnosis in inpatient psychiatry. It is therefore imperative for the pharmacist on the team to collect information on whether the patient actually took their prescribed medications, and to review the medication administration record (MAR) for PRNs that were administered, along with their indications.

Drug name	Why was it started?	On anything else at the same time?	Maximum daily dose taken	Duration of trial	What did it help with?	Adverse effects noticed	Why was it stopped?	How often was it missed?

FIGURE 7-1. Example chart used for collecting past medication trial information.

Additionally, one can review nursing documentation to assess the patient's response to PRNs. Reviewing the use of PRNs can help determine if changes need to be made to the standing medication orders or if additional medications need to be scheduled.

Lab draws, vital signs, and imaging are collected less frequently in an acute inpatient psychiatry unit than in a general medical or intensive care unit; however, it is still vital to review these items daily or as they become available. When collecting drug level results, to allow for their proper assessment, pharmacists should also make note of how long the patient has been on the medication, how long after the last dose the level was drawn, and whether any interacting medications were recently administered. In most inpatient psychiatric practices, hours of sleep will be recorded as an additional objective measurement to collect and review.

Physician progress notes can also be helpful to review on a daily basis, as they are likely to include descriptions of symptoms. Pharmacists should pay special attention to the mental status exam included in these notes in order to see what symptoms are improving, which are worsening, if any new symptoms have appeared, or if psychiatric adverse effects may be emerging.

Unique to psychiatry is often the patient's legal status. Patients can be admitted voluntarily (much like in other areas of the hospital), or they may be legally required to stay in the hospital. They can also participate in care and take medications on a voluntary basis (during which time they also have the right to decline treatments and tests), or they may be court-ordered to take medications or allow certain tests (during which time staff can force these interventions even if a patient declines them). The process, timing, details, and terminology for involuntary admissions and medication administration vary from state to state. It is important to be knowledgeable of state laws and standards regarding the ability to administer treatment and medications against a patient's will. Potential resources to locate these state laws and standards are found in references 11 through 13.[11-13]

Table 7-2 provides a more detailed overview of what information can be collected during chart review and **Table 7-3** provides examples of data that may be collected in an interview.

TABLE 7-2

Examples of Data That Can Be Collected During Chart Review in Preparation for Patient Interview

Data to Collect During Chart Review	Rationale for Collecting Specific Data
Chief complaint/reason for admission	Understanding what brought the patient to the hospital can help the pharmacist determine which symptoms are most problematic and need to be prioritized. It can also help the pharmacist determine the patient's level of insight and their interest in seeking treatment (eg, Did the patient self-present or did family or emergency services bring the patient in?).
History of present illness	Knowing details, including timeline of the symptoms a patient has previously experienced can help with determining the symptoms that have been most concerning, where they are in their disease progression (eg, first episode of psychosis vs treatment-resistant schizophrenia), and the factors that may be contributing to the current need for admission.

Legal/Commitment status	Determining if this patient is in treatment voluntarily or is court-ordered will help to identify important considerations when developing medication plans. If court-ordered, the pharmacist will want to know what medications can be forced (if needed) and when the orders expire.
Past diagnoses	Past medical and psychiatric history are important in understanding the full picture of what might be going on with the patient. It can highlight comorbidities that could influence treatment decisions or help steer the pharmacist toward or away from certain medications.
Family history	Psychiatric disorders can be genetic, so understanding what illnesses family members have can aid in diagnosis and help with psychoeducation. If a family member has responded well to certain medications, it is possible the patient will too.
Support system outside of the hospital	Understanding a patient's support system allows the pharmacist to know what support or barriers exist that could influence the patient's ability to adhere to follow-up plans. For example: Can someone help coordinate frequent visits for appointments or labs? Can they help patients manage complex daily medication regimens? Can they financially support the patient if copays are burdensome?
History of violence	Occasionally, patient's symptoms present in an aggressive way, so it is important to be aware of any history of violence so you can take precautions and remain safe. Knowing the circumstances surrounding aggressive behavior can help the pharmacist assess if there might be a current threat. Knowing this history helps determine if it is safe to interview the patient on your own, or if it would be better with the team. Always check with nursing staff prior to interviewing, as circumstances may have recently changed. It should also be noted that most patients with schizophrenia are not aggressive and are more often the victims of violence.[8]
The Interprofessional Plan of Care (IPOC), including provider treatment plans and goals of therapy	It is important for the pharmacist to be aware of the goals and plans of other members of the treatment team to ensure all recommendations align and any discrepancies are addressed proactively.
Nursing assessments	Nursing notes contain valuable information on how the patient behaves when not meeting with the treatment team. They may also include patients' goals, concerns, responses to medications, or potential side effects.
Mental Status Exam	This is the psychiatric interview.[14] This will give insight into the patient's thought process, thought content, cognitive status, and insight into their illness and their judgment. *Note this is different than the mini-mental state exam (MMSE) used to screen for cognitive impairment*
Current and past medications used to treat their mental illness	Understanding what has been used previously can help guide the next steps in the treatment plan.

Recent medication fills from external pharmacy data	Determining adherence to current medication regimens will help the pharmacist assess if the treatment has not worked or if barriers should instead be addressed.
PDMP Review	It is important to know if the patient is on any controlled substances to understand if controlled substances may be contributing to the current presentation and to prevent the patient from going into withdrawal. The PDMP can also aid in determining what outpatient pharmacy a patient uses, particularly if the patient is unable to provide this information.
History of LAI antipsychotic	Knowing someone's history of LAI use can clue a pharmacist into patient preferences and alert the pharmacist to potential difficulties with adhering to a daily medication regimen. If the patient has recently received a LAI antipsychotic, the drug concentration will need to be considered when developing a treatment plan.
PRN medications received while in the emergency department	If a patient has been using multiple PRN medications for agitation or aggression, the pharmacist may want to delay the interview or complete the interview with a team for reasons of safety. It can also be helpful to determine if the patient might be somnolent and unable to participate in an interview as the result of the recent medications. Knowing what PRN medications a patient used and the patient's response can also provide guidance on what medications to use as part of an ongoing treatment plan.
Patient characteristics: age, weight, comorbidities	Knowing patient characteristics can help with medication selection and dosing. For example, if someone has diabetes, we may be less likely to use a high-metabolic risk antipsychotic.
Allergies/adverse reactions to past psychotropic medications	Knowing how a patient has reacted to previous medications can help determine which medications are reasonable to try and which should be avoided.
Insurance status	Knowing if a patient has insurance and if so, what type, helps to determine which medications may be options once a patient is discharged. If something is not available to the patient as an outpatient, it does not make much sense to use it inpatient unless it is intended only for short-term, inpatient use.
Review of labs	Renal function tests and liver function tests (LFTs) can help guide the pharmacist's dosing recommendations for medications. A history of diabetes or elevated glucose may also help in selecting a medication. Baseline lipid panel, glucose levels, CBC, and pregnancy tests (as applicable) will allow the pharmacist to appropriately monitor antipsychotic therapy. Thyroid-stimulating hormone (TSH) levels can be used to rule out hypo/hyperthyroidism that could contribute to psychiatric symptoms.
Review of urine drug screen (UDS)	Knowing the UDS results helps rule out substance-induced psychosis or potential for withdrawal-related psychosis.
Pharmacogenomic testing	While not routinely recommended or obtained, it is important to gather any available pharmacogenomic results so they may be interpreted and incorporated when developing a plan.

KEY POINT

Obtaining a detailed history of past psychotropic medication trials, including indication, duration of use, maximum daily dose, and the reason surrounding discontinuation can help the pharmacist provide patient-centered treatment recommendations.

TABLE 7-3

Patient Interview: Examples of Data That Can Be Collected During the Patient Interview

- What does your medication help you with?
- What are your personal goals of medication therapy?
- What did your doctor tell you your mediation was for?
- When was the last time you took your medication?
- How often do you miss your medication?
- Have you experienced any bothersome side effects that have kept you from wanting to take your medications?
- Are you interested in a 2-week or monthly LAI form of your medication?
- Do you have any difficulty obtaining your medications? If yes, is it secondary to finances or transportation (ability to pick up your medication)?
- Do you take any over-the-counter medications? Herbal medications?
- Do you use cannabis? If so, do you typically use products higher in THC or CBD? By what route or how do you use it?
- Do you smoke cigarettes or use other nicotine products? Do you drink caffeinated beverages (eg, coffee, soda)? Do you drink alcohol, wine, or beer? If yes, how much and how often do you use it? What is the earliest or latest time you consume it? Do you use any illicit or nonprescription substances? Do you use prescription substances (eg, opioids, benzodiazepines, stimulants) that were not prescribed to you?

Interview/Discussion with family:
- How would you describe the patient's willingness to take medications?
- Have you witnessed the patient miss any doses of medication?
- Have you noticed any recent changes in behavior? For example, is the patient more isolated or paranoid? Has the patient been keeping up with his/her hygiene (eg, grooming, showering)?
- Are you aware of any illicit substance use?

Approaching the collect step of the PPCP using a biopsychosocial framework allows the pharmacist to consider the multitude of factors that influence the patient's illness presentation and course. The APA (American Psychiatric Association) Practice Guidelines for the Treatment of Patients with Schizophrenia recognize the importance of a holistic approach, recommending that clinicians include biological (symptoms, substance use, treatment history, physical health), psychological (goals, preferences), and social (culture) assessments, among others, when working with patients with mental illness.[15] Doing so sets practitioners up to build rapport with those they serve and allows them to individualize treatment strategies to improve outcomes. By gathering all of this information, pharmacists are in a better position to engage in shared decision-making and can provide more effective education that is tailored to the individual.[15] Such information also aids pharmacists in implementing multiple strategies to decrease implicit bias, such as perspective taking, partnership creating, cultural understanding, and individuating. **Figure 7-2** highlights factors to consider when preparing a biopsychosocial formulation for a patient with schizophrenia.

Biological:
- Gender
- Age
- Genetics
- Pathophysiology, symptoms
- Comorbid conditions, physical function
- Medications, substance use
- Diet, exercise

Psychological:
- Goals, preferences
- Beliefs, understanding of illness
- Stress, coping skills
- Personality
- Lifestyle
- Choice, autonomy
- Cognitive function

Social:
- Socioeconomic status
- Family, community, culture
- Social support
- Access to care
- Living situation
- Education
- Stigma

FIGURE 7-2. Biopsychosocial model of health for a patient with schizophrenia.

KEY POINT

Approaching the collect step of the PPCP using a biopsychosocial framework allows the pharmacist to consider the multitude of factors that can influence the patient's illness presentation and course.

The following fictitious patient case scenario will follow the inpatient care of a patient admitted to our facility with schizophrenia. This will be used to illustrate how the PPCP, clinical reasoning, and critical thinking were integrated to provide optimal care to this patient.

The Case of Arlo J.: Overview

A 25-year-old white male, Arlo J. (AJ), is voluntarily admitted to inpatient psychiatry for worsening paranoia that people are out to get him. He carries a diagnosis of schizophrenia for the past 3 years, but prior to that, he had been treated for major depressive disorder with psychotic features in his early 20s. He was brought to the emergency department by his family for increasing isolation, refusing to leave the house, not showering in almost one week, and barely eating because he believes his food is being poisoned. Recently, he self-reduced and sometimes skipped his quetiapine dose and reports his paranoia is getting worse. He reports he has had more difficulty sleeping because voices are keeping him up at night. During the interview, he pauses as if he is hearing something and seems very distracted at times. He denies any visual hallucinations. He reports having been tried on multiple antipsychotics in the past. Some initial information obtained during medical record review includes:

Past Medical History:
Deep vein thrombosis (DVT)—Provoked; therapy completed
Schizophrenia, paranoid type
Insurance:
Private insurance: He is dependent on his parent's insurance.

CLINICAL REASONING, CRITICAL THINKING, AND THE PHARMACISTS' PATIENT CARE PROCESS FOR THE CARE OF ARLO J.

The following series of tables delineates the inpatient pharmacy utilization of the PPCP as it is applied to the care of AJ. For each step, from Collect to Monitor, the pharmacist's clinical reasoning is described along with examples of how the critical thinking standards can be applied to optimize the pharmacist's clinical reasoning. Clinical reasoning is described in terms of the conclusions drawn along with case information or premises on which the conclusions are based. Critical thinking intellectual standards are expressed in the form of past-tense statements, because the case analysis was performed in reflection following the clinical encounter. An exception to this past-tense format of critical thinking statements is with the Collect step, where the future-tense is used to illustrate how the standards can be applied in preparation for the clinical encounter. As a reminder, the critical thinking standards are embodied in the mnemonic "Clear ROAD for Logic." They are clarity, relevance, significance, objectivity, fairness, accuracy, precision, depth, breadth, and logic.

Collect

As previously described, during this step, the pharmacist collects the subjective and objective information about the patient in order to understand the relevant medical, psychiatric, medication history, and clinical and legal status of the patient. This will include information from the medical record review conducted by the pharmacist in preparation for interprofessional team rounds and verified with the patient during either the team or one-on-one interview. It will also include assessments, such as an abnormal involuntary movement scale (AIMS) assessment, performed by the pharmacist or medical team.

COLLECT: Medications	
Conclusions	Rationale
Review currently ordered inpatient medications and compare it to the patient's most recent home medication list. [Referred to as Medication Reconciliation]. *(Collected during the chart review)*	It is important to know what medications a person is currently taking (both scheduled and as needed). Knowing the medications a patient was recently taking as an outpatient allows the pharmacist to assess whether the inpatient regimen is complete, if dosing is correct (or if reasonable adjustments were made), and if anything has been discontinued that could worsen symptoms or lead to withdrawal. This also helps the pharmacist identify any transcription errors, for example, if divalproex sodium 500 mg—Take three tablets (1500 mg) at bedtime was prescribed as only one tablet (500 mg) at bedtime; this gives an opportunity for the pharmacist to intervene.

Recent adherence to medication regimen. *(Collected during the chart review and patient interview)*	Knowing whether someone has regularly been taking their medication allows the pharmacist to assess if the medication is working. If the patient remains symptomatic, it is important to know if the drug needs to be changed (increased dose or new medication) or if a conversation regarding barriers to taking the medication would be more impactful.
Collect past antipsychotics. *(Collected during the chart review and patient interview)*	Knowing which medications a patient has taken in the past and their response helps the pharmacist develop a treatment plan for current symptoms. Furthermore, knowing why a patient stopped a medication (eg, because it was not working or if it was secondary to side effects), will help the pharmacist develop a patient-specific plan to increase the likelihood of adherence after discharge. Lastly, quantifying how many antipsychotics and at what doses the patient took in the past will help the pharmacist determine if the patient meets the criteria for treatment resistance, which will impact antipsychotic selection.[16]
Collect indication or reason medications were prescribed. *(Collected during the chart review and patient interview)*	Knowing why a medication was prescribed by the provider will help the pharmacist know what symptoms the prescriber was targeting and what diagnosis the patient has received in the past. This is important information to collect as the prescriber may have documented a different reason than the patient reports the medication was prescribed for. This knowledge will help the pharmacist in developing a patient-specific treatment plan with **clear** instructions for patient education. For example, a patient may be prescribed olanzapine at bedtime for schizophrenia per the provider, but may report during a medication history that the medication "helps with sleep."
Determine what the patient feels the medication has helped with. *(This is typically best to collect during a patient interview rather than chart review, as there may be nuance or changes over time.)*	Knowing the patient's thoughts on their medication can help illuminate what symptoms have been targeted and can help build rapport with the individual *(partnership creating)*. Additionally, knowing what the patient believes it was prescribed for and what symptoms it has helped with in the past, will help the pharmacist educate the patient in **clear** patient-friendly language. Using the patient's language can aid in their understanding, can help the patient feel heard, and strengthen the pharmacist–patient relationship. For example, some patients may deny or disagree with the diagnosis of schizophrenia; but will report medication helps with "voices" or "organizing their thoughts," others may also say it helps with sleep.

Critical Thinking Checks for the Collect: Medications

During the completion of a medication reconciliation for this patient, it was important to collect **applicable** information **free from confusion** that will enable the pharmacist to draw **rational** conclusions on target symptoms for medications, medication effectiveness, adverse effects, adherence, barriers to access or adherence, and the patient's overall views on taking medications. It is also important to **verify** the patient report with collateral sources for **accuracy** and for greater **details** as needed.

- During the patient interview, AJ expressed he did not like taking medications that made him "shake" (also referred to as extrapyramidal symptoms or EPS). He said if a medication actually took his "voices" away, he would be willing to consider a new medication. He reports he reduced the dose of his current quetiapine for two reasons: to reduce his next day sleepiness and because he was still hearing voices when taking it. So he thought he would see if there would be any differences if he took less or skipped a dose.

- AJ's mother was contacted for collateral information, and she confirmed during a previous trial of haloperidol, he had a hand tremor, which caused difficulty drinking liquids without spilling. While he seemed less distracted on that medication, his frustration with the tremor led him to stop. On his current regimen, he still seemed to get distracted and occasionally conversed, although no one was around.

The use of effective, **fair-minded**, and empathetic communication skills with patients, including paranoid patients, is essential to build rapport and to ensure that all information is **accurate** from both the pharmacist's and patient's viewpoint. Utilizing **clarifying** questions during the interview and succinctly summarizing the patient's responses back to them for validation can help ensure we are relaying **exact** information to the medical team regarding the patient's desires for medication treatment. This method of communication also helps the pharmacist to avoid assumptions and biases.

- AJ never described his medications as helping to treat schizophrenia. Rather, he explained he wanted a medication to get rid of the "voices." Therefore, when gathering information on medications trialed in the past, the pharmacist asked if the medications had been helpful in reducing the "voices" instead of asking if they were helpful in treating schizophrenia. AJ also reported that he previously stopped his haloperidol due to "shakiness." The pharmacist clarified whether the shakiness was an internal feeling of restlessness (akathisia) or a physical movement that he could not control (tremor). He explained his hand shook. As a final step, the pharmacist summarized the conversation, saying "It sounds like you would be interested in exploring new medication options with the goal of finding one that got rid of the voices. Is that correct?"

 KEY POINT

When interviewing a patient in an acute psychiatric crisis, thought content and process should be taken into account and attempts should be made to obtain collateral information to confirm the accuracy of information provided by the patient.

 KEY POINT

Utilizing clarifying questions during the interview and succinctly summarizing the patient's responses back to the patient for validation can help ensure we are relaying exact information to the medical team regarding the patient's desires for medication treatment.

Collected Current Medication and Updated Medication Reconciliation Information Entered into the Medical Record

This information was obtained by reviewing outside pharmacy fill history and interview with the patient, and inpatient orders on admission.

Current home medication regimen:
- Quetiapine 200 mg—Take two tablets at bedtime—Indication (per chart): Schizophrenia; Indication (per patient): voices, sleep, and his worries about people's intentions. *Reports he takes intermittently, sometimes only takes one tablet at bedtime; last dose was 3 days ago;* reports some next-day sleepiness after taking and increased appetite.
- Benztropine 0.5 mg BID—Indication (per chart): EPS; Indication (per patient): to prevent the "shakes". *Reports still taking as prescribed, last dose this morning;* reports dry mouth
- Clonazepam 0.5 mg BID—Indication (per chart and patient): anxiety. *Reports still taking as prescribed, last dose evening before admission;* no ADRs

Inpatient orders on admission:
- Quetiapine 100 mg at bedtime (restarted, dose adjusted)
- Benztropine 0.5 mg BID (restarted)
- *Note: Clonazepam was not restarted, based on UDS results*
- Nicotine 14 mg/24 hr patch (new on admission)

Collected Past Psychiatric Medication Trials and ADRs [Example Using a Medication History Table]

This information was obtained primarily through interview with the patient, but also by reviewing past discharge summaries and outpatient visit notes.

Drug	Indication concurrent meds	Max dose and duration	Helped with	Adverse effects	Why was it stopped?
Haloperidol	Started for "voices". Coprescribed with fluoxetine and benztropine.	Maximum dose 10 mg/day; 6 months.	Helped with voices, but did not fully go away.	"Shakiness" [EPS]	Stopped because of "shakiness".
Risperidone	Depression augmentation/ depression with psychotic features. Coprescribed with escitalopram and benztropine.	4 mg; 2 years off and on.	Paranoia improved	Sexual dysfunction	Switched to paliperidone palmitate injection.
Paliperidone palmitate	Voices, schizophrenia. Coprescribed with benztropine.	156 mg monthly; several consecutive months.	Voices improved, but did not fully go away.	None reported	Did not like getting injections; felt it was not fully helping.
Quetiapine	Voices, schizophrenia. Coprescribed with benztropine.	400 mg at bedtime; about one year.	Paranoia improved; voices mostly unchanged.	Sedation	Still prescribed, not helping.

Fluoxetine	Depression Coprescribed with haloperidol and benztropine.	40 mg daily	Unsure, maybe helped with some anxiety.	None reported	Not working
Escitalopram	Depression, anxiety. Coprescribed with risperidone and benztropine.	10 mg daily	Unsure	Sexual dysfunction	Discontinued when diagnosis was changed to schizophrenia.
Venlafaxine XR	Depression, anxiety	150 mg daily	Unsure	Worsened insomnia	Unsure

COLLECT: Allergies, Vital Signs, Labs, and Other Objective Information

Conclusions	Rationale
Verify the patient's allergies. Report specific effects that the patient experienced. Determine if it is an allergy versus a side effect. *(Collected during the chart review and the interview)*	Documenting specific allergy information can help determine if it is a true allergy versus a side effect. For example, many patients will report allergies to antipsychotics but describe a dystonic reaction (swollen tongue, stiff jaw, torticollis) or other adverse effect.
Collect vital signs, height and weight, body mass index (BMI), and pertinent labs (eg, lipid panel, glucose, A1C, absolute neutrophil count (ANC), creatinine clearance). *(Collected during the chart review)*	It is important to review vital signs to monitor for orthostasis and/or tachycardia, which may be an adverse effect of certain antipsychotics. Tachycardia on admission may be related to agitation or anxiety. If available, looking at trends over time can be helpful for assessing vital signs.
	Determining baseline BMI will help in selection of an antipsychotic based on individual metabolic risk.
	The Center for Medicaid Services requires monitoring of lipid panel and glucose or A1C since antipsychotics have been associated with weight gain and metabolic adverse effects. Therefore, it is important to determine if baseline metabolic monitoring (lipid panel, A1C or glucose) has been completed. If it has not been obtained, this provides an opportunity for the pharmacist to make an intervention and request the lipid panel and A1C or glucose to be checked at baseline[15,17] On occasion, to reduce risk of harm to the nursing staff if a patient is extremely agitated, the treatment team may delay ordering laboratory work until the patient is calmer and more agreeable.
	If the team is considering clozapine therapy as an option, there will be a need to establish a baseline ANC prior to starting therapy[18]
	Lastly, it is important for the pharmacist to determine the patient's creatinine clearance to know if any medications (including nonpsychiatric medications) need to be avoided or adjusted based on renal function. Most antipsychotics are hepatically cleared, but paliperidone palmitate does require dosage adjustment in renal impairment and is contraindicated if the creatine clearance is below 50 mL/min.[19]

Collect AIMS score. *(Can be collected during the chart review or pharmacist can perform exam)*	Antipsychotics carry a risk of tardive dyskinesia, a long-term irreversible adverse effect of antipsychotics. Therefore, it is important to determine a baseline AIMS score for future comparison if a patient develops any abnormal involuntary movements. If a patient has tardive dyskinesia at baseline, this will impact the decision of which antipsychotic to initiate.
Collect UDS. *(Collected during the chart review, results can be confirmed during patient interview)*	Collecting the UDS results will help the pharmacist determine if the patient recently used any substances (eg, cocaine) that could be contributing to psychosis.[20] If a patient is on prescription medications such as opioids or benzodiazepines, UDS may be used to confirm the patient is taking them before restarting them as an inpatient. However, the pharmacist needs to be aware of the limitations of the UDS, and which medications (eg, oxycodone, clonazepam) may exhibit false-negatives.[21] The pharmacist should also be aware of medications that can exhibit false-positive results.[22]
Collect results of the Mental Status Exam. *(Collected during the chart review, results can be confirmed during patient interview)*	Reviewing the Mental Status Exam[14,23] helps the pharmacist understand the patient's thought process, thought content, mood, and insight and judgment regarding their illness. During interview, pharmacists can determine if they agree with the documented observations on appearance, speech, and affect.

Critical Thinking Checks for the Collect Plan for Arlo J.'s Allergies, Vital Signs, Labs, and Other Objective Information

When gathering information on allergies, it is important for the pharmacist to obtain **explicit** descriptions of reactions in order to **accurately** determine if the reported allergy is a **true** allergy or an adverse reaction.

- For example, a review of the medical record showed AJ reported an allergy to haloperidol. In discussion with the patient, he reported that when he took haloperidol, he developed "shakiness" (eg, a tremor). This is actually an EPS reaction, referred to as drug-induced parkinsonism, which is more frequently seen with high-potency first-generation antipsychotics (FGAs) like haloperidol. EPS is not a contraindication to prescribing haloperidol or other antipsychotics in the future. This reaction may have been dose-related or may be minimized with the use of an anticholinergic medication like benztropine. Often, when haloperidol has been listed as an allergy in the medical chart, it may be related to a different EPS called dystonia, where the patient reports a thick tongue, jaw tightness, and/or difficulty swallowing. This dystonic reaction is treated with diphenhydramine or benztropine. The use of diphenhydramine may also impact the perception that it was an allergy when it was actually an adverse reaction. Dystonia (tonic contraction of muscles, often in the head and neck) is most common in younger males.[24,25] Practitioners may be more hesitant to prescribe high-potency FGAs to someone with a history of a dystonic reaction versus a parkinsonism reaction. Based on this finding about AJ's reaction to haloperidol, it will be important to update the listed "allergy" to "intolerance."

- Acquiring a **deep** understanding of the potential implications of a patient's reactions to medications, as exemplified above, can be critical for effective diagnostic and therapeutic reasoning.

It is critical for the pharmacist to collect the most **relevant, accurate, and precise** information regarding labs, vital signs, and weight.

- Vital signs and weight are usually manually entered into the electronic medical record. Given many medications are weight-based and may be calculated based on the information in the chart, it is important for the unit-based pharmacist to confirm the weight is **accurate** and prevent errors if a weight was inadvertently entered as kilogram instead of pounds.
- It is also critical for the pharmacist to know the **validity** of a UDS and potentials for false-positives and false-negatives, including the hospital laboratory's limitations.[22]
- In the case of AJ many antipsychotics are associated with weight gain.[26] Therefore, it is important for the pharmacist to view the trend in weight since initiation of antipsychotic therapy. Many antipsychotics can cause orthostasis (including quetiapine and clozapine) and it is important to assess blood pressure and if the patient was evaluated for orthostatic hypotension (by measuring blood pressure in a supine, sitting, and standing position).[27]

KEY POINT

When gathering information on allergies, it is important for the pharmacist to obtain explicit descriptions of reactions in order to accurately determine if the reported allergy is a true allergy or an adverse reaction.

KEY POINT

It is critical for the pharmacist to know the validity of a urinary drug screen and potentials for false-positives and false-negatives, including the hospital laboratory's limitations.

Collected Allergies, Vital Signs, Labs and Other Objective Information Entered into the Medical Record

Allergies: Haloperidol (extrapyramidal symptoms) → pharmacist changed from "allergy" to "intolerance"

Vital signs: BP: 118/77 HR: 98 RR: 20 Temp 98.7F

Pertinent labs: LFTs: WNL

A1C: 5.4%

Glucose: 89 mg/dL

Lipids: Cholesterol, total = 168 mg/dL, HDL = 43 mg/dL, LDL = 94 mg/dL, and TG = 155 mg/dL

Urine Drug Screen: Opi (-), BZD (-), ETOH (-), PCP (-), AMP (-), MAMP (-)

Weight: 159 lb; Height: 69 in

AIMS: zero

Pertinent mental status exam findings:

Appearance: poor hygiene with hair and beard disheveled, wearing wrinkled pajamas midday

Behavior: poor eye contact, frequently looks to other parts of the room, cooperative

Speech: normal tone and volume, frequent pauses

Mood: "fine"

Affect: flat

Thought process: tangential, thought blocking, occasional loose associations

Thought content: delusions of persecution (being poisoned), auditory hallucinations, no suicidal ideation/homicidal ideation (SI/HI)

Insight: good

Judgment: good

Abbreviations: BP = blood pressure; HR = heart rate; RR = Respiratory rate; LFTs = liver function tests; WNL = within normal limits; HDL = high-density lipoprotein; LDL = low-density lipoprotein; TG = triglycerides; OPI = opioids; BZD = benzodiazepines; PCP = phencyclidine; AMP = amphetamines; MAMP = methamphetamine; lb = pounds; in = inches; AIMS = abnormal involuntary movement scale; SI = suicidal ideation; HI = homicidal ideation

COLLECT: Social History	
Conclusions	Rationale
Evaluate current use of nicotine, alcohol use, illicit substances, including marijuana	Smoking cigarettes can cause enzyme induction of cytochrome P450 (CYP) 1A2, which can affect the serum concentrations of certain antipsychotics, including clozapine, olanzapine, and asenapine.[28–30]
	Assess if illicit substances could be contributing to current symptoms (eg, cocaine or methamphetamine intoxication can contribute to psychosis; marijuana potentially increases risk of early onset of schizophrenia; alcohol withdrawal can be associated with hallucinations).[20,31–34]
Determine what social support the patient has and what their current living situation is.	Knowing what kind of support a person has outside of the hospital can help the pharmacist understand what assistance the patient may need or barriers the patient may face. For example, stigma from loved ones or lack of access to reliable transportation should be considered when developing a treatment plan.
	A person's living situation may also contribute to decisions on what medications to use. For example, if someone does not have a secure place to keep medications, a LAI antipsychotic might be beneficial. If someone struggles with adherence, but lives in a supportive setting, more complicated regimens may be possible.

Critical Thinking Checks for the Collect Plan for Arlo J.'s Social History

When obtaining a social and educational history for a patient, it is important to consider what information is **pertinent** and **impactful** to the disease state, current presentation, and potential future plans.

- Substance use may worsen symptoms, prevent medications from being effective, or may lead to drug interactions. Diet and exercise may contribute to a risk of adverse effects. Social support may enhance or inhibit adherence. Having detailed information can allow the pharmacist to think **deeply** to assess these **interrelationships** in order to develop a **fair and logical** plan.

Some information may be subjective or lack verifiable data. **Clarity** should be sought when possible by confirming this type of information with family, friends, records, or labs.

Collected Social History Entered into the Medical Record

Substance use:
Denies smoking marijuana. Drinks "occasionally" one or two Saturdays per month. Does not drink more than three 12-oz beers in one evening. Smokes ½ to 1 pack of cigarettes per day. Denies e-cigarette or chewing tobacco use. Denies other illicit substances.

Education:
Completed high school, and 2 years of community college before his first episode of psychosis.

Dietary habits:
Does not eat vegetables regularly. Eats a banana most days. Prefers to eat out at fast food restaurants (burgers, fries, and milkshakes).

Exercise:
When stable, reports going to the gym 2 to 3 times/week.

COLLECT: Current Symptoms/Presentation of Schizophrenia

Conclusions	Rationale
Collect current untreated or undertreated symptoms. *(Collected during chart review, patient interview, discussions with family/friends, and discussions with the interprofessional team)*	Recognition of what symptoms are present will guide the pharmacist in assessment and planning stages. It is important to gather information from outside sources (family, friends, roommates, etc.) and to also collaborate with members of the interprofessional team to gather their perspectives. Gathering information from the patient regarding their insight and experience with the symptoms will also be vital.
Determine how symptoms impact the patient's life. *(Collected during patient interview and discussions with family/friends)*	Gathering information on how symptoms impact various aspects of a patient's life will help when determining goals and priorities. Consideration should be given to social and occupational/academic functioning, relationships, independence, and overall quality of life.
Gather information on the patient's desired outcomes. *(Collected during patient interview)*	In order to guide future treatment goals, it is essential to collect information regarding the patient's personal goals and desires so that they may be incorporated. Such goals may relate to desired symptom reduction, avoidance of certain adverse effects, or improvements in certain aspects of life.

Critical Thinking Checks for the Collect Plan for This Patient's Schizophrenia Current Symptoms/Presentation

Early in a hospitalization for acute psychosis, the pharmacist has to determine the **accuracy** of the information the patient will be able to provide. Additionally, if the patient is paranoid, the pharmacist needs to be cautious as the patient may not trust them nor be willing to share information. To build a trusting relationship with the patient, it is important for the pharmacist to be **fair-minded**: to be nonjudgmental and refrain from any biases.

When considering the patient's age, disease prognosis, and response and intolerability of medications, it is important to think **broadly**, to take into consideration what medications they may be willing to take, and the effectiveness, safety, and adherence to the treatment plan. It is important to be **fact-based** and avoid **anchoring bias or framing effect** by collecting our own information from the medical record prior to developing a treatment plan.

In **fairness** to the patient, a patient-centered care approach allowing the patient, even if experiencing psychosis or paranoia, to make a choice in their therapeutic plan can increase cooperation, buy-in, and long-term adherence.

It is critical for the pharmacist to focus on collecting the most **relevant** information regarding vital signs, allergies, and labs. This will include the patient's weight, due to the metabolic risk of antipsychotics.

 KEY POINT

To build a trusting relationship with the patient, it is important for the pharmacist to be fair-minded: to be nonjudgmental and refrain from any biases.

Collected Current Symptoms/Presentation of Schizophrenia Entered into the Medical Record

Current symptoms include auditory hallucinations, persecutory delusions (belief that food is poisoned), thought disorganization (thought blocking, loose associations), and negative symptoms (isolation). These symptoms have impacted his ability to sleep, obtain proper nutrition, participate in activities of daily living (eg, showering), and maintain social interactions with family. He also experiences anxiety as the result of his hallucinations and delusions. His goal is to reduce his voices without experiencing movement-related adverse effects.

Example Collect Statement for Arlo J.

AJ is a 25-year-old male who presented with worsening psychosis (voices/paranoia), increased isolation, and reduced self-care in the context of reducing his quetiapine dose. He has a past medical history of DVT (provoked; therapy completed) and schizophrenia, paranoid type. His inpatient orders on admission were quetiapine (100 mg at bedtime, indication: schizophrenia), benztropine (0.5 mg BID, indication: EPS), and nicotine 14 mg/24 hr patch (new on admission). He was taking clonazepam (0.5 mg BID, indication: anxiety), but it was not restarted based on UDS results that were negative for all substances including benzodiazepines.

He reports he did not feel like the quetiapine was working, even at the higher dose. He also reported significant sedation with the quetiapine. He reports previously taking haloperidol, which caused EPS, but he did not like to take it, because it "made him shaky and stiff." He also took risperidone tablets by mouth in the past and paliperidone long-acting injection. He reports his voices were "manageable" but never fully went away. He did not like the pain of the injection, but is willing to take an injection again if needed. He did not like being "shaky" and said the benztropine helped, but he often feels like he has a "cotton mouth" with this medication. AJ cannot recall if he had shakiness on quetiapine and reports he has only taken the benztropine in combination with the quetiapine together.

He denies any current symptoms of depression or suicidal ideation. He reports he gets anxious when the voices tell him to do something, for example, jump out of a moving car. He reports continued anxiety related to fears that people are out to harm him and that people are poisoning his food. He is only willing to accept packaged foods from nursing staff or unopened juices or bottled water. He reports having taken escitalopram, fluoxetine, and venlafaxine in the past for depression. AJ states he has continued to take his clonazepam as prescribed, because it reduces his anxiety related to his voices. As the team collects more history, it appears his anxiety is related to his symptoms of psychosis and he does not meet the criteria for a generalized anxiety disorder (GAD).

His reported allergy to haloperidol, changed to intolerance based on reaction: extrapyramidal symptoms. Weight: 159 lb, height: 69 in; BP, RR, temp, LFTs, lipids, A1C, glucose: WNL.

Pertinent Mental Status Exam findings include poor hygiene with hair and beard disheveled, wearing wrinkled pajamas midday; poor eye contact, frequently looks to other parts of the room, cooperative; normal speech tone and volume with frequent pauses; mood "fine"; affect flat; thought process tangential, thought blocking, occasional loose associations; delusions of persecution (being poisoned), auditory hallucinations; no suicidal or homicidal ideation; insight good; judgment good.

He denies smoking marijuana, drinks no more than three beers once to twice monthly, smokes ½ to one pack of cigarettes per day, and denies other illicit substances. He prefers to eat out at fast food restaurants (burgers, fries, and milkshakes), does not eat vegetables regularly, but eats a banana most days. When stable, he reports going to the gym two to three times/week. He is currently covered on his parents' private insurance policy.

Assessment of Collected Information

During the Assess phase of the PPCP, the acute care psychiatric pharmacist will evaluate subjective and objective information collected during the collect phase. During this step, it is important to keep in mind the symptomatology of the patient and the **validity** of the information obtained. To fully assess the data collected, ideally, information should be **verified for accuracy** with pharmacy records, outside provider notes, or family/caregiver/facility input, and collateral information obtained to confirm the patient's report to ensure it is **undistorted**. In **fairness** to the patient, we should take into consideration the patient's motivation for taking and discontinuation of medications and their personal goals of treatment. When assessing the information obtained, it is important to take into account past medication responses and the side effects that patients find most concerning. Also, in **fairness** to the patient, we want to make sure we are making decisions **specific** to this patient's needs and **free of bias** from past experiences with other patients with schizophrenia.

ASSESS: Schizophrenia and History of Anxiety	
Conclusions	Rationale
Schizophrenia: Currently uncontrolled	AJ reports hearing voices and worrying his food has been poisoned. His family reports lack of motivation.
	He reports having reduced/discontinued his quetiapine. Pharmacy records indicate that his quetiapine was last filled over 6 weeks ago, also indicating he is not taking it as prescribed.
Schizophrenia: Meets criteria for treatment-resistant schizophrenia	AJ tried at least two antipsychotics including haloperidol, paliperidone, and quetiapine at adequate dosages and for an adequate period of time, and still reports continuing to hear voices when treated with the above antipsychotics. Therefore, he meets the criteria for treatment-resistant schizophrenia.[15,16]

Schizophrenia: Patient is sensitive to EPS side effects of antipsychotics; does not currently exhibit symptoms of tardive dyskinesia	AJ reports an "allergy" to haloperidol. He was prescribed benztropine for EPS in the past. He subjectively reported did not like the "shakiness." His AIMS score was zero.
Schizophrenia: Patient is not currently experiencing metabolic adverse effects of antipsychotics	AJ's BMI and weight are not indicative of obesity or malnutrition at baseline and his lipids and A1C are WNL.
Anxiety: Unclear historical diagnosis; does not currently meet the criteria for GAD; therefore, no standing medication needed at this time.	Reported anxiety and use of clonazepam is related to paranoia and uncontrolled schizophrenia more so than a GAD.
Anxiety: Cannot determine clonazepam adherence based on UDS results alone.	AJ reports adherence to clonazepam and taking his dose daily as prescribed (subjective data). Review of PDMP records indicate clonazepam was filled within the past 14 days, which supports that he was filling and picking it up regularly (objective data). This conflicts with his UDS, which is negative for benzodiazepines (objective data).
	However, in this case, we cannot make a definite determination regarding adherence to clonazepam based on UDS results alone. Clonazepam frequently is a "false negative" on many hospital UDS that are screening for nonconjugated forms of oxazepam or metabolites of nordiazepam, thus it does not provide an accurate picture of adherence.[22] We also need to take into consideration refill history, patient report, and weigh the risk of benzodiazepine withdrawal if he was indeed taking it daily and we do not restart it.

Critical Thinking Checks for Assessing This Patient's Schizophrenia

When assessing information prior to determining a plan, it is important to think **deeply** and **broadly** and with an **objective**, **fair-minded** perspective, to arrive at a **clear** and **accurate** diagnostic understanding and to determine **exact** symptoms to treat, to help assure optimal care is provided to the patient.

- In the case of AJ to reduce risk of **diagnosis momentum bias** the pharmacist reviewed past outpatient notes and noted he was originally diagnosed with depression with psychotic features, even in the absence of depressive symptoms. Three years ago, the diagnosis was changed to schizophrenia. The assessment of the current target symptoms the patient was experiencing, which included psychosis, voices and paranoia, and the denial of any mood symptoms, is consistent with schizophrenia.

- The continued diagnosis of depression with psychotic features may also represent an unconscious racial/ethnic bias. Data support the notion that Black patients are more frequently diagnosed with schizophrenia, while White patients are more frequently diagnosed with a mood disorder.[35-37] This is likely the result of racial biases versus biological differences and can contribute to misdiagnosis, which can delay appropriate treatment. In this case, AJ spent several years being treated with antidepressants instead of antipsychotics before his diagnosis was updated and effective treatments targeted at his symptoms of psychosis were offered. It is important for pharmacists to be aware of the **complex** ways race and ethnicity may contribute to diagnosis, treatment, assessment, and access to care, so that they may critically evaluate their impacts on patient care.

Critical Thinking Checks for Assessing This Patient's Schizophrenia

- Recognition of the correct diagnosis also provides **clarity** on how to approach the mood and anxiety symptoms AJ has reported. Treating those as separate diagnoses in the past did not yield positive results (eg, antidepressants did not relieve symptoms). It is important to note that depressive symptoms in persons with schizophrenia may improve, as psychosis improves with antipsychotic treatment alone, and it has been suggested to reassess depressive symptoms after psychosis improves/resolves rather than immediately starting an antidepressant.[38]

To evaluate this patient's past treatment properly, the past medical records were reviewed to consider all **relevant** and **significant** information needed, including past antipsychotic trials (dose, duration), side effects and current risk for side effects. This evaluation is important to support a **credible and reasonable** pharmacotherapy plan.

- For AJ, we were confident that since he was experiencing symptoms despite having at least two adequate trials of antipsychotics at adequate doses and adequate duration, that he met the criteria for treatment-resistant schizophrenia[16]
- To be **fair** and **objective**, it will be important to be aware of potential biases of providers and caregivers that might negatively impact drug selection. For example, some providers and social workers are hesitant to prescribe clozapine because of perceived barriers to access, before even offering it as an option to the patient and caregiver.

 KEY POINT

When assessing information prior to determining a plan, it is important to think deeply and broadly and with an objective, fair-minded perspective, to arrive at a clear and accurate diagnostic understanding, to determine exact symptoms to treat, and to help assure optimal care is provided to the patient.

Critical Thinking Checks: Clonazepam Adherence and Anxiety

To make sure our assessment was **clear, accurate,** and **precise**, we took a **broad** perspective, evaluating information collected from the patient, the PDMP, and the **validity** of the hospital UDS. We also used information from the provider's assessment to **clarify** his diagnosis.

- The patient continued to report adherence to clonazepam despite a negative UDS.
- Before concluding that he was not taking clonazepam at home, other plausible hypotheses were considered. We learned the UDS at our hospital only tests for free or nonconjugated forms of oxazepam or nordiazepam metabolites, a common limitation of many general UDS.[21,22] Clonazepam often tests negative as it is primarily reduced to 7-aminoclonazepam, and does not have an oxazepam or conjugated metabolite; therefore, it does not cross-react with this specific immunoassay screen.[22]
- Using **logic** and knowledge of medicinal chemistry, the pharmacist **reasonably** concluded the UDS results did not **accurately** reflect his adherence to clonazepam and presented as a false-negative. In **fairness** to the patient, this information was presented to the team to support the idea that he was most likely indeed taking his clonazepam.
- As the team collects more history, it becomes **clearer** that his anxiety is related to his symptoms of psychosis and does not meet the **objective** criteria for GAD.

ASSESS: Smoking Cessation	
Conclusion	**Rationale**
Nicotine Use Disorder: 1. At risk for nicotine withdrawal due to inability to smoke while an inpatient 2. Candidate for smoking-cessation therapy postdischarge with potential consequences for medication therapy	1. Smoking is not permitted in an inpatient setting and given that the inpatient psychiatric is a locked unit, patients cannot leave and smoke outside. In AJ's case, suddenly going from ½–1 pack per day down to no cigarettes can lead to nicotine withdrawal, which can lead to discomfort and agitation. Accordingly, his inpatient orders included nicotine 14 mg/24 hr patch. 2. It will be appropriate to assess AJ's desire to quit smoking postdischarge. If he is precontemplative about stopping his use of cigarettes, it will be critical to assess the potential impact of the decreased CYP1A2 activity that may result from smoking cessation, on planning for his medication therapy.[28–30]

Critical Thinking Checks: Smoking Cessation

Thinking **deeply** to understand the **implications** of not being able to smoke in an inpatient unit is critical for AJ's care. These implications include the risk for nicotine withdrawal and the possibility that his withdrawal symptoms could be misperceived as being related to his acute psychosis, the possibility that he may desire smoking cessation therapy postdischarge, and the potential effects on drug therapy due to the role of cigarette smoking in enzyme induction.

ASSESS: Drug Therapy Problems	
Conclusions	**Rationale**
Need additional therapy/ineffective drug Dosage too low: quetiapine	AJ self-reduced his quetiapine dose from 400 mg at bedtime to 200 mg at bedtime. Typical doses of quetiapine in schizophrenia are 400 to 600 mg per day; thus, 200 mg per day is subtherapeutic. Furthermore, based on his report and family's report, the current antipsychotic regimen does not appear to be working for treating his voices and schizophrenia symptoms.
Unnecessary drug therapy: benztropine	During AJ's physical exam, no extrapyramidal symptoms were noted. AJ had been prescribed benztropine since he was on risperidone, paliperidone, and haloperidol in the past. It is possible benztropine was carried forward and never discontinued, even after risperidone and haloperidol were discontinued.
Unknown adherence: clonazepam	Most general drug screens commonly detect metabolites of oxazepam and nordiazepam, not clonazepam. It is common to see a false-negative report for benzodiazepines for clonazepam.[21,22]

Unnecessary drug therapy versus risk for adverse drug reaction	The patient reports taking clonazepam regularly at home, which is supported by PDMP records. Given the limitations with UDS results for clonazepam, it is most likely this was a false negative. The indication for long-term use remains unclear, especially since the treatment team ruled out a diagnosis of GAD. However, given his chronic use prior to hospitalization, not resuming could result in benzodiazepine withdrawal and leave his symptoms of anxiety (likely related to his symptoms of schizophrenia) untreated. Continuation of current clonazepam is indicated but consider recommending further evaluation of current anxiety to determine if continuation or dose optimization of clonazepam is indicated.
Dosage too low: Nicotine	Based on AJ's report of smoking ½ to 1 pack per day, the dose of 14 mg/24 hr is too low based on his current cigarette usage. This could increase his risk or nicotine withdrawal and agitation if not adequately treated, which could be perceived as related to his acute psychosis instead of nicotine withdrawal. For someone who smokes $\geq$10 cigarettes per day, the recommended nicotine replacement transdermal dose is 21 mg/24 hr patch.[39]

Critical Thinking Checks for Assessing Arlo J.'s Drug Therapy Problems

Given the complexities associated with AJ's diagnoses, clinical status, and therapy, there are numerous considerations for the assessment of AJ's drug therapy problems that require **deep** thinking to draw the **clear**, **accurate**, **precise**, and **fair-minded** conclusions that will be critical for therapeutic planning and implementation and for expressing the conclusions in a manner that can be clearly understood by other stakeholders.

- Before concluding that he was not taking clonazepam at home, other **plausible** hypotheses were considered. Before making recommendations to adjust doses of quetiapine or nicotine, the **relevance** of patients' reports and concerns were taken into account.
- Additionally, the **interrelationships** of all of his symptoms, medications, and disease states were taken into consideration. An example of a concept map that can be useful to help grasp these interrelationships is shown in **Figure 7-3**.

Example Assess Statement for Arlo J.

AJ is a 25-year-old male presenting with worsening psychotic symptoms including voices and paranoia and decreased activities of daily living.

1. Schizophrenia—Uncontrolled with an acute exacerbation of symptoms of psychosis. Currently undertreated.

   Patient is currently reporting positive symptoms of schizophrenia including hearing voices and paranoia. He is observed to be responding to internal stimuli. These symptoms are affecting his sleep, his eating, and overall ability to function. Although he is currently prescribed the antipsychotic quetiapine, he is taking a suboptimal dose (200 mg), despite being prescribed 400 mg.

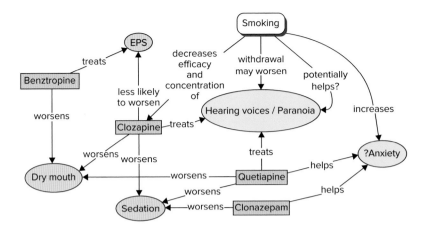

FIGURE 7-3. Concept map depicting interrelationships between this patient's symptoms, medications, and disease states.

Per history obtained, he has trialed multiple antipsychotics at adequate doses, for adequate duration, and reports his symptoms never fully go away. He has also discontinued past medications secondary to adverse effects. Given he has trialed more than two antipsychotics, without adequate response, he meets criteria of treatment-resistant schizophrenia; and a trial of clozapine is warranted.[15,16]

AJ could benefit from selecting an antipsychotic with improved efficacy toward treating his symptoms of hallucinations and paranoia, while minimizing side effects. He also could benefit from counseling focused on the importance of medication adherence.

Drug therapy problems:

1. Dosage too low: quetiapine
2. Needs additional therapy: treatment-resistant schizophrenia
3. Unnecessary drug therapy: benztropine
4. Risk for inappropriate adherence

2. Agitation/Anxiety/Benzodiazepine use—Uncontrolled, acute on potentially chronic, yet unclear indication.

During an acute decompensation of schizophrenia, it is difficult to assess if he has a history of GAD versus if his anxiety and agitation are secondary to his symptoms of psychosis. At this point in treatment, we do want to minimize his anxiety and agitation and reduce risk of potential benzodiazepine withdrawal.

The patient reports taking his clonazepam to help with anxiety and when feeling paranoid. Despite a negative UDS for benzodiazepines, it is possible that he was indeed taking his clonazepam based on his report and refill history as clonazepam can cause a false negative. Unfortunately, we did not have access to a more sensitive liquid chromatography mass spectrometry (LCMS) laboratory report to confirm this in a timely manner. Therefore, in his case, the risk of benzodiazepine withdrawal if clonazepam is not restarted if he was indeed taking it, outweighs the concern of restarting him on a benzodiazepine if he was not actually taking it.

If his anxiety and agitation are primarily driven by his symptoms of psychosis and paranoia and we adequately treat his schizophrenia, it is possible that his anxiety may improve and a benzodiazepine may no longer be indicated (nor would a first-line treatment for GAD such as an SSRI). If clonazepam is no longer indicated, we will need to develop a slow tapering plan.

Drug therapy problem:

Unnecessary drug therapy versus risk for potential adverse drug reaction: clonazepam

3. History of DVT—Provoked; therapy completed.

Inpatient psychiatry differs from other acute medical floors in that patients are mostly ambulatory and encouraged to leave their rooms. Inpatient psychiatry usually has a dayroom, where patients are encouraged to eat, play games, watch television, and interact with other patients. They are also encouraged to attend group educational meetings. Thus, routine DVT prophylaxis is not indicated for all patients. While inpatient, observe if AJ remains in his room primarily in bed versus if he is ambulatory; and determine if DVT prophylaxis for him is indicated.

4. Smoking/nicotine use disorder/nicotine withdrawal—nicotine withdrawal is acute, symptomatic, and undertreated in the presence of a chronic, moderate nicotine use disorder.

AJ reports smoking ½ to 1 pack of cigarettes per day. On day one of admission, he has not expressed an interest to quit smoking; however, because he will be unable to smoke while hospitalized, he is at risk for nicotine withdrawal, which could impact/worsen his agitation. The currently prescribed dose of nicotine 14 mg/24 hr transdermal daily is too low based on his current cigarette usage.[39]

Smoking cessation would be beneficial for him given his history of DVT. Furthermore, if he plans to resume smoking after discharge, this will need to be taken into account as it can impact the serum concentrations of antipsychotics metabolized via CYP1A2 pathway.[28–30]

Drug therapy problem:

Dosage too low: Transdermal nicotine

The conclusions drawn in the Assess step of the PPCP process serve as the basis for the therapeutic decision-making that will occur in the Plan step.

Plan, Implement, and Monitor

PLAN: Goals	
Conclusions:	Rationale: Information or Premise to Support the Conclusion
For Schizophrenia: 1. Within 1 to 2 weeks at a target dose of antipsychotic, voices/hallucinations will be minimized to a point where the patient no longer reports distress and paranoia will have decreased to the point the patient is comfortable eating unpackaged food.	1. AJ currently reports hearing voices and is visually seen responding to internal stimuli, which supports that he is acutely experiencing positive symptoms of schizophrenia and has an indication to start an antipsychotic.

2. Within 1 to 2 weeks at a target dose of antipsychotic, decrease negative symptoms of psychosis to the point the patient is able to maintain appropriate hygiene, and leave his room unprompted at least once per day. Once appropriate for groups, attend at least one patient group activity per day within 7 to 14 days of starting a therapeutic dose of a new antipsychotic.

3. Consistently take medications as prescribed, missing no more than 20% of scheduled doses throughout the admission and no more than 48 hours of consecutive doses.

4. Decrease risk of EPS or will not experience EPS. The patient's score on the Modified Simpson Angus Scale should remain below 3 throughout the admission.

5. For a minimum of 48 hours prior to discharge, avoid the need for PRN antipsychotics or benzodiazepines to treat psychosis, agitation, or anxiety.

2. Current symptoms of schizophrenia that are impacting quality of life and ability to safely discharge are auditory hallucinations, delusions that his food is being poisoned, limited self-care, and isolation. Positive symptoms are typically faster to respond to medications than negative symptoms, with improvement starting to be seen within one week, on average.[40] Negative symptoms may take longer to treat, so the goal is to see some improvement but not full resolution prior to discharge.

3. Nonadherence to medications was a precipitating factor for this admission, so it is important that he regularly takes his medications during his stay to get into the habit of daily medication and to ensure medications remain at steady-state levels to allow for proper assessment of effects. Due to clozapine's short half-life, if it is discontinued for more than 2 days, it must be retitrated.[41]

4. AJ has previously stopped medications due to adverse effects, including "shakiness" (EPS), and is currently reporting bothersome adverse effects (dry mouth) so it is important to minimize risks through medication selection, regular monitoring, and efficient management. Utilization of clozapine should help reduce EPS symptoms. Patient also reports dry mouth; discontinuing benztropine may help reduce dry mouth; however, clozapine is very anticholinergic and may cause/worsen this adverse effect.

5. He is currently requiring one to two PRNs per day to manage severe, distressing voices that cause anxiety. These symptoms will need to decrease before he is able to be safely discharged.

For Anxiety/Benzodiazepine Use:

1. Prevent benzodiazepine withdrawal such that symptoms on the Clinical Institute Withdrawal Scale—Benzodiazepines (CIWA-B) will remain below 20 throughout the admission.

2. Maintain the anxiety severity under the patient's goal level of 3/10 for at least 48 hours prior to discharge.

1. One of the first rules of medicine is medicine, is "first do no harm."[42] If this patient was indeed taking clonazepam daily, and this is withheld on admission, he would be at risk of benzodiazepine withdrawal, which could lead to hallucinations, paranoia, agitation, insomnia, and even seizures, which could be fatal.[43] If clonazepam is restarted and he was not actually taking it, we may start an unnecessary medication and increase risk of sedation; however, the consequences of this are less severe than the complications of benzodiazepine withdrawal.

2. AJ continues to report anxiety secondary to his hallucinations and delusions, so it is important to provide patient-centered treatments.

For Smoking/Nicotine Use Disorder/ Nicotine Withdrawal:	
1. Patient will experience minimal symptoms of nicotine withdrawal while hospitalized. 2. Patient will accept counseling on benefits of smoking cessation and risks of continued smoking.	1. Smoking is not permitted in an inpatient setting. Suddenly going from ½—1 pack per day down to no cigarettes can lead to nicotine withdrawal, which can lead to discomfort and agitation. 2. Smoking can also induce CYP1A2, which may decrease the level of some antipsychotics including clozapine, making them less effective.[28–30] Because this does not align with his treatment goals, AJ expressed a desire to permanently quit smoking.

Critical Thinking Checks for Developing This Patient's Goals

The SMART goals were developed with **clear** understanding of the patient's diagnosis and consideration of all members of the interprofessional treatment team and the patient.

The SMART goals were developed with the intention of achieving the best possible outcomes for this patient's individual needs, incorporating the patient's **clear** understanding of what is achievable for meeting his healthcare wants and needs.

The SMART goals set for this patient is **clearly** stated including their timeframe and expected outcomes.

The SMART goals were developed in consideration of the most **significant** factors affecting this patient's health and the most **significant** expected outcomes.

The SMART goals were developed with a **fair and objective** consideration and participation of the patient, with a **clear** patient awareness of the importance of continued monitoring of his clozapine. Additionally, the goals were developed with the patient without the undue influence of emotions or biases and in a manner that empowers him to self-manage his health and health behaviors.

The SMART goals were developed with **deep** consideration of this patient's future outcomes and access to care, clozapine, and labs.

The SMART goals make **logical** sense based on disease pathophysiology, a full assessment of the patient, clinical guidelines, potential therapeutic strategies, and what is realistically achievable for this patient.

 KEY POINT

SMART goals are developed with a fair and objective consideration and participation of the patient, with a clear patient awareness of the importance of continued monitoring of his clozapine Additionally, the goals were developed with the patient without the undue influence of emotions or biases and in a manner that empowers him to self-manage his health and health behaviors.

Based on the pharmacists' knowledge of guidelines and monitoring, they logically and critically evaluate the pros and cons of different therapeutic options and discusses them with the team, the patient, and the caregivers. Conclusions are drawn based on the patient's input on desired outcomes and adverse effects to avoid, and critically thinking about access to medications and about which medications can yield the best outcomes.

PLAN: Schizophrenia

Goals:

1. Within 1 to 2 weeks at a target dose of antipsychotic, voices/hallucinations will be minimized to a point where the patient no longer reports distress and paranoia will have decreased to the point the patient is comfortable eating unpackaged food.

2. Within 1 to 2 weeks at a target dose of antipsychotic, decrease negative symptoms of psychosis to the point the patient is able to maintain appropriate hygiene, and leave his room unprompted at least once per day. Once appropriate for groups, attend at least one patient group activity per day within 7 to 14 days of starting a therapeutic dose of a new antipsychotic.

3. Consistently take medications as prescribed, missing no more than 20% of scheduled doses throughout the admission and no more than 48 hours of consecutive doses.

4. Decrease risk of EPS/Will not experience EPS. The patient's score on the Modified Simpson Angus Scale should remain below 3 throughout the admission.

5. For a minimum of 48 hours prior to discharge, avoid the need for PRN antipsychotics or benzodiazepines to treat psychosis, agitation, or anxiety.

Conclusions	Rationale: Information or Premise to Support the Conclusion
Initiate clozapine 12.5 mg at bedtime and titrate by 12.5 to 25 mg/day as tolerated.	Due to its risk for severe orthostatic hypotension, clozapine needs to be initiated low and titrated slowly. In the inpatient setting, since we can assess vital signs and dizziness daily, we may increase the dose on a daily basis.
	Initiation of clozapine will target reduction of positive symptoms of schizophrenia (hallucinations and paranoia), and also help improve the negative symptoms (Goals 1 and 2). Clozapine will also be less likely to cause EPS than most other antipsychotic options (Goal 4).
	Clozapine was also chosen in consideration of the long-term benefit of the medication and the likelihood that it would be efficacious in managing symptoms without the need for PRNs (Goal 5).
Discontinue benztropine	Discontinuation of benztropine, an anticholinergic medication, will help reduce AJ's current complaint of dry mouth, which is likely caused by benztropine.
	Furthermore, benztropine is used primarily to treat the EPS adverse effects of antipsychotics. At this time, benztropine is no longer indicated as he is being switched to clozapine, which has a very low risk of EPS (Goal 4). Furthermore, clozapine is also extremely anticholinergic, so continuation of benztropine will increase risk of anticholinergic adverse effects (eg, constipation, dry mouth, tachycardia).
Cross titrate from quetiapine to clozapine. Continue quetiapine 100 mg nightly until the patient is at 100 mg nightly of clozapine, then discontinue quetiapine.	Since clozapine needs to be started well below typical therapeutic doses and slowly titrated, cross-titrations are often helpful so that patients have some therapeutic antipsychotic exposure when starting clozapine. Although AJ was prescribed quetiapine 400 mg nightly, he was inconsistently taking it and often only took 200 mg. Since his last dose was three days prior to admission, 100 mg would be an appropriate dose to restart inpatient therapy and to provide during the cross-titration.

	In addition to AJ feeling that quetiapine was not effective and causing adverse effects, there is little evidence to support the routine use of antipsychotic polypharmacy, so quetiapine will be reduced and ultimately discontinued. The plan to cross-titrate was chosen to help minimize the use of PRN medications for agitation while titrating clozapine to a therapeutic dose, which will target reduction of positive symptoms of schizophrenia (hallucinations and paranoia), and also help improve the negative symptoms (Goals 1, 2, and 5).
Educate on the use of clozapine, including the importance of adherence.	Clozapine requires significant patient education to ensure safe and appropriate use. Patients should be made aware of common and severe adverse effects and what to do should they occur. They should be provided with information on the required blood testing and given resources for follow-up. Patients should also be counseled on the importance of adherence, since clozapine needs to be retitrated if more than 48 hours of doses are missed (Goal 3).

 KEY POINT

Clozapine requires significant patient education to ensure safe and appropriate use. Patients should be made aware of common and severe adverse effects and what to do should they occur.

One approach for supporting therapeutic decision-making and expressing its reasoning is to create an argument map that begins with the assessment and ends with the conclusion of which therapy to recommend. An argument map supporting the recommendation of clozapine for this patient is shown in **Figure 7-4**. This map describes the structure of the argument including conclusions that were drawn secondary to the assessment that support the SMART Goal.

Critical Thinking Checks: Schizophrenia

As the pharmacist on an inpatient interprofessional team, a key service we provide is providing a **comprehensive** and **well-founded** recommendation to help the psychiatric team choose an antipsychotic medication that a patient can access, is willing to take, will help with the target symptoms, have reduced or tolerable side effects, and have minimal interactions with their other medications. At times, the pharmacist may bring an **alternative perspective** after discussion with the patient, which may ultimately change the team's initial pharmacotherapy plan.

Knowledge of AJ's relevant medication history and symptoms allowed for the development of a **logical** medication plan backed by treatment guidelines and medication receptor binding profiles. Thinking **broadly** and **deeply** about the patient's goals, concerns, and social supports enabled the development of **clear** and **fair-minded** recommendations.

By **objectively** evaluating relevant information, the pharmacist was able to avoid common forms of bias. When considering clozapine for a patient, providers often raise concerns about an individual's interest in a medication with the potential for significant adverse effects (possibly driven by **confirmation bias**) and their ability to adhere to the complex treatment and monitoring requirements. While it is important to be mindful of common barriers to treatment, **framing effect** and **groupthink** can lead to **inaccurate** conclusions and dismissal of this medication option if concerns are not considered and evaluated using **clear** and **objective** information **specific** to the individual receiving treatment.

The pharmacist's understanding of the **complexities** of schizophrenia and the medications used to treat it allowed for a **comprehensive** evaluation of treatment options. While multiple options existed, clozapine was chosen as it aligned best with the patient's goals of decreasing auditory hallucinations and persecutory delusions while avoiding adverse effects he had experienced with other medications. His ability to participate in weekly monitoring was verified.

Recommendation **Clozapine** **Initial dose day 1: 12.5 mg at bedtime** **Titrate by 12.5 to 25 mg/day to a minimum target dose of 250 or 300 mg/day**				
Patient has tried at least two antipsychotics at therapeutic doses for adequate time and reported continuing to continue to experience paranoia and voices.	Clozapine is indicated for treatment-resistant schizophrenia and is supported/ recommended by both the Canadian Psychiatric Association's 2017 Guidelines and the American Psychiatric Association's 2020 Guidelines.[15,44]	Clozapine has a low risk of EPS. Therefore, we can discontinue benztropine. Clozapine does cause dizziness, sedation, and anticholinergic side effects, so we need to monitor in this patient who has reported these side effects with other antipsychotics.	There are no absolute contraindications to clozapine for this patient. All second-generation antipsychotics carry risk of venous thromboem-bolism. Patient reports smoking, therefore, CYP1A2 drug–drug interaction will need to be considered when discussing target dose, if he decides not to stop smoking after discharge.	Assumption to verify: Patient is willing and able to get weekly blood draws.
SMART Goal				
Within 1 to 2 weeks at a target dose of clozapine, voices/hallucinations will be minimized to a point where the patient no longer reports distress,paranoia will have decreased to the point that the patient is comfortable eating unpackaged food, and negative symptoms will have improved to the point that the patient is able to maintain appropriate hygiene and leave his room unprompted at least once a day.				
Assessment				
Uncontrolled schizophrenia with contributing factors that include inappropriate adherence to quetiapine and manifesting as inadequate control of symptoms. Drug therapy Problem: Need for additional therapy				

FIGURE 7-4. Argument map for the recommendation of clozapine for this patient.

KEY POINT

By objectively evaluating relevant information in the development of a comprehensive and well-founded recommendation to help the psychiatric team choose an antipsychotic medication, the pharmacist is able to avoid common forms of bias.

PLAN: Anxiety/Benzodiazepine Use

Goals:

1. Prevent benzodiazepine withdrawal such that symptoms on the Clinical Institute Withdrawal Scale—Benzodiazepines (CIWA-B) will remain below 20 throughout the admission.

2. Maintain the anxiety severity below the patient's goal level of 3/10 for at least 48 hours prior to discharge.

Conclusions	Rationale: Information or Premise to Support the Conclusion
Refer patient for GAD assessment; no antidepressant indicated at this time	Based on recent provider evaluations, AJ does not meet criteria for GAD; therefore, first-line treatment with an antidepressant is not indicated. It is anticipated the treatment of schizophrenia will improve mood, anxiety, and paranoia symptoms (Goal 2).
Restart clonazepam 0.5 mg BID with plan to taper	While cross-titrating antipsychotic medications, AJ would be at risk for subtherapeutic drug concentrations and subsequent increases in symptoms. This could worsen his anxiety and agitation, making it reasonable to have medications available to help manage such symptoms. Additionally, based on the assessment of his recent benzodiazepine use, the patient would be at risk for benzodiazepine withdrawal if the medication were to be held or discontinued during the admission.[43] Given the serious and potentially fatal consequences of withdrawal, the benefits of resuming his outpatient regimen outweigh risks. Additionally, stopping clonazepam abruptly may put him at risk for clonazepam-withdrawal catatonia.[45] This would not only complicate his presentation, but it would also make treating schizophrenia difficult due to the deleterious effects antipsychotics can have on catatonia.[46] Clonazepam was restarted to reduce risk of benzodiazepine withdrawal and to help manage anxiety and agitation (Goals 1 and 2). During hospitalization, his clonazepam was reduced to 0.25 mg in the morning and 0.5 mg at bedtime. In the future, a slow taper should be continued if he is unable to tolerate the pharmacodynamic interaction between this and other sedating medications (clozapine) or if his symptoms of anxiety resolve once his persecutory delusions are reduced.

Critical Thinking Checks: Anxiety/Benzodiazepine Use

The decision not to begin an antidepressant for this patient was based on a **deep** understanding of the factors contributing to his presentation and the way additional medications may interact with current treatments. Relying on **critical**, **objective**, and **accurate** information regarding the patient's symptoms and diagnosis aided the pharmacist in avoiding **anchoring bias**, which may have otherwise led to the decision to treat an anxiety disorder.

By **clarifying** the patient's history of benzodiazepine use through **verifiable** dispense data, the pharmacist was positioned to consider the risks and benefits of resuming treatment. While long-term use might not be indicated, the **implications** of suddenly stopping treatment make it not only **reasonable** but necessary to resume treatment during this admission. By taking into account **pertinent** pharmacodynamic and pharmacokinetic information, the pharmacist prioritized avoiding harm to the patient.

PLAN: Smoking/Nicotine Use Disorder/Nicotine Withdrawal

Goals:
1. Patient will experience minimal symptoms of nicotine withdrawal while hospitalized.
2. Patient will accept counseling on benefits of smoking cessation and risks of continued smoking.

Conclusions	Rationale: Information or Premise to Support the Conclusion
Minimize nicotine withdrawal by increasing nicotine patch dose to 21 mg/24 hr daily	Based on report of smoking 10+ cigarettes per day, the recommended initial dose of nicotine patch is 21 mg daily to avoid symptoms of nicotine withdrawal (Goal 1).
Offer nicotine transdermal at discharge	As AJ's symptoms of schizophrenia begin to improve, we will continue to educate him on the benefits of smoking cessation, treatment options, and the impact of smoking on his medications postdischarge (Goal 2).
	Per the Joint Commission hospital-based inpatient psychiatric services (HBIPS) tobacco measures, this patient was identified as a tobacco user within the past 30 days, and therefore was offered an FDA-approved smoking cessation product nicotine transdermal patches.[47] Dose of transdermal nicotine 21 mg/24 hr was determined because the patient smokes at least ½ pack (>10 cigarettes) per day.[39] Although the psychiatric risk of varenicline is less than originally thought, the psychiatry providers were more comfortable starting nicotine replacement therapy over varenicline in this patient with decompensated schizophrenia.[48]

Critical Thinking Checks: Smoking Cessation

By having **clarity** regarding AJ's outpatient smoking habits, the pharmacist was able to **anticipate** that he may experience nicotine withdrawal while inpatient, since he would not have access to cigarettes. **Understanding the relationship** between nicotine withdrawal, mood, and agitation allowed for recognition of the **significant** impact this may have on his symptoms and the importance of providing treatment during his inpatient stay. Medications were chosen using a **deep** understanding of available literature.

In **fairness** to the patient, the pharmacist avoided making assumptions regarding his desire to stop smoking long term. However, the **impact** of smoking on AJ's new antipsychotic plan was noted, so **reasonable** adjustments could be made if he decided to resume his use of cigarettes upon discharge.

IMPLEMENT/MONITOR → Psychiatric	
1. Clozapine for uncontrolled schizophrenia secondary to ineffective medications or not taking medications.	
2. Clonazepam to reduce risk of benzodiazepine withdrawal and treat agitation and anxiety.	
3. Nicotine replacement therapy for nicotine withdrawal	
Conclusions	**Rationale: Information or Premise to Support the Conclusion**
Implement: • Enroll the provider and patient in the Clozapine Risk Evaluation Mitigation Strategy (REMS) system[18] • Obtain and review baseline ANC • Obtain C-reactive protein (CRP), troponin, and electrocardiogram (ECG) • Start clozapine 12.5 mg at bedtime and titrate to target dose (Initial dose day 1: 12.5 mg at bedtime. Titrate by 12.5 to 25 mg/day to a minimum target dose of 250 or 300 mg per day.) • Prior to discharge, confirm availability of clozapine at local pharmacy • Restart clonazepam at home dose of 0.5 mg twice daily	*Implement:* To ensure access to clozapine, the pharmacist needs to confirm the patient and provider have been enrolled in the clozapine REMS to prevent any delay in treatment. The pharmacist works with the provider to ensure compliance with clozapine REMS.[18] Per program regulations, patients can obtain medication through the period of time before the next ANC check is due. For newly started patients, only one week of medication is authorized at a time. To adhere to REMS requirements, the pharmacist must confirm the patient's baseline ANC is above 1.5 k/µL prior to initiating clozapine. Results must be current (no more than one week old). For this patient, suggest ECG, CRP, and troponin at baseline given patient's history of DVT and clozapine's risk of myocarditis and cardiomyopathy.[41] Not every pharmacy is enrolled in the clozapine REMS and has the ability to monitor clozapine or dispense clozapine. To be proactive, the pharmacist must work with the patient to identify a pharmacy that is able to dispense clozapine to ensure a smooth transition of care and reduce risk of relapse if someone cannot access their medication postdischarge. Clonazepam was restarted at home dose of 0.5 mg twice daily to reduce risk of withdrawal, and to help with agitation and anxiety. As his psychosis begins to improve, consider reducing dose by 0.25 mg per day prior to discharge.
Education to Patient: • Educate patient and family on role of clozapine for treatment-resistant schizophrenia • Educate patient on the importance of diet, exercise, and metabolic risk of clozapine	*Education:* Clozapine can cause several adverse effects. Patients should be aware of these risks, what to watch for, and what can be done to prevent or treat them.

• Educate patient on common adverse effects with clozapine, including sedation, dizziness, constipation, and drooling. • Educate patient on importance of blood draws and risk for neutropenia • To ensure ease of access, have patient teach back locations of pharmacies and how often he needs to get his blood drawn. • Confirm patient and family know where blood monitoring is available. Work with social worker to ensure this information is provided on discharge paperwork. • Educate patient on risk of continued smoking and impact on clozapine efficacy • Educate patient on the symptoms of anxiety and the goal of reducing clonazepam dosing.	Follow-up for required weekly blood work requires additional planning to ensure the logistics work out and the patient can access the care they need. While the patient's goal is to not return to smoking upon discharge, it is important that he understand the risks and impact of it in case he changes his mind. This will enhance agency and allow him to proactively seek care for monitoring and dose adjustments.
Education to Provider: • Educate provider on clozapine REMS • Inform the provider they can only write a prescription for a 7-day supply at discharge • Ensure provider provides a laboratory order for CBC with Differentials weekly at discharge • Educate provider about potential benzodiazepine taper strategies	*Education:* Provider education is important as there are several requirements that are unique to clozapine. Incorrect prescribing or failure to obtain required bloodwork can lead to delays in care, so it is important to be proactive and ensure the provider is aware of all required steps.
Monitor: • Monitor for adverse effects daily during rounds. For every adverse effect identified by the patient or treatment team, develop a management plan that results in the patient feeling comfortable continuing the treatment regimen. – Common adverse effects include weight gain, metabolic syndrome, constipation, drooling, and sedation. • Monitor for efficacy (reduction in hallucinations and delusions; improvement in agitation and self-care) while titrating and for at least 1 to 2 weeks after reaching the target dose. • While inpatient, complete weekly lab work for clozapine initiation. Within one week of discharge, complete required lab work, obtain refill of clozapine, and continue to complete follow-up with weekly lab work as indicated. • Monitor for symptoms of nicotine and benzodiazepine withdrawal. • Reassess if patient has any change in desire to quit smoking postdischarge. • Work with team regarding patient's plan to reinitiate smoking and include in discharge communication to outpatient provider that clozapine may require further adjustment.	*Monitor:* To continue to minimize adverse effects, the pharmacist should screen for common adverse effects of clozapine (eg, dizziness, sedation, dry mouth, drooling, constipation) each day while rounding on the patient.[41] Weekly ANC is required for the first 6 months of therapy, as per the clozapine REMS requirements to obtain refills and to continue clozapine.[18] On the inpatient unit, the pharmacist can ensure the order is in the day prior to blood work is due, and then review to ensure ANC has remained WNL to continue clozapine titration. The ANC must be reviewed by a pharmacist in the clozapine REMs prior to dispensing the clozapine. AJ has support from his family to provide transportation to the lab and pharmacy. He has insurance that will cover these costs. For antipsychotic metabolic monitoring, while inpatient, the pharmacist should ensure a baseline weight, lipid panel, and A1C were obtained. While inpatient, the pharmacist can also monitor for early weight gain.[15,17] Effective communication with the outpatient provider is important for optimizing the transition of AJ's care to the outpatient setting.

KEY POINT

Clozapine remains an effective antipsychotic for treatment-resistant schizophrenia and requires pharmacist involvement to ensure proper monitoring for severe neutropenia and other common side effects (eg, weight gain, constipation, orthostasis).

Critical Thinking Checks for Arlo J.'s Implementation and Monitoring Plan for Schizophrenia, Clozapine, and Resuming Clonazepam

The decision to start clozapine took into account all of the **complexities** to access and monitor clozapine and this patient's ability and willingness to adhere to treatment.

- The pharmacist looked at **alternative perspectives** prior to advocating for clozapine and presented a **rational** argument to the team and patient as to why this was the ideal treatment for AJ at this time.

When developing an implementation and monitoring plan, the pharmacist must think with a **broad** and **fair-minded** mindset that is inclusive of all stakeholders in the patient's care. For example, involving the patient and his support system in the implementation of the PPCP is important to increase chances of success postdischarge. On an inpatient treatment team, the pharmacist works alongside the psychiatrist to ensure implementation of the treatment plan and compliance with the clozapine REMS. They also work alongside social workers for discharge planning to ensure access to blood work and clozapine postdischarge.

- Recognizing an interruption in blood monitoring or not picking up a clozapine prescription can be an early warning sign of reduced adherence or future decompensation. A theory as to why some patients are successful on clozapine therapy is their frequent contact with the healthcare system.

Clear and concise education regarding the **explicit** need for clozapine blood monitoring and rationale as to why we had to find a different pharmacy (short-term) than his preferred pharmacy will help his engagement in the treatment plan.

- Proper education regarding the treatment options, adverse effects, and monitoring requirements helped AJ and his family understand the benefits and risks of each agent under consideration. It was important to take into consideration his past medication experiences and adverse effects while educating him on the risks with clozapine versus other antipsychotics. During the counseling session, the pharmacy team outlined the benefits, risks, and monitoring requirements of clozapine versus other antipsychotics. He was encouraged to ask questions and share which treatment choices he was most open to trying.

The decision to restart clonazepam was considered **deeply** and took into account the **applicability** of the UDS results, and that we could **not be free from doubt** as to whether or not he was taking his clonazepam at home. In **fairness** to the patient, we accepted his report that he was taking his clonazepam and resumed it to minimize risk of withdrawal.

KEY POINT

Involving the patient and his support system in the implementation of the PPCP is important to increase chances of success post-discharge.

Arlo J.'s Discharge

Prior to discharge, the patient reported no hallucinations. He was again willing to eat regular food and was not concerned that his food or drink were being poisoned.

At discharge, he had improved insight into his illness and was willing to continue to take medications to manage his psychiatric and medical conditions.

The patient was ultimately discharged on:

1. Clozapine 200 mg tablet—Take 1.5 tablets (300 mg) at bedtime
2. Clonazepam 0.5 mg tablet—Take 0.5 tablet (0.25 mg) in the morning and one tablet (0.5 mg) at bedtime with instructions to outside provider to consider a continued taper and ultimately a discontinuation.
3. Nicotine transdermal patch 21 mg/24 hr—Apply one patch daily

He was given instructions to follow-up with getting his blood drawn (for ANC) within 7 days of discharge, and a psychiatrist appointment was scheduled 2 weeks after discharge.

CONCLUSION

Managing schizophrenia in an acute psychiatric setting when the patient has uncontrolled symptoms and is paranoid can be a difficult and complex process, requiring excellent critical thinking and clinical reasoning in each step of the PPCP. This is particularly important if the patient is not trusting of the treatment team. However, one must remember that we should still take patient preferences into account, if feasible, and offer and advocate for evidence-based treatments with the best chance of success.

Pharmacists serve a vital role on the interprofessional acute psychiatric care team by providing evidence-based recommendations in consideration of drug–drug interactions and comorbid disease states, and they make recommend dosage adjustments based on the symptoms patients are experiencing and the side effects that they are reporting. Furthermore, although education sessions with the patient could be delayed during the admission until psychiatric symptoms have improved, by providing this education, pharmacists can help improve medication adherence as the patient understands the rationales, goals, and dosing of each medication.

Summary Points

- Patients receiving care in an acute care inpatient psychiatry unit may present with a variety of disease states, among them being schizophrenia. The role of pharmacists in this setting is diverse and includes applying their critical thinking and clinical reasoning skills to medication reconciliation, recognizing and managing drug therapy problems, input into pharmacotherapy plans, monitoring adverse effects, pharmacokinetic monitoring, and provider, patient, and caregiver education.
- In approaching the Collect step for the schizophrenia patient, using a biopsychosocial framework allows the pharmacist to consider and evaluate the multitude of factors that can influence the patient's illness presentation and course. To help assure accuracy of collected information when interviewing a patient in an acute psychiatric crisis, it is important for pharmacists to build a fair-minded, trusting relationship with the patient and to refrain from any biases. The patient's thought content and process should be taken into account, and attempts should be made to obtain collateral information to confirm the accuracy of information provided by the patient.
- When assessing collected information, it is important to think deeply and broadly and with an objective, fair-minded perspective, to arrive at a clear and accurate

diagnostic understanding and to determine exact symptoms to treat that will help assure optimal care is provided to the patient. It is important to recognize that nonadherence is common in patients with schizophrenia due to lack of insight, and negative views toward medication; thus, pharmacists can help identify barriers to adherence and work with patients to find a medication they are willing to continue.

- In the Plan step, SMART goals are developed with a fair and objective consideration and participation of the patient, without the undue influence of emotions or biases, and in a manner that empowers the patient to self-manage their health and health behaviors. In the development of a therapeutic plan for the patient, a key service provided by pharmacists on an inpatient interprofessional team is to apply their critical thinking skills and their understanding of the complexities of schizophrenia and medications to develop a comprehensive and well-founded recommendation that will help the psychiatric team choose an optimal treatment plan. Also, including the patient's input and perspective when choosing a medication may help improve adherence and long-term outcomes.

- To help assure successful implementation of the plan, there must be clarity to assure the patient has a firm understanding of the actions needed to achieve disease state goals. Clozapine, in particular, requires significant patient education about its adverse effects to ensure safe and appropriate use. Provider education is also important, as there are several requirements that are unique to clozapine. Communication should occur in a fair-minded, clear, and concise manner to ensure the participation of the patient and his family and to increase the chances of the plan's success postdischarge.

Abbreviations

ADR	Adverse Drug Reaction
A1C	Glycated Hemoglobin
AIMS	Abnormal Involuntary Movement Scale
AMP	Amphetamine
ANC	Absolute Neutrophil Count
APA	American Psychiatric Association
BID	Twice Daily
BMI	Body Mass Index
BP	Blood Pressure
BZD	Benzodiazepine
CBC	Complete Blood Count
CBD	Cannabidiol
CIWA-B	Clinical Institute Withdrawal Scale
CRP	C-Reactive Protein
CYP	Cytochrome P450
DVT	Deep Vein Thrombosis
ECG	Electrocardiogram
EPS	Extrapyramidal Symptoms
ETOH	Ethyl Alcohol
FDA	U.S. Food and Drug Administration
FGA	First Generation Antipsychotics
GAD	Generalized Anxiety Disorder

HBIPS	Hospital-Based Inpatient Psychiatric Services
HDL	High-Density Lipoprotein
HR	Heart Rate
IPOC	Interprofessional Plan of Care
kg	Kilograms
LAI	Long-Acting Injectable
lbs	Pounds
LCMS	Liquid Chromatography Mass Spectrometry
LDL	Low-Density Lipoprotein
LFT	Liver Function Tests
MAMP	Methamphetamine
MAR	Medication Administration Record
MMSE	Mini Mental State Exam
Opi	Opioids
PCP	Phencyclidine
PDMP	Prescription Drug Monitoring Program
PGY1	Postgraduate Year One
PGY2	Postgraduate Year Two
PPCP	Pharmacists' Patient Care Process
PRN	As Needed
REMS	Risk Evaluation Mitigation Strategy
RR	Respiratory Rate
SAMHSA	Substance Abuse and Mental Health Services Administration
SI/HI	Suicidal Ideation/Homicidal Ideation
SSRI	Selective Serotonin Reuptake Inhibitor
THC	Tetrahydrocannabinol
TG	Triglycerides
TSH	Thyroid Stimulating Hormone
UDS	Urine Drug Screen
WNL	Within Normal Limits

References

1. Silvia RJ, Lee KC, Bostwick JR, et al. Assessment of the current practice of psychiatric pharmacists in the United States. *Ment Health Clin*. 2020;10(6):346-353.

2. Stimmel GL. Psychiatric pharmacy. *Am J Health Syst Pharm*. 2013;70(4):366-367.

3. Dopheide JA, Werremeyer A, Haight RJ, Gutierrez CA, Williams AM. Positioning psychiatric pharmacists to improve mental health care. *Ment Health Clin*. 2022;12(2):77-85.

4. Cates ME, Woolley TW. Effects of a psychiatric clinical rotation on pharmacy students' attitudes toward mental illness and the provision of pharmaceutical care to the mentally ill. *Ment Health Clin*. 2018;7(5):194-200.

5. Diefenderfer LA, Iuppa C, Kriz C, Nelson LA. Assessment of pharmacy student attitudes and beliefs toward patients with mental illnesses on inpatient psychiatric units. *Ment Health Clin*. 2020;10(1):1-5.

6. Doan K, Shabo L, Crouse EL. The impact of pharmacy candidates' understanding of psychiatry on personal mental health concerns and patient treatment. *Curr Pharm Teach Learn*. 2022;14(1):56-61.

7. Frick A, Osae L, Ngo S, et al. Establishing the role of the pharmacist in mental health: implementing Mental Health First Aid into the doctor of pharmacy core curriculum. *Curr Pharm Teach Learn*. 2021;13(6):608-615.

8. *Diagnostic and Statistical Manual of Mental Disorders*. 5th ed. American Psychiatric Association; 2022.

9. Citrome L. New second-generation long-acting injectable antipsychotics for the treatment of schizophrenia. *Expert Rev Neurother.* 2013;13(7):767-783.

10. Crismon M, Smith T, Buckley PF. Schizophrenia. In: DiPiro JT, Yee GC, Posey L, Haines ST, Nolin TD, Ellingrod V, eds. *Pharmacotherapy: A Pathophysiologic Approach.* 11th ed. McGraw Hill; 2020. https://accesspharmacy.mhmedical.com/content.aspx?bookid=2577&sectionid=224358695. Accessed October 07, 2022.

11. Mental Health Policy: Involuntary Commitment (Assisted Treatment) Standards (50 states)—Treatment Advocacy Center. Available at https://mentalillnesspolicy.org/national-studies/state-standards-involuntary-treatment.html.

12. Civil Commitment and the Mental Health Care Continuum: Historical Trends and Principles for Law and Practice. Substance Abuse and Mental Health Services Administration (SAMHSA). Available at https://www.samhsa.gov/sites/default/files/civil-commitment-continuum-of-care.pdf.

13. Hedman LC, Petrila J, Fisher WH, Swanson JW, Dingman DA, Burris S. State laws on emergency holds for mental health stabilization. *Psychiatr Serv.* 2016;67(5):529-535.

14. Norris D, Clark MS, Shipley S. The mental status examination. *Am Fam Physician.* 2016;94(8):635-641.

15. *The American Psychiatric Association Practice Guideline for the Treatment of Patients with Schizophrenia.* 3rd ed. Washington, DC: American Psychiatric Association; 2021.

16. Correll CU, Howes OD. Treatment-resistant schizophrenia: definition, predictors, and therapy options. *J Clin Psychiatry.* 2021;82(5):MY20096AH1C.

17. Centers for Medicare & Medicaid Services. *Inpatient Psychiatric Facility Quality Reporting Program Manual.* Version 4.1; 2018.

18. The Clozapine Risk Evaluation and Mitigation Strategy. Available at www.newclozapinerems.com. Accessed August 11, 2022.

19. Paliperidone palmitate (Invega Sustenna) prescribing information, Janssen Pharmaceuticals, Inc.

20. Tang Y, Martin NL, Cotes RO. Cocaine-induced psychotic disorders: presentation, mechanism, and management. *J Dual Diagn.* 2014;10(2):98-105.

21. Kale N. Urine drug tests: ordering and interpreting results. *Am Fam Physician.* 2019;99(1):33-39.

22. Moeller KE, Kissack JC, Atayee RS, Lee KC. Clinical interpretation of urine drug tests: what clinicians need to know about urine drug screens. *Mayo Clin Proc.* 2017;92(5):774-796.

23. Voss RM, M Das J. Mental status examination. In: *StatPearls.* Treasure Island, FL: StatPearls Publishing; September 16, 2021.

24. Winslow RS, Stillner V, Coons DJ, Robison MW. Prevention of acute dystonic reactions in patients beginning high-potency neuroleptics [published correction appears in Am J Psychiatry 1986 Sep;143(9):1204. Robinson MW [corrected to Robison MW]]. *Am J Psychiatry.* 1986;143(6):706-710.

25. Addonizio G, Alexopoulos GS. Drug-induced dystonia in young and elderly patients. *Am J Psychiatry.* 1988;145(7):869-871.

26. Musil R, Obermeier M, Russ P, Hamerle M. Weight gain and antipsychotics: a drug safety review. *Expert Opin Drug Saf.* 2015;14(1):73-96.

27. Gugger JJ. Antipsychotic pharmacotherapy and orthostatic hypotension: identification and management. *CNS Drugs.* 2011;25(8):659-671.

28. Haslemo T, Eikeseth PH, Tanum L, Molden E, Refsum H. The effect of variable cigarette consumption on the interaction with clozapine and olanzapine. *Eur J Clin Pharmacol.* 2006;62(12):1049-1053.

29. Lowe EJ, Ackman ML. Impact of tobacco smoking cessation on stable clozapine or olanzapine treatment. *Ann Pharmacother.* 2010;44(4):727-732.

30. Tsuda Y, Saruwatari J, Yasui-Furukori N. Meta-analysis: the effects of smoking on the disposition of two commonly used antipsychotic agents, olanzapine, and clozapine. *BMJ Open.* 2014;4(3):e004216.

31. Roncero C, Daigre C, Grau-López L, et al. An international perspective and review of cocaine-induced psychosis: a call to action. *Subst Abus.* 2014;35(3):321-327.

32. Masood B, Lepping P, Romanov D, Poole R. Treatment of alcohol-induced psychotic disorder (alcoholic hallucinosis)-a systematic review. *Alcohol.* 2018;53(3):259-267.

33. Wood E, Albarqouni L, Tkachuk S, et al. Will this hospitalized patient develop severe alcohol withdrawal syndrome? The rational clinical examination systematic review [published correction appears in JAMA. 2019;322(4):369]. *JAMA.* 2018;320(8):825-833.

34. Marconi A, Di Forti M, Lewis CM, Murray RM, Vassos E. Meta-analysis of the association between the level of cannabis use and risk of psychosis. *Schizophr Bull.* 2016;42(5):1262-1269.

35. Schwartz RC, Blankenship DM. Racial disparities in psychotic disorder diagnosis: a review of empirical literature. *World J Psychiatry.* 2014;4(4):133-140.

36. Gara MA, Minsky S, Silverstein SM, Miskimen T, Strakowski SM. A naturalistic study of racial disparities in diagnoses at an outpatient behavioral health clinic. *Psychiatr Serv.* 2019;70(2):130-134.

37. Olbert CM, Nagendra A, Buck B. Meta-analysis of Black vs. White racial disparity in schizophrenia diagnosis in the United States: do structured assessments attenuate racial disparities? *J Abnorm Psychol.* 2018;127(1):104-115.

38. Ceskova E. Pharmacological strategies for the management of comorbid depression and schizophrenia. *Expert Opin Pharmacother.* 2020;21(4):459-465.

39. American Family Physicians Pharmacologic Product Guide: FDA-approved medications for smoking cessation. Updated January 17, 2019. Available at https://www.aafp.org/dam/AAFP/documents/patient_care/tobacco/pharmacologic-guide.pdf. Accessed August 2, 2022.

40. Hrdlicka M, Dudova I. Atypical antipsychotics in the treatment of early-onset schizophrenia. *Neuropsychiatr Dis Treat.* 2015;11:907-913.

41. Clozaril. Prescribing Information. Novartis Pharmaceuticals Corporation. https://www.accessdata.fda.gov/drugsatfda_docs/label/2010/019758s062lbl.pdf. Accessed August 14, 2022.

42. Hughes G. First do no harm; then try to prevent it. *Emerg Med J.* 2007;24(5):314.

43. Lader M, Kyriacou A. Withdrawing benzodiazepines in patients with anxiety disorders. *Curr Psychiatry Rep.* 2016;18(1):1-8.

44. Remington G, Addington D, Honer W, Ismail Z, Raedler T, Teehan M. Guidelines for the pharmacotherapy of schizophrenia in adults. *Can J Psychiatry.* 2017;62(9):604-616.

45. Brown M, Freeman S. Clonazepam withdrawal-induced catatonia. *Psychosomatics.* 2009;50(3):289-292.

46. Sienaert P, Dhossche DM, Vancampfort D, De Hert M, Gazdag G. A clinical review of the treatment of catatonia. *Front Psychiatry.* 2014;5:181.

47. Specifications Manual for Joint Commission National Quality measures v2020A. Tobacco Treatment Measures. Available at https://manual.jointcommission.org/releases/TJC2020A/TobaccoTreatmentMeasures.html. Accessed August 10, 2022.

48. Anthenelli RM, Benowitz NL, West R, et al. Neuropsychiatric safety and efficacy of varenicline, bupropion, and nicotine patch in smokers with and without psychiatric disorders (EAGLES): a double-blind, randomised, placebo-controlled clinical trial. *Lancet.* 2016;387(10037):2507-2520.

8

Inpatient and Outpatient Pediatric Care— Nephrology Service

Christine Tabulov

CHAPTER AIMS

The aims of this chapter are to:
- Use the Pharmacists' Patient Care Process (PPCP), clinical reasoning, critical thinking, and patient-specific factors for assessing and resolving drug therapy problems on a multidisciplinary pediatric nephrology service.
- Within the PPCP, identify common drug therapy problems that may be faced in the pretransplant and posttransplant phases of the care of a pediatric nephrology patient.

KEY WORDS

• Pediatrics • nephrology • kidney transplant • clinical reasoning • clinical problem solving • medication-related problems • critical thinking • PPCP

INTRODUCTION

Pediatric pharmacy practice provides many opportunities for pharmacists to manage a wide range of age populations from neonates to adulthood.[1] As valuable members of healthcare teams, pediatric pharmacists help prevent medication errors, educate patients and caregivers, and provide pharmacotherapy recommendations based on the child's age, pharmacokinetics, and development.[1–5] They also perform weight-based or body surface area-based calculations to ensure the dose is appropriate for the child. Pediatric pharmacists may practice as general pediatric pharmacists, but can also specialize in various areas of pediatric care, such as critical care, neonatology, hematology/oncology, and transplant. The Joint Commission recommends 24-hour pediatric pharmacy services, which led to an increase in the demand for pharmacists trained in pediatrics.[1,4–6]

It is recommended for those who decide to pursue a pediatric pharmacy career to complete at least a postgraduate year 1 (PGY1) residency. Postgraduate year 2 (PGY2) training is also strongly recommended as it allows the pharmacist to gain more exposure with specific pediatric populations, such as neonatal intensive care, pediatric intensive care, and hematology-oncology.[1,4,5,7] For this vulnerable population, it is critical that pediatric pharmacists utilize their extensive knowledge in providing competent care through the application of effective clinical reasoning and critical thinking using the Pharmacists' Patient Care Process (PPCP).[8]

OUR PRACTICE—A PEDIATRIC NEPHROLOGY SERVICE

Our practice is a pediatric nephrology service located in a tertiary, academic medical center. The pediatric nephrology pharmacist provides medication management and education during various phases of care for the pediatric kidney transplant patient. These phases of care include *pretransplant* evaluation at the transplant center, *perioperative* care in the pediatric intensive care unit and general pediatric floor, and *posttransplant* care at outpatient follow-up visits. Members of the service round daily and include a pediatric nephrologist, pediatric pharmacist, nurses, nutrition staff, case management staff, and learners (eg, interns). Patients in our service include children with chronic kidney disease (CKD)/end-stage renal disease, kidney transplant recipients, and other renal disorders. This chapter will focus on the pediatric nephrology pharmacist's role in pediatric kidney transplant management.

 KEY POINT

Pediatric kidney transplant involves knowledge about three different phases of care (pretransplant, perioperative, posttransplant) to optimize patient outcomes.

Our transplant patients receive either deceased or living donor kidney transplants, with our center averaging around one to three transplants per month. Transplant centers are required to document clinical pharmacist participation for the accreditation standards by the United Network for Organ Sharing (UNOS) and the Centers for Medicare & Medicaid Services (CMS).[9-11] The pediatric nephrology pharmacist participates in several aspects of care for these patients, including attending multidisciplinary medical review board (MRB) meetings that discuss if a patient is eligible to be added to the transplant list after an initial evaluation. The pharmacist also participates in patient care rounds, performs patient education, and participates in discharge meetings.[9,12-14] Most centers allow a pediatric patient to receive a kidney transplant once he or she is 10 kg.[15-17] The age of patients in our pediatric kidney transplant patient population range from infants to 21 years of age. Transplants may come from a living or deceased donor, with deceased donors being most common.

 KEY POINT

Some examples of where a pediatric nephrology pharmacist can positively impact patient care by using the PPCP include attending multidisciplinary review board meetings, participating in patient care rounds, performing patient education, and attending discharge planning meetings.

UTILIZING CRITICAL THINKING SKILLS IN OUR PRACTICE

For the pediatric nephrology pharmacist, critical thinking must be utilized throughout the entire patient care process in both inpatient and outpatient care. The pharmacist must consistently question and reflect on information gathered to ensure it is factual and reliable.[18] When developing a treatment plan, the pharmacist must assure that decisions are evidence-based, patient- and family-centered, and that cognitive biases have been identified and addressed.[18] Proper application of critical thinking standards will also be valuable for the development and maintenance of an effective relationship with the patient and/or caregiver or parent that will enable the pharmacist to best understand a patient's clinical status and healthcare needs. In turn, this understanding will enable the development of the best strategy for optimal immunosuppression therapy while limiting potential side effects and complications.[9] **Table 8-1** lists some of the questions pharmacists on our pediatric nephrology service can ask themselves to help assure effective critical thinking and clinical reasoning through the application of the intellectual standards of critical thinking: clarity, relevance, significance, objectivity, fairness, accuracy, precision, depth, breadth, and logic—embodied in the "Clear ROAD to Logic" mnemonic described in Chapter 1.

TABLE 8-1

Sample Standards-Based Questions That Can Be Applied to Assure That Intellectual Standards for Thinking Are Met as the Pharmacist Provides *Care on a Pediatric Nephrology Service*

Clarity (explicit, unambiguous, intelligible, free from confusion or doubt)	• Have I clearly collected all necessary information from the patient/caregiver and electronic health record about medication use and side effects? • Have I clearly written my thought process in the electronic health record so other members of the healthcare team can understand my reasoning? • Have I clarified any discrepancies between medication information in the chart and the medications the patient is actually taking? • Have I evaluated the patient's therapeutic drug monitoring levels and clearly correlated changes with recent treatment or dietary modifications?
Relevance (pertinent, applicable, germane)	• What collected information during the medication history/reconciliation interview is relevant? • Is it clear I am following relevant institutional protocols and governing body recommendations? • Am I able to locate any relevant pediatric-specific literature to support my pharmacotherapy recommendation? • Am I extrapolating appropriate relevant adult literature and applying it appropriately to my pediatric patient?
Significance (important, nontrivial, necessary, critical, required, impactful)	• What significant information have I collected from the parent/caregiver, patient (if appropriate), and other provider's notes? • Have I determined what information is most clinically significant and applied it to develop an effective treatment plan?

Objectivity (fact-based, unbiased)	• Is my judgment influenced by biases (eg, race, sexual gender, religious or political beliefs)? • Have I checked my biases to ensure I am objective? • Am I aware of how my emotions may impact my work? • Have I established appropriate patient-provider boundaries?
Fairness (unbiased, equitable, impartial)	• Have I fairly considered the patient's, the parents'/caregivers', and the providers' perspectives? • Have I displayed empathy during my consideration of these various perspectives? • Am I able to use my professional judgment to assess patients who are on their second kidney transplant in a fair and unbiased manner?
Accuracy (verifiable, valid, true, credible, undistorted)	• What information collected should I spend some extra time to ensure it is clear and accurate? • What questions can I ask to ensure accuracy of the information the patient is telling me?
Precision (exact, specific, detailed)	• Have I created this regimen in a patient-specific manner to minimize the risk of nonadherence? • When providing patient education, what level of detail should be provided to the patient? • What educational delivery method is appropriate for this patient (eg, handout, teach-back method)? • What stage of development is the patient at (sensory-motor, preoperational, concrete operational, formal operational)?[19,20]
Depth (roots, fundamentals, complexities, interrelationships, cause/effect, implications)	• What medical complexities and pharmacokinetic considerations must be thought of when determining proper therapy, dosing, and considerations regarding side effects? • What psychological and social factors are impacting the management of the transplanted organ?
Breadth (comprehensive, encompassing, alternative perspectives)	• What are appropriate questions to ask to determine psychological impacts in relation to the transplanted organ? • Who is the family member or caregiver of the patient that may be impacted by changes to medication therapy? • Are there perspectives and insights from other members of our interprofessional team that should be considered in my decision-making?
Logic (reasonable, rational, without contradiction, well-founded, sound)	• How do I know when my hypotheses are reasonable? • Have I identified alternative explanations? • What steps do I need to take to evaluate alternative explanations associated with my hypothesis? • Is this patient's treatment plan reasonable based on age, pharmacokinetics, and developmental changes?

 KEY POINT

The pediatric nephrology pharmacist utilizes critical thinking to ensure patient-specific pharmacotherapy needs are identified while ensuring side effects and complications are minimized.

APPLICATION OF THE PPCP IN OUR PRACTICE DURING THE THREE PHASES OF KIDNEY TRANSPLANTATION

Pretransplant Phase

During the pretransplant phase, the pediatric nephrology pharmacist will perform an assessment on the pharmacologic and nonpharmacologic risks in a patient-specific manner to assist the multidisciplinary team at the MRB meeting in deciding if a patient is eligible for transplant. Pharmacologic risks are evaluated by reviewing the patient's medication list, drug–drug and drug–food interactions, medication allergies, hormonal contraception, current use of immunosuppressants or immunomodulators, drug absorption issues (eg, requires gastric tube administration for medications), and herbal supplement or nutraceutical utilization.[9,12] For example, a child with epilepsy who is on medications that can interact with the immunosuppression regimen may be at increased risk for supratherapeutic or subtherapeutic immunosuppressant levels. The pharmacist will run a drug interaction report to determine if the antiepileptic medications will interfere with the immunosuppressant regimen. Upon review of this report, the pharmacist will either recommend to the MRB alternative antiepileptic medication(s) the patient can switch to after consultation with the patient's neurologist, or will determine a plan with the current antiepileptic medications that will ensure immunosuppression is both efficacious and safe. The pharmacist will also screen for nonpharmacologic risks, such as psychosocial factors that may impact the patient's transplant management. These include health literacy gaps, inadequate family support, and nonadherence.[9,21] An example of a nonpharmacologic risk would be if the patient's parents are not present to help the child with the complex medication regimen. During the MRB meeting, it is crucial that the pharmacist listens to input from the child psychologist or social worker to identify if there is a legal guardian (eg, grandparent, aunt, uncle) to help the child with his or her medication regimen to ensure success of the transplant.

Perioperative Phase

The perioperative phase begins once the patient is listed on the transplant waiting list and continues until discharge from the inpatient kidney transplant care. During the perioperative transplant phase, the pediatric nephrology pharmacist will collect patient-specific information, such as previous pertinent acute 24-h events (eg, procedures, significant changes in clinical status [stable vs. unstable], current problem[s], vital signs [blood pressure, heart rate, respiratory rate, temperature], weight, complete metabolic panel [CMP], complete blood count [CBC], iron panel, urine output, and microbiology [blood culture, urine culture, etc.]). Medication information is also collected, including but not limited to dose (eg, in units and unit/kg or unit/m^2 as applicable), route, frequency, administration times, and therapeutic drug monitoring levels (eg, for tacrolimus) with timing of the blood draws. During the Assess phase, the pharmacist will perform medication reconciliation (pretransplant to pediatric intensive care unit to general pediatric floor to discharge). The pharmacist will also evaluate the need for dosage adjustments based on the pediatric patient's current renal function and on patient-specific factors, such as hypertension, therapeutic drug monitoring levels, and adverse effect management.[9,22] The pharmacist will document the assessment and treatment plan in the patient's electronic health record in accordance with CMS Conditions of Participation and

UNOS policies.[9-11] The treatment plan will be effectively communicated within the electronic health record and on daily patient rounds with the various medical teams responsible for care of the patient, such as the pediatric critical care, general pediatrics, and transplant teams.

Posttransplant Phase and Ambulatory Setting

The posttransplant phase, which begins once the patient is discharged from the inpatient setting, is key to the success of the transplanted kidney.[23] The pediatric nephrology pharmacist plays an essential role throughout the life of the transplanted kidney, which for some patients can be lifelong.[9,12,14,23] Collecting information about immunosuppression medications, patient-specific needs, and laboratory parameters are examples of information collected by the pharmacist in this phase.[12] During the Assess step, the pharmacist will determine if a patient's transplant medications need to be modified. The pharmacist can also assess if a patient is beginning to experience kidney transplant rejection, and determining any need for opportunistic infection management.[24] The pharmacist will then work with the pediatric nephrologist to develop a plan for medication-related changes, provide education to implement the medication management plan, and follow-up with the patient at later clinic visits.[23]

In all phases of transplant care, the pediatric nephrology pharmacist's involvement in the patient care process starts with collecting information that will be assessed to form the basis for the development of SMART goals with the patient/caregiver, and the plan to meet the goals. The treatment plan is communicated effectively to the patient, caregiver, and to other healthcare providers. A monitoring and follow-up plan are also developed and communicated with the pediatric nephrology transplant team. Described below will be a patient case in which all PPCP steps are performed in a systematic and deliberate clinical problem-solving process in which clinical reasoning and critical thinking are applied by the pediatric nephrology pharmacist to optimize transplant care.

THE COLLECTION OF PATIENT INFORMATION IN OUR PRACTICE

In our practice, the Collect step starts with a chart review that will help ensure effective patient/caregiver interviews for all phases of transplant care and effective multidisciplinary rounding in the perioperative phase. Information gathered in the Collect step is vital for gaining an understanding of the complexities of pediatric kidney transplant medication management. Examples of the type of information that is collected during a chart review during various phases of transplant care are shown in **Table 8-2**. Details of chart information collected in the pre- and posttransplant phases will be described in a case study later in the chapter. The timing of the chart review will vary based on the transplant phase. It is best practice for the pretransplant phase and for the posttransplant ambulatory care setting to review the chart within 48 hours before and the morning of the appointment prior to speaking with the patient and caregiver(s). During the perioperative phase, it is best practice to review the chart before and during patient care rounds to ensure information collected is the most up-to-date.

 KEY POINT

Pediatric kidney transplant patients require completion of a thorough patient history to appreciate the complexities of kidney transplant medication management.

TABLE 8-2

Examples of Data That Can Be Collected During Chart Review During Various Phases of Pediatric Kidney Transplant Care

Data to Collect During Chart Review	Rationale for Collecting Specific Data
Patient characteristics: age, weight, comorbidities	When providing safe and effective dosing recommendations for pediatric patients, it is crucial to know the age and weight of the patient. Patient comorbidities will be helpful in identifying other pharmacotherapy needs for the patient and can also explain variability in lab results.
Date of transplant and how many days since transplant	Collecting date of transplant, and how many days since transplant is critical in managing a pediatric transplant patient's pharmacotherapy because pharmacotherapy needs for immunosuppression dosing and antimicrobial prophylaxis may change. For example, appropriate therapeutic drug monitoring values can change based on the timeframe from after transplant (eg, tacrolimus level goals decrease when further out from transplant—refer to institution-specific protocol).
Characteristic of the transplant—deceased donor; living donor; EBV; CMV; and HLA status	Collecting information about the type of kidney transplant performed is important for the pediatric nephrology pharmacist to know, as it will help with formulating recommendations for immunosuppression.
Labs: renal function panel, hepatic function, complete blood cell count, iron studies	Labs can assist with dosing of medications, monitoring for side effects, and monitoring how the patient is responding to the transplant. It is important to be aware that age can influence some lab results (eg, younger ages have lower serum creatinine).[25]
Immunosuppression medication levels (eg, tacrolimus, sirolimus)	Immunosuppression monitoring is critical in making sure the immunosuppression is safe and effective for the pediatric patient. It is also important to collect the times that the patient is taking the immunosuppression medications (eg, tacrolimus, mycophenolate mofetil immediate release (IR), prednisone) as this is critical for prevention of organ rejection.
Vital signs (eg, HR, BP, RR, pain)	Vital signs are important to collect as immunosuppression medications can cause side effects that can impact vital signs. Vital signs vary by patient age.[26]
Insurance coverage and potential barriers for discharge medication planning	The pharmacist should be aware of the potential barriers for filling a patient's prescriptions in the outpatient setting.[9] For example, only certain pharmacies carry immunosuppression medications (eg, tacrolimus and mycophenolate) or compounded medications for pediatric patients.[27] It will also be important to determine if the pharmacy is contracted with the patient's insurance carrier. Furthermore, it can be critical to be proactive when arranging discharge medications (ideally a week in advance) to ensure medications are provided to the patient when discharged, to prevent delays in therapy that might occur if the patient and caregiver were to pick up the medications on their own.

With a thorough chart review completed, the Collect step continues with a patient interview. **Table 8-3** describes examples of data that can be completed during the interview.

Pharmacist-provided pediatric transplant management and our practice are examined below with an in-depth analysis of a fictitious case of a pediatric patient undergoing a new kidney transplant. There will be two parts, with the first part being a mini-case covering a patient in the pretransplant phase and the second part a mini-case with the same patient in the posttransplant phase in an ambulatory setting. This analysis will depict the clinical reasoning and critical thinking that occurs during each PPCP step, with the primary goal being to empower the reader to understand how the PPCP, clinical reasoning, and critical thinking can be combined to optimize patient-centered care for a pediatric kidney transplant patient.

The Case of Chris A.: Overview of the Pretransplantation Phase

Chris A. (CA) is a 12-year-old male who presents to the pediatric nephrology clinic with his parents for pretransplantation evaluation. His past medical history includes Stage 5 CKD secondary to polycystic kidney disease and he is currently on hemodialysis every Monday, Wednesday, and Friday. CA and his parents are interested in him being listed for a kidney transplant to help improve his quality of life after being on hemodialysis for 5 years.

Past medical history:

- CKD (Stage 5 on Hemodialysis MWF)
- Hypertension
- Anemia of CKD
- Controlled metabolic bone disease secondary to CKD
- Seasonal allergies
- Insurance coverage: Commercial

TABLE 8-3

Patient Interview: Examples of Data That Can Be Collected During the Patient Interview

Caregiver's and patient's (as age-appropriate) description of the following topics:
- Current pain description (perioperative, posttransplant/ambulatory care)
  – Duration, intensity, location, pain pattern
  – Description of pain sensations: nociceptive (sharp, stabbing, dull, aching) vs. neuropathic (burning)
- Activity levels (pretransplant, perioperative, posttransplant/ambulatory care)
  – Confirming if patient can get out of bed and walk around as able
- Eating ability (pretransplant, perioperative, posttransplant/ambulatory care)
  – Patient ability to eat appropriate amount of food. Also determine the patient's ability to take oral medications
- Caregiver and patient's perception of the impact of the patient's condition on their quality of life (pretransplant, perioperative, posttransplant/ambulatory care)
  – Overall life satisfaction
- Complete medication review (pretransplant, perioperative, posttransplant/ambulatory care)
  – Current medications: dose, route, frequency, indication, dosage form, missed doses, identified side effects, perceived efficacy, palatability
  – Past medications used for transplant management: indication, length of time, dosing, rationale for discontinuation
  – Insurance coverage, access issues, copayment costs

CLINICAL REASONING, CRITICAL THINKING, AND THE PPCP FOR THE CARE OF CHRIS A.

Systematic problem solving for CA will be depicted in a sequence of tables describing the pharmacist's clinical reasoning and critical thinking from the Collect to Monitor steps of the PPCP. Clinical reasoning will be described in terms of conclusions along with their associated rationale, and critical thinking will be described in terms of selected critical thinking intellectual standards applied to help optimize the pharmacist's clinical reasoning. For the Collect step, these intellectual standards are articulated in the future tense to illustrate critical thinking applied in preparation for data collection. In the remaining PPCP steps, the standards are articulated in the past tense in reflection after the clinical encounter. The critical thinking standards are represented in the mnemonic "Clear ROAD for Logic": clarity, relevance, significance, objectivity, fairness, accuracy, precision, depth, breadth, and logic.

Collect

In this step, the pediatric nephrology pharmacist collects subjective and objective information in order to understand the patient's medical and medication history, and current clinical status. This will include information from a chart review in preparation for bedside rounds or clinical visits, and verified with the caregiver and/ or patient (as appropriate) during the session.

 KEY POINT

When collecting information to create a pharmacotherapy recommendation for a pediatric transplant patient, it is best practice to collect information from the chart and the healthcare team and verify the information with the caregiver and patient, as appropriate.

COLLECT (Pretransplant): Current Medications and Immunizations	
Conclusions	Rationale: Information or Premise to Support the Conclusion
Perform a full and complete medication review with the patient and/or caregiver during the pretransplant evaluation. *(To be collected during the chart review and the interview.)* Match each medication with its indication. Evaluate adherence, any current side effects, and drug interactions. Collect information on insurance coverage. *(To be collected during the chart review and the interview.)*	• Though the focus will be on the nephrology medications during this visit, it is important the pediatric nephrology pharmacist has a good understanding of the complete medication regimen. • Confirming the indication with each medication can help identify any medications that might not be indicated any longer or possible duplications of therapy. • Identifying possible drug–drug and drug–food interactions, or possible side effects are fundamental roles of the pediatric nephrology pharmacist. • Assessment of adherence to past medication regimens can help determine if a patient will be compliant with their kidney transplant medication regimen. • The pediatric nephrology pharmacist works with case management staff and/or social work staff to ensure the patient will have adequate insurance coverage for transplant medications.

Determine if immunizations are up-to-date. (*To be collected during chart review.*)	• It is imperative to assure the patient's immunization records are up-to-date as pediatric transplant patients may be at increased risk for complications and morbidity as the result of posttransplant immunosuppression.[17,28] Vaccination recommendations vary by transplant center.

Critical Thinking Checks for the Collect Plan for This Patient's Current Immunizations and Medications

To ensure I collect the necessary information, I will need to **clearly** communicate to the caregiver and/or patient (as appropriate) and that I understand what they are communicating to me.

• As the pediatric nephrology pharmacist, I need to ensure that I communicate clearly the expectations for the medication management of the kidney transplant. For example, I must ensure that I communicate in a manner that best matches the patient and parents' health literacy and pause during my communication to ask if there are any questions. I need to make sure I collect information appropriately about previous medication regimens by asking open-ended questions to CA and his parents, so I can get as much **precision** (detail) as possible including information on his history of adherence to medication regimens. This is to uncover any adherence issues that may compromise the success of posttransplant medication therapy. I must also demonstrate **breadth** in the collection of immunization data and confirm that all live vaccines have been administered, since live vaccines are not recommended posttransplant as they can cause serious vaccine-induced disease.

It is imperative that I collect sufficiently **accurate** and **precise** (detailed) information to ensure that the information I have is sufficient to draw **logically** sound conclusions about any pharmacy-related concerns and about contraindications to renal transplant for CA.

• I will be collecting information required to draw sound conclusions about medication nonadherence, medication allergies or intolerances, current use of anticoagulants or antiplatelets, and use of medications with significant drug–drug interactions with immunosuppressants commonly used in the posttransplant (eg, tacrolimus, mycophenolate mofetil IR). I collect immunization data to ensure vaccines are up-to-date before the patient becomes immunosuppressed posttransplant.

It is also imperative that I engage with other medical professionals involved in CA's care in a **fair-minded** and **objective** manner.

• For example, after this pretransplant visit, I will attend an MRB meeting to collect more information from the patient case discussion to gain the perspectives and insights from other medical professionals involved in CA's care that may be important for my decision-making.

I will need to ensure I think **deeply** about CA's medications and conditions.

• It is vital as a pediatric nephrology pharmacist that I understand the complexities of interrelationships among his conditions and medications. Additionally, it is important for me to understand what aspects of the CKD will most likely be corrected posttransplant such as hypertension, hyperphosphatemia, vitamin D deficiency, and anemia.

Collected Current Medication and Immunization Information Entered into Health Record

Current medication regimen:

• Amlodipine 10 mg PO daily. Indication: hypertension (controlled). The patient takes daily; no ADRs reported

- Calcium acetate 1334 mg PO three times daily with meals. Indication: hyperphosphatemia. The patient takes three times daily with meals; no ADRs reported
- Cholecalciferol 2000 IU PO daily. Indication: vitamin D deficiency secondary to CKD. The patient takes daily; no ADRs reported
- Epoetin alfa 4000 units IV three times weekly. Indication: anemia of CKD. The patient takes three times weekly on dialysis days (MWF) at the dialysis unit; no ADRs reported
- Ferrous sulfate 325 mg (65 mg elemental iron) PO daily. Indication: anemia of CKD (controlled). The patient takes daily; no ADRs reported
- Loratadine 10 mg PO daily. Indication: seasonal allergies. The patient takes daily; no ADRs reported

Current immunizations:

- COVID-19 vaccine: up-to-date
- Diphtheria, Tetanus, & Acellular Pertussis vaccine: up-to-date
- *Haemophilus influenzae* type B vaccine: up-to-date
- Hepatitis B vaccine: up-to-date
- Human papillomavirus vaccine: up-to-date
- Inactivated poliovirus vaccine: up-to-date
- Influenza vaccine: up-to-date
- Measles, mumps, rubella vaccine: up-to-date
- Meningococcal vaccine: up-to-date
- Pneumococcal vaccine (PCV13 & PPSV23): up-to-date
- Rotavirus vaccine: up-to-date
- Varicella vaccine: up-to-date

COLLECT (Pretransplant): Allergies, Vital Signs, Labs	
Conclusions	Rationale: Information or Premise to Support the Conclusion
Verify and document allergy status of the patient and specific reaction the patient experienced. *(To be collected during the chart review and the interview.)*	• Verifying all allergies is an important step for patient safety. Clarifying the allergic reaction will also help assess if patient has a true allergy or a drug intolerance.
Collect the patient's current vital signs, height, weight, and pertinent labs. *(To be collected during the chart review and the interview.)*	• Vital sign review can identify if further follow-up is needed from pediatrician or other pediatric specialties to ensure appropriateness for kidney transplant.[9] • Monitoring height and weight of pediatric patients is vital, especially for a patient with CKD.[9,29] Also, certain medications used in pediatric kidney transplant can cause weight gain.[9,30] • Reviewing pertinent labs based on comorbidities, infectious disease parameters, and current medications are important to identify drug therapy problems related to dosing concerns or reduced kidney function.

Collect ABO compatibility, Panel of Reactive Antibody (PRA), Crossmatch, and HLA Tissue Typing. *(To be collected during chart review after labs are drawn.)*	• If kidney transplant donor and recipient have incompatible blood types, transplantation is typically contraindicated.[31] • A patient with a higher PRA can have a decreased likelihood of finding a suitable kidney and is at higher risk of rejection.[32] • A positive crossmatch is likely a contraindication for pediatric kidney transplant. A risk of positive crossmatch is increased with history of blood transfusions and retransplantation.[33] • HLA tissue typing can help determine suitability of match for kidney transplant donor and recipient.[32,33]

Critical Thinking Checks for the Collect Plan for This Patient's Allergies, Vital Signs, and Labs

When reviewing labs and tissue typing, it is important to obtain **accurate** and **precise** information to ensure that the patient is an appropriate candidate for kidney transplant.

- CA had labs drawn that will determine his candidacy for kidney transplant. These labs include, but are not limited to PRA, blood typing, HLA typing and crossmatching, vaccination titers, and infectious disease serologies (eg, CMV, EBV). It is also imperative to ask CA and his parents about previous blood transfusions and previous transplants as these can increase the chance of a positive crossmatch. This information should be collected prior to the MRB meeting. This information will then be utilized when there is a call to the pediatric nephrologist for a potential match to ensure the patient will receive the best organ possible.

When reviewing labs, it is vital to distinguish **significant** labs that can impact medication therapy (eg, higher PRA, EBV status, etc.).

- There are some key laboratory markers that can impact dosing of medications, such as PRA and EBV status. In addition, obtaining a CMP and CBC is important because this can impact medications being chosen for therapy (eg, induction agent) and if the patient is able to be prescribed the necessary medications for posttransplant. For example, the presence of leukopenia would necessitate a switch from sulfamethoxazole/trimethoprim to pentamidine. Leukopenia and EBV mismatch status (Donor +/Recipient −) would also prompt a reduction of the mycophenolate mofetil dose. Finally, once the pediatric nephrologist receives a call that there is a match for the transplant, crossmatching and HLA tissue typing can help determine the induction therapy the patient will receive.

It is also important that I think **deeply** to determine the complexities of how these labs relate to his CKD, particularly given its dynamic nature, so I can appropriately collect the labs needed to make an **accurate** assessment of his pharmacotherapy plan.

- I need to be mindful when evaluating CA's labs that they are reflective of the current status of his CKD. These labs will likely change once he gets transplanted. So, once the patient is in the perioperative phase, I need to remember to ask the pediatric nephrologist to obtain new labs.

Collected Allergies, Vital Signs, And Lab Information Entered into Health Records:

Allergies: NKDA

Vital signs: Height: 5'2" (157.5 cm), Weight: 103.6 lb (47 kg), HR: 82, BP: 100/75; RR: 12

Labs:

CMP: Na: 140; K: 4.3; Cl: 108; BUN: 78; SCr: 5.4; Blood glucose: 87; Phos: 5.9; Mg: 2.1; Ca: 8.6; Albumin: 2.7; PTH: 186; Vitamin D: 30

GFR (Modified Bedside Schwartz Equation): 12 mL/min/1.73 m^2

Iron studies: Iron 60 mcg/mL; Total Iron Binding Capacity (TIBC): 270 mcg/dL; Transferrin Saturation (TSAT): 30%

CBC: Within normal limits (WNL) except Hemoglobin 9.4 g/dL

Immunization titers: Normal

No history of blood transfusions or transplants

CMV: +; EBV: −

Example Collect Statement for CA

CA is a 12-year-old male who presents for pretransplant evaluation. CA and his parents are hoping that having a kidney transplant will improve his quality of life after being on hemodialysis for the past five years. Parents report no issues with adherence to previously prescribed medication regimens and no side effects. CA has commercial insurance that offers low copays for immunosuppressant medications and insurance is in contract with local pharmacy. CA has no known medication allergies. Medications include amlodipine for hypertension (controlled), calcium acetate for hyperphosphatemia (controlled), cholecalciferol for vitamin D deficiency secondary to CKD (controlled), epoetin alfa and ferrous sulfate for anemia of CKD (not controlled), and loratadine for allergic rhinitis (controlled). Current labs are appropriate for a patient who has CKD on hemodialysis. He has a low hemoglobin of 9.4 g/dL. He has positive CMV status and negative EBV status.

Assessment of Collected Information

During the Assess step, the pediatric nephrology pharmacist evaluates all subjective and objective data acquired during the Collect step to provide a comprehensive assessment of the patient's current health status, to identify and prioritize drug therapy problems, and to determine if there are any contraindications to kidney transplant from a pharmacy perspective. It is imperative to understand what conclusions you are making to recognize how the information collected is related to the patient's eligibility for a kidney transplant listing. Appropriate critical thinking standards must be used during this process to ensure a complete and accurate assessment of the patient. (See Table 8-1 and Chapter 1.)

When assessing the patient's current medical conditions, it is important to consider if these are related to the CKD and if these medical conditions would be resolved after the kidney transplant. Caregiver and patient treatment goals should also be considered. Each medication should be assessed for efficacy, adherence patterns, current side effects, and any concerns the caregiver or patient may have. Examples of caregiver/parent or patient concerns may include cost of medications, dosing frequency, or administration problems (eg, taste of medication, swallowing large capsules). This approach provides a more complete history when identifying drug therapy problems along with their contributing factors and aids the pharmacist in problem prioritization. During the pretransplant evaluation, the pediatric nephrology pharmacist will also evaluate if there are any pharmacy contraindications to kidney transplantation, such as nonadherence and lack of adequate social support.

 KEY POINT

When assessing each medication, it is crucial to identify concerns from the caregiver and patient to ensure effective implementation of the plan.

ASSESS (Pretransplant): Chronic Kidney Disease Associated Conditions and Medication Therapy	
Conclusions	Rationale: Information or Premise to Support the Conclusion
Controlled hypertension secondary to CKD: Not a pharmacy contraindication to kidney transplant.	Blood pressure is 100/75 mm Hg. Goal blood pressure: less than 50th percentile (normal blood pressure) using the appropriate table as in the American Academy of Pediatrics (AAP) Hypertension Guidelines.[34] Amlodipine is an appropriate antihypertensive with CKD as it is not nephrotoxic and is at its maximum dose of 10 mg PO daily. There are no reported side effects or issues with adherence.
Uncontrolled anemia of CKD: Not a pharmacy contraindication to kidney transplant. Drug Therapy Problem: Epoetin alfa *dosage too low*	The patient's hemoglobin is 9.4 g/dL. Target hemoglobin is 11 to 13 g/dL.[35] Currently on epoetin alfa and ferrous sulfate. The epoetin alfa dose was recently increased by 25% 39 days ago to 4000 units (~85 units/kg) IV three times weekly on dialysis days, but it is not achieving the minimal hemoglobin level of 11 g/dL and patient has iron studies within normal limits. Appropriate ferrous sulfate dose. No side effects reported with these medications.
Controlled metabolic bone disease secondary to CKD	The patient's phosphorus is 5.9 mg/dL, which is within normal limits.[36] The patient is currently on calcium acetate, which is being effective in lowering his phosphate levels. Corrected calcium is 9.6 g/dL, which is within normal limits. Parathyroid hormone is 186 pg/mL, which is expected for dialysis patients. No side effects or missed doses reported. Vitamin D is 30 ng/ml, which is within normal range.[36] The patient's dose of cholecalciferol was recently increased to 2000 IU PO daily for treatment dosing of vitamin D deficiency. No side effects or missed doses reported.

 KEY POINT

When assessing for drug therapy problems in a pediatric patient, it is important to remember to reference age-specific lab ranges and vital signs.

Critical Thinking Checks for Assessing This Patient's Chronic Kidney Disease Associated Conditions and Medication Therapy

In my determination of this patient's drug therapy problems, I have analyzed the most **significant** patient information and have based my conclusions on a sufficiently **broad** and **deep** analysis of the **relevant** literature.

- Literature was utilized to ensure medication dosing is safe. There are limited guidelines available in the pediatric population, which were used to evaluate the antihypertensive treatment of CA. Pediatric literature is also commonly based on smaller population sizes (less than 100 patients) and lower levels of evidence (eg, retrospective studies, case reports). Therefore, sometimes extrapolation from adult literature is warranted. When evaluating CA's CKD-associated conditions, recommendations were extrapolated from guidelines based on the adult population.

To evaluate this patient's CKD, I needed to evaluate all information that is **relevant** for supporting my assessment of his candidacy for kidney transplant, and I needed to ensure that it is **accurate** and **precise** to draw valid conclusions.

- This included my evaluations of CA's CKD-associated conditions (including relevant lab values) and his medication safety, efficacy, and adherence. Evaluations from other team members will also need to be taken into consideration.

Also, I needed to make sure my assessment was **fair** and **objective** to avoid any biases.

- In order to perform a proper assessment of CA's kidney transplant candidacy, I needed to ensure I analyzed the information collected from the interview, chart review, and multidisciplinary meeting free of any biases and consider the perspectives of CA and his family in a **fair-minded** empathetic manner. He has a diagnosis of Stage 5 CKD, and is currently on hemodialysis to support his kidney function. A kidney transplant would help his quality of life based on his current diagnosis. I need to also ensure that I avoid potential biases that may impair my **objective** thought process, such as the **framing** and **bandwagon** effects, so I can make an informed decision from a pharmacy perspective to advocate for the listing of CA for a kidney transplant at the MRB meeting.

Due to the patient's complexity, it can be helpful to draw a concept map to see how the Stage 5 CKD and medications interact with one another. Concept maps can be used to help understand the interrelationships (**Figure 8-1**) and make a thorough assessment.

Example Pretransplant Assess Statement for CA

CA is a 12-year-old male presenting for a pretransplant evaluation due to his Stage 5 CKD on hemodialysis every Monday, Wednesday, and Friday.

(1) Uncontrolled anemia of CKD: The patient's hemoglobin is 9.4 g/dL. Target hemoglobin is 11 to 13 g/dL.[35] Iron studies are within normal limits; therefore, it can be concluded that there is enough iron present in the body for erythropoiesis. Currently on epoetin alfa 4000 units (~85 units/kg) IV three times weekly given on dialysis days during the dialysis session through the dialysis access port. The dialysis port allows for easier administration and helps minimize pain from subcutaneous administration. Epoetin alfa's half-life also allows for three times weekly administration. There is room to go up on dose by 25%. No reported adverse effects. No missed doses.

(2) Controlled hypertension secondary to CKD: Blood pressure is currently 100/75 mm Hg, below the 50th percentile (normal blood pressure according to the AAP Hypertension Guidelines).[34] Currently taking amlodipine 10 mg PO daily with no adverse drug events.

(3) Controlled metabolic bone disease secondary to CKD: The patient's phosphorus is 5.9 mg/dL and corrected calcium is 9.6 mg/dL, which is within normal limits.[36] Currently on calcium acetate. Parathyroid hormone is 186 pg/mL, which is in the expected range for dialysis patients of 150 to 600 pg/mL. No side effects or missed doses reported. Vitamin D is 30 ng/mL, which is within normal range of greater than 20 ng/mL.[36] Cholecalciferol was initiated last month at 2000 IU PO daily for vitamin D deficiency. No side effects or missed doses reported.

(4) Kidney transplant candidacy: This patient has no contraindications to kidney transplant from a pharmacy perspective. There are no reports of medication nonadherence, medication accessibility issues, major drug–drug interactions, issues with drug absorption, or medication allergies.[9]

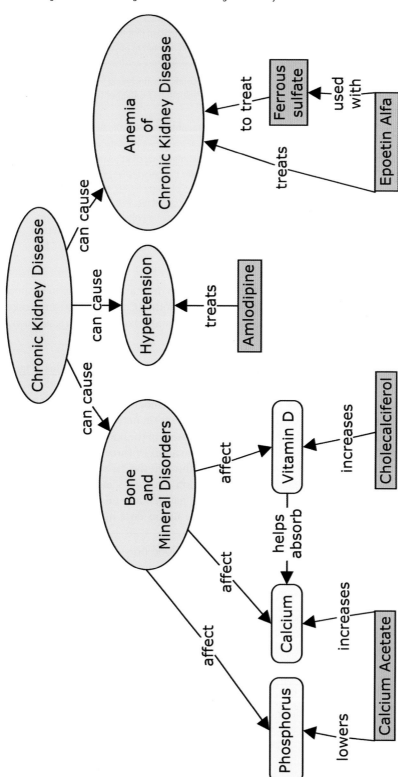

FIGURE 8-1. Concept map illustrating the interrelationships of Chris A.'s medications and chronic kidney disease.

Other recent labs are reported as WNL. No issues with adherence or access to medications.

Drug therapy problem:

- *Dosage too low:* Epoetin alfa dose is too low for the desired response of Hgb greater than 11 g/dL.[35]

These conclusions drawn in the Assess step will serve as the basis for the goal-setting and therapeutic decision-making in the Plan step that follows.

Plan, Implement, and Monitor

PLAN (Pretransplant): Goals	
Conclusions	Rationale: Information or Premise to Support the Conclusion
Goal: Increase hemoglobin to 11-13 g/dL within the next four weeks.	Current hemoglobin: 9.4 g/dL. Goal: 11-13 g/dL.[35]

Critical Thinking Checks for Developing This Patient's Goals
The SMART goals are **clearly** stated including timeframes and expectations.
The SMART goals were developed **fairly and objectively** without the undue influence of emotions or biases in conjunction with patient-specific needs.
The SMART goals were developed **logically** based on the complexity of CKD pathophysiology, possible therapeutic plans, and patient-specific goals.
Creating SMART goals for CA were important to ensure success with his kidney transplant. Having his anemia corrected would help increase his quality of life while he is waiting for a kidney transplant match. As the pediatric nephrology pharmacist, I need to make sure these SMART goals are obtainable for CA and his parents.

PLAN: Anemia of Chronic Kidney Disease	
Goal: • Increase hemoglobin to 11-13 g/dL within the next four weeks.	
Conclusions	Rationale: Information or Premise to Support the Conclusion
Increase epoetin alfa dose to 5000 units (~100 unit/kg—rounded for easier volume measurement) IV three times weekly on dialysis days: Monday, Wednesday, and Friday.	The current epoetin alfa regimen is 4000 units three times weekly. There is room to increase the dose by 25%, which is expected to increase hemoglobin levels between 11-13 g/dL within the next four weeks as the onset of action is 10 days, with peak effect of 2 to 6 weeks.

Chapter 1 describes therapeutic reasoning as the pharmacist empowers the patient in selecting goals of therapy and helps the patient select among the top offered plans. Based on the pharmacist's knowledge, experience, and evidence-based practice, potential strategies and supporting arguments are formed. Conclusions are typically formed in a patient-specific manner to help patients reach their specific goals. An argument map may be used to develop and show the premises for supporting an argument. An example of a map for supporting the argument for a recommendation of epoetin alfa is shown in **Figure 8-2**, which depicts the

Recommendation			
Epoetin alfa 5000 units IV three times weekly on dialysis days (MWF)			
No contraindications to kidney transplant from a pharmacy perspective.	No issues with adherence to past medications.	There is room to increase the dose by 25%, which is expected to increase hemoglobin levels to between 11-13 g/dL within the next four weeks.	Assumption to verify: Commercial insurance will cover epoetin alfa.
SMART Goal			
Increase hemoglobin to between 11-13 g/dL within the next four weeks.			
Assessment			
Patient currently has Stage 5 CKD that is overall well-controlled, except for uncontrolled anemia of CKD: Hemoglobin level is 9.4 g/dL with appropriate adherence to current epoetin alfa therapy. Drug therapy problem: Dose too low.			

FIGURE 8-2. Argument map for epoetin alfa dosing recommendation.

underlying structure of the argument, starting with inferences drawn to generate the Assessment, which supports inferences drawn for the SMART Goal, which underlies the premises—including one of the assumptions—that collectively help support the recommendation for epoetin alfa.

IMPLEMENT/MONITOR (Pretransplant): Uncontrolled Anemia of Chronic Kidney Disease	
Conclusions	Rationale: Information or Premise to Support the Conclusion
Implement: Recommend: Epoetin alfa 5000 IU intravenously three times weekly administered as an IV bolus using a dialysis access port during the dialysis sessions on Monday, Wednesday, and Friday. *Monitor:* • Monitor hemoglobin weekly. If patient has not received a kidney transplant and the hemoglobin does not increase by at least 1 g/dL, consider 25% dose increase at week four of the new dose. • If patient receives a kidney transplant, stop therapy and monitor hemoglobin and hematocrit (H&H). If H&H low, then restart therapy.	*Implement:* Administering epoetin alfa through the dialysis access port allows for easier administration and decreased pain that may be seen with the subcutaneous route. Epoetin alfa may be administered anytime during the dialysis session. It is recommended to use the intravenous form for hemodialysis.[38] *Monitor:* Onset of action is 10 days, with peak effect of 2 to 6 weeks. Although rare, monitor for thrombosis.[37] Epoetin alfa therapy may not be needed posttransplant.

Critical Thinking Checks for This Patient's Implementation and Monitoring Plan

I have **clearly** communicated the plan to the caregiver and/or patient in an empathetic manner that discusses the plans and goals of therapy, whether or not the patient receives a kidney transplant.

To ensure successful implementation of the plan, I have determined the most **significant** issue that would need to be corrected for a patient with CKD; however, I am aware that anemia of CKD is not a contraindication to kidney transplant.

It is very important when discussing the medication plan that may be used in the posttransplant setting and any changes to the pretransplant medication regimen will be to engage CA and his parents with **fair-minded** approach that is empathetic and receptive to open discussion and questions from the CA and his parents. I need to be mindful of the lifestyle change this family will endure with an increased number of medications and frequencies throughout the day. I need to focus on what is best for CA and his health and do my best as his pharmacist to make sure he is getting the best care possible.

It was illustrated above how the PPCP, clinical reasoning, and critical thinking were integrated to optimize patient care provided by the pediatric nephrology pharmacist in the pretransplantation phase of a pediatric kidney transplant for CA. As previously mentioned, the pediatric nephrology pharmacist is involved in three different phases of care, including pretransplant, perioperative, and ambulatory care setting (posttransplant). Now the same process will be applied to illustrate the care provided to CA, posttransplant, in the ambulatory care setting.

The Continued Case of Chris A.: Overview of the Posttransplant Phase in the Ambulatory Care Setting

CA is a 12-year-old male who has received a deceased donor kidney transplant (DDKT) and is here for a routine posttransplant follow-up visit. He is currently posttransplant day #21. He is a negative crossmatch, Kidney Donor Profile Index (KDPI) score = 5%, PRA = 5%. CMV: D+/ R+. EBV: D+/R−.* He received two doses of basiliximab for induction. He has a chief complaint of increased diarrhea that started 4 days ago. There has been nothing done yet to treat the diarrhea. *(D = donor, R = recipient, + = seropositive, − = seronegative)

Diet: Regular diet. No issues with eating.

Past medical history:

- CKD (Stage 5 on Hemodialysis MWF)—Now resolved
- Hypertension
- Anemia of CKD
- Hyperphosphatemia
- Seasonal allergies

Tacrolimus level today is 12 ng/mL (initial goal per EBV mismatch protocol 10 to 12 ng/mL)

Weight: 50 kg

Height: 5'2" (157.5 cm)

Gastrointestinal panel: Negative, CBC: WNL, CMP: WNL

Vital signs: WNL

Insurance coverage: Commercial

Collect

In this step, the pediatric nephrology pharmacist collects the subjective and objective information from the chart review in preparation for the ambulatory care visit. This information is verified with the caregiver and/or patient during the visit. Visits will also include therapeutic drug monitoring and a patient interview discussing medication adherence and adverse effects, vaccination recommendations, and comorbid disease state management. The pediatric nephrology pharmacist can also provide supplemental patient and caregiver education on a case-by-case basis.

 KEY POINT

Consistent education is recommended to empower the patient and caregiver to be successful with the transplant medication regimen.

COLLECT (Posttransplant): Current Medications and Immunizations	
Conclusions	Rationale: Information or Premise to Support the Conclusion
Perform a full and complete medication review with the patient during the transplant ambulatory care visit. *(To be collected during chart review and patient interview.)* Match each medication with its indication. Evaluate efficacy and any current side effects and drug interactions. Verify adherence to each medication. Ensure appropriate timing of medication administration. *(To be collected during chart review and patient interview.)*	• Though the focus will be on the transplant medications during this visit, it is vital the pediatric nephrology pharmacist has a good understanding of the complete medication regimen.[24] • Confirming the indication with each medication can help identify any medications that might not be indicated any longer or can identify possible duplications of therapy. In addition, reviewing the institution's protocol will be helpful in determining if medications (eg, opportunistic infection prophylaxis) are still indicated.[24] • Identifying possible drug–drug interactions or drug–food interactions is critical for the pediatric nephrology pharmacist (eg, for tacrolimus). This is especially important when a patient is starting any new medications (eg, prescription medications, over-the-counter products, herbal supplements). • Identifying possible side effects and adherence patterns are fundamental roles of the pediatric nephrology pharmacist.
Reinforce medication education provided in the pretransplant and perioperative transplant settings to ensure caregiver and patient understand the indication and purpose, proper dosing, use, timing, missed doses, and side effects. *(To be completed during patient interview)*	• Reinforcing the purpose and use of the medications with caregiver and patient (if appropriate) to help with adherence and understanding of the entire medication regimen. • Timing of medications is critical to ensure appropriate immunosuppression. If medications are not given on a strict schedule, it can increase the risk of rejecting the transplanted kidney. • Some transplant medications (eg, tacrolimus) require therapeutic drug monitoring to ensure appropriate immunosuppression. The caregiver and patient (if appropriate) should understand why the levels are taken.
Determine if immunizations are up-to-date. *(To be collected during chart review and patient interview.)*	• Since transplant patients are considered immunocompromised, it is important that the patient's immunization status is up-to-date to ensure the best possible immunity.[28] Transplant patients are at greater risk of complications and morbidity associated with preventable infections.

KEY POINT

Pharmacists can play a role during the pretransplant phase to identify any discrepancies in a patient's immunization records to minimize risk of posttransplant complications and morbidity.

Critical Thinking Checks for the Collect Plan for This Patient's Current Immunizations and Medications

During the transplant medication review for this patient, it will be important to collect information with sufficient **accuracy** and **precision**.

- Collecting accurate and precise information on medication efficacy and safety will enable me to determine that CA's transplant medication regimen is optimal for him. I also need to ensure I collect information that will enable me to assess CA's adherence by evaluating if there are any factors negatively impacting his medication use experience (taste, smell, insurance coverage).

- Another example where precision of collected information is vital for solid organ transplant patients is for patients who present with diarrhea. Diarrhea is a common condition in these patients, and there are several potential causes that pharmacists must be knowledgeable about. These include infectious and noninfectious (eg, medication) causes. For patients such as CA who present with diarrhea following a transplant, it is recommended in guidelines[39] that clinicians obtain a detailed clinical history to accurately determine its cause.

A critical part of my practice is optimizing medication use. It is critical that I center my communication to the caregiver's and patient's needs to ensure that I **clearly** understand the caregiver and patient and that they understand me.

- I need to have a clear understanding of the complete medication regimen, clearly reinforce the purpose of the medications, and communicate clear instructions on any changes to a patient's medication plan, especially during the first three months of the posttransplant phase where medication changes can occur on a weekly basis. Since CA is 12 years old, it is appropriate for me to communicate the changes to him and his parents. I ask at each visit how the patient is taking his medications and use that information to compare to what is documented on CA's medication sheet. This sheet encompasses the drug name, drug strength, drug dose, the number of pills per dose, how many times a day the dose is given, and the times the medications are supposed to be given.

Transplant patients have complex medication regimens. It is crucial for me to think **deeply** as the caregiver, patient, and I discuss the patient's medication usage following the transplant medication sheet, so that I can gather the **relevant** information needed for me to **clearly** understand the complexity of the patient's and caregiver's medication use experience.

When collecting information about the medication regimen and immunization status, it is important to ensure that I am being **objective** and free from my own biases.

I also need to consider how the medications, food, and their timing interact with one another, so it is important for me to understand the **depth** of interrelationships and complexities of these different factors.

- I need to determine if CA is taking his regimen according to the plan presented to him after transplant. He is taking his medications at the appropriate scheduled times, and I have documented the timing of his medications in the electronic health record. I also need to ask him if he is consistently taking his medications at the same time each day and if he is taking his medications consistently with respect to meals so I can determine if and how his food intake may be affecting the bioavailability of any of his medications.

Collected Current Medication and Immunization Information Entered into Health Records

Current medications:

- Tacrolimus capsule 4 mg PO q12h (0.15 mg/kg/day). Indication: immunosuppression; no ADRs or missed doses—doses have been given on time (takes at 8 AM and 8 PM)
- Mycophenolate mofetil IR tablet 500 mg (~300 mg/m²/dose) PO every 12 hours. Indication: immunosuppression; ADR: patient has been experiencing diarrhea (two stools daily) and no missed doses—doses were given on time (takes at 8 AM and 8 PM)
- Prednisone tablet 15 mg PO every 12 hours. Indication: immunosuppression; no ADRs or missed doses—doses were given on time (takes at 8 AM and 8 PM)
- Valganciclovir tablet 450 mg PO every 12 hours. Indication: cytomegalovirus (CMV) prophylaxis; no ADRs or missed doses—doses were given on time (takes at 8 AM and 8 PM)
- Trimethoprim/Sulfamethoxazole tablet 160 mg/800 mg PO daily. Indication: *Pneumocystis jiroveci* pneumonia (PJP) prophylaxis; no ADRs or missed doses—doses were given on time (takes medication at 8 AM)
- Nystatin suspension 100,000 units/mL—500,000 units PO (swish and swallow) after meals and before bedtime. Indication: candidiasis prophylaxis; no ADRs or missed doses; complains of funny taste—doses were given on time (8:30 AM, 12:30 PM, 8:30 PM, 10:00 PM)
- Famotidine tablet 20 mg PO every 12 hours. Indication: gastrointestinal prophylaxis while on steroids; no ADRs or missed doses—doses were given on time (8:00 AM and 8:00 PM)
- Loratadine tablet 10 mg PO daily. Indication: seasonal allergies. The patient takes daily at 8:00 AM; no ADRs

Current immunizations:

- COVID-19 vaccine: up-to-date
- Diphtheria, Tetanus, & Acellular Pertussis vaccine: up-to-date
- *Haemophilus influenzae* type B vaccine: up-to-date
- Hepatitis B vaccine: up-to-date
- Human papillomavirus vaccine: up-to-date
- Inactivated poliovirus vaccine: up-to-date
- Influenza vaccine: up-to-date
- Measles, mumps, rubella vaccine: up-to-date
- Meningococcal vaccine: up-to-date
- Pneumococcal vaccine (PCV13 & PPSV23): up-to-date
- Rotavirus vaccine: up-to-date
- Varicella vaccine: up-to-date

COLLECT (Posttransplant): Allergies, Vital Signs, and Labs

Conclusions	Rationale: Information or Premise to Support the Conclusion
Verifying patient's allergy status is a particularly important part of medication management. It is crucial that specific reactions are reported into the electronic health record. *(To be collected during chart review and the interview.)*	• An important patient safety step is to verify all allergies on a regular basis. Knowledge of the allergic reaction will help assess if true allergy or drug intolerance.

Collect patient's current vital signs, height, weight, and pertinent labs. *(To be collected during chart review and the interview.)*	• Blood pressure, temperature, and weight are important to monitor in a kidney transplant patient, especially within the first 3 months posttransplant in which rejection episodes and infection are at the highest risk. Patient and caregivers are expected to monitor and record these values at home.
	• Weight and lab values (eg, basic metabolic panel, magnesium, phosphorus, CBC, tacrolimus level) are important factors in the dosing of medications (eg, tacrolimus)
	• Labs to consider recommending to the physician for a patient presenting with diarrhea include *C. difficile*, bacterial stool pathogens, and CMV PCR testing.[39]
Collect patient's current tacrolimus level goal. *(To be collected during chart review.)*	• Collecting the patient's tacrolimus goal will be helpful during therapeutic drug monitoring. The patient's tacrolimus goal is influenced by time posttransplant, EBV mismatch status, and any infectious complications. It is imperative to ensure the tacrolimus level is drawn appropriately (~30 minutes prior to the next scheduled dose) and to confirm the time of last dose, which will ideally be 11.5 hours before.

 KEY POINT

Keeping track of times that a pediatric transplant patient takes his or her medications is important to ensure therapeutic drug monitoring is performed correctly.

Critical Thinking Checks for the Collect Plan for This Patient's Allergies, Vital Signs, and Labs

When verifying CA's allergies, it is imperative that I am **precise** and **accurate** to accurately distinguish between a drug allergy and side effect. This is performed in the same manner as in the pretransplant phase.

When collecting labs, vital signs, and height and weight, I need to determine the **relevance** of this information to my assessment of the transplant medications.

• I need to review labs such as, but not limited to, the CBC, CMP, and infectious disease serologies. In addition, I need to monitor trends in vital signs, weight, and height. This information will be vital in the Assess step to see if I need to make any adjustments to medication dosages or frequencies.

COLLECT (Posttransplant): Social History

Conclusions	Rationale: Information or Premise to Support the Conclusion
Complete a full social history on the patient. *(To be collected during chart review and the interview.)*	• It is important to consider and collect information on the child's social history as part of the biopsychosocial model. This may include personal information about the living situation, health behaviors, caregiver and personal choices, and financial stability/concerns. Examples of specific information to collect include living environment, parent or caregiver information, current school grade and where child goes to school (after transplant, typically children are home-schooled according to transplant center's protocol), dietary habits, and exercise habits. In addition, collecting information on the tiers of copays of the patient's insurance is imperative to ensure the family is able to afford the medications.

Critical Thinking Checks for the Collect Plan for This Patient's Social History

To ensure I understand the social history of the patient, I must communicate in a **clear** manner to ensure the caregiver and patient understand me and that I understand them. If I identify any communication barriers, it is imperative that I address them in the best way I can.

I will need to gather **relevant** and **precise** information about CA's social history to maximize his transplant medication regimen adherence by ensuring that there are no barriers to acquiring the medications, the medication costs are affordable, and to determine if there are any problems with medication regimen adherence that should be addressed.

I will also need to ensure I am **objective** and **fair** when collecting a patient's social history as this may be a sensitive subject and it is vital that I obtain **accurate** and **precise** information on social factors that may affect his medication usage. I will ensure my interaction will encourage open communication, suspend premature judgment, and avoid any biases.

- CA has a strong support system with both of his parents being involved in his posttransplant care. He also has access to insurance that provides low copays, so his family does not endure a high financial burden from his chronic medications. It is imperative to inquire about social history on each visit, since this can change at any time, and it is better to have a proactive approach to address any problems to avoid any missed doses. Missed doses can result in increased risk of transplant rejection. My **clear** communication can help me develop rapport with CA and his family.

Example Collect Statement for Chris A.

CA is a 12-year-old male who is posttransplant day #21 after DDKT. He received two doses of basiliximab for induction. He is negative crossmatch, KDPI score = 5%, PRA = 5%, CMV: D+/ R+ and EBV: D+/R−. He has a chief complaint of increased diarrhea that started 4 days ago. CA and his parents are here in clinic for a routine posttransplant follow-up and did not alert the transplant center of the increased diarrhea prior to this visit. The stool is described as "mushy but not too loose." He is taking his medications as prescribed on an 8 AM and 8 PM schedule (tacrolimus, mycophenolate mofetil IR, and prednisone for immunosuppression), valganciclovir for CMV prophylaxis, and famotidine for gastrointestinal prophylaxis while on steroids. He also takes trimethoprim/sulfamethoxazole for PJP prophylaxis and loratadine daily for seasonal allergies at 8 AM. In addition, CA and his parents are reporting that the nystatin suspension tastes funny. He is still taking his Nystatin 4 times daily (after meals and before bedtime—8:30 AM, 12:30 PM, 8:30 PM, 10:00 PM). There are no other current concerns regarding his transplant medications. He has been taking his medications on time. CA has no known medication allergies. His tacrolimus level goal is 10 to 12 ng/mL per institution protocol and previous levels have been within goal and drawn correctly. His tacrolimus level today is 12 ng/mL. Health conditions include DDKT (uncontrolled) and allergic rhinitis (controlled). He had a previous history of Stage 5 chronic kidney on hemodialysis; however, this has been resolved with his kidney transplant. Vital signs are stable and he is not on any antihypertensive medications. His labs are within normal limits. Vaccinations are up-to-date.

Assessment of Collected Information

During the Assess phase, the pediatric nephrology pharmacist reviews all subjective and objective information obtained during the Collect step to provide the best explanation of the patient's current status. During this time, it is important to understand what types of conclusions you are working toward to recognize how the information collected is related to the kidney transplant. Many of the various healthcare concerns can be impacting each other and it is important to understand these dynamics when working to develop a proper treatment regimen for this patient. It is vital to use critical thinking standards during this process to ensure a full and complete assessment of the patient's situation. (See Table 8-1 and Chapter 1.) When assessing each current medical condition, it is important to consider the impact of other conditions, other medications, and related patient treatment goals. Additionally, it is important to complete a full medication review ensuring each medication listed is linked to a current health-related problem and make note of unnecessary drug therapy. Each medication should be assessed for indication, efficacy, the patient's adherence patterns, timing of medications, current side effects, and any concerns the patient might have regarding each medication. Examples of patient concerns can include the dosing frequency or administration problems (eg, tastes funny). As the pediatric nephrology pharmacist focuses on the kidney transplant regimen, the assessment should include a review of previously prescribed medications and reasons for discontinuation. This provides the pediatric nephrology pharmacist with a more complete history when identifying drug therapy problems along with their contributing factors and helps to determine their order of priority.

 KEY POINT

It is crucial that the pediatric nephrology pharmacist reviews all the medications and disease states the patient has due to the immunosuppression regimen having an increased risk of drug–drug and drug–disease interactions.

ASSESS (Posttransplant): Drug Therapy Problems—ADRs—Diarrhea, Medicine Palatability	
Conclusions	Rationale: Information or Premise to Support the Conclusion
The patient's mild-to-moderate diarrhea is more likely caused by mycophenolate mofetil IR usage than by tacrolimus usage or by infectious causes. Drug Therapy Problems: • *Adverse drug reaction:* Intolerance to mycophenolate mofetil IR. (diarrhea) • *Needs additional therapy:* Need for relief of diarrhea	A common adverse effect of mycophenolate mofetil IR is diarrhea, which is dose-dependent and likely from enterocyte damage.[39-41] As stated above in the Collect section, The Diagnosis and Management of Diarrhea in Solid-Organ Transplant Recipients: Guidelines from the American Society of Transplantation Infectious Diseases Community of Practice Guidelines state it is imperative to identify the cause of diarrhea and directly manage it. Causes of diarrhea in solid organ transplant patients include bacterial, viruses, parasitic, immunosuppressant medications, nonimmunosuppressant medications (antibacterial, antiarrhythmic, antidiabetic, laxatives, proton pump inhibitors, and protease inhibitors), and other causes (graft-versus-host-disease, inflammatory bowel disease, posttransplant lymphoproliferative disorder, colon cancer, malabsorption).[39] Calcineurin inhibitors, such as tacrolimus, may cause diarrhea due to the increased gastrointestinal motility associated with its macrolide effect.[39] There is uncertainty reported in the literature for gastrointestinal side effects of calcineurin inhibitors.[41] It has also been reported that tacrolimus levels can increase in patients experiencing diarrhea.[42]

Diarrhea unlikely from tacrolimus	Calcineurin inhibitors, such as tacrolimus, may cause diarrhea due to the increased gastrointestinal motility associated with its macrolide effect.[39] However, there are limited reports of tacrolimus-induced diarrhea so this is likely not a cause for CA.[41,42] Further monitoring of tacrolimus levels is indicated since levels can increase in patients experiencing diarrhea.
Diarrhea unlikely from infectious causes	It is recommended by AST Diarrhea guidelines that *C. difficile*, bacterial pathogens, and CMV PCR testing should occur.[39] Gastrointestinal panel and infectious tests came back negative, which suggests diarrhea is likely unrelated to infectious causes.
The patient is experiencing a palatability problem with nystatin oral suspension. Drug Therapy Problem: • *Adverse drug reaction:* Nystatin has poor taste for the patient.	Nystatin suspension is reported to have a banana-flavored taste.[43] This can cause an adverse taste experience for some children.

 KEY POINT

The pediatric patient population has limited guidelines to guide therapy. It is common to extrapolate recommendations from adult primary literature while considering pediatric-specific factors (eg, pharmacokinetics) to determine if the findings are clinically appropriate for a specific pediatric patient.

Critical Thinking Checks for Assessing This Patient's Diarrhea/Drug Therapy Problems

I need to ensure that I am communicating with the patient in a **clear** manner by asking **accurate**, precise questions so that I gather a detailed history related to what may be causing their diarrhea.

I will need to ensure the subjective and objective information I have on the diarrhea is **relevant** for my clinical decision-making.

Since this patient's diarrhea may be from several causes, I **deeply** considered a sufficiently **broad** array of alternative explanations in coming to what I believe to be the most **logical** explanation of the cause of CA's diarrhea.

• It was imperative to have an appropriate assessment of the diarrhea CA is presenting with. I needed to consider different potential causes of his diarrhea, such as medications (eg, mycophenolate mofetil IR) or illness. I needed to make sure I collected enough information on his diarrhea to ensure I was not missing anything from his clinical picture to make sound conclusions.

Given the complexity of this patient, who has several factors that can be leading to his diarrhea, it can be useful to create a concept map to help grasp some of the interrelationships that contribute to the complexity (see **Figure 8-3**). Understanding these interrelationships can be useful to create a comprehensive assessment of this patient, which is expressed in the Assess statement below.

 KEY POINT

When creating a pharmacotherapy plan for a complex patient, such as a pediatric kidney transplant patient, a concept map is helpful to identify how the medications, disease states, and patient-specific factors relate to one another.

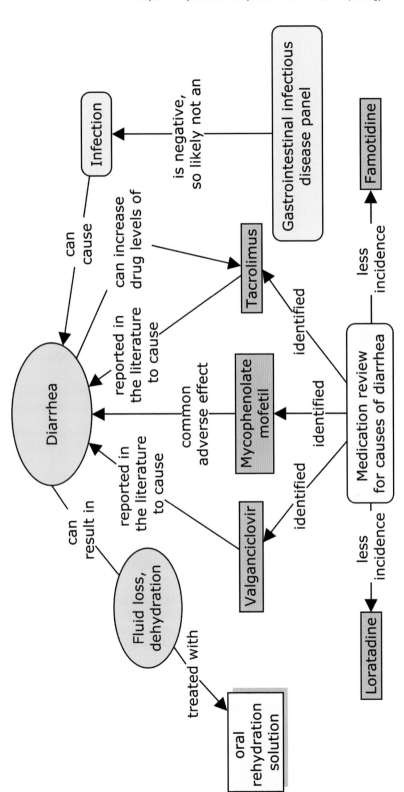

FIGURE 8-3. Concept map to aid the clinical reasoning about the potential causes of Chris A.'s diarrhea.

Example of the Posttransplant Assess Statement for Chris A.

CA is a 12-year-old male who is posttransplant day #21 after DDKT. CA and his parents are here in clinic for a routine posttransplant follow-up. He is noted to be experiencing diarrhea for the past four days, described as "mushy but not too loose." A common adverse effect of mycophenolate mofetil IR is diarrhea, which can be dose-dependent and is likely from enterocyte damage.[39-41] Other potential causes of diarrhea in solid organ transplant patients include bacteria, viruses, parasites, immunosuppressant medications, nonimmunosuppressant medications (antibacterial, antiarrhythmic, antidiabetic, laxative, proton pump inhibitor, and protease inhibitor), and other causes (graft-versus-host-disease, inflammatory bowel disease, posttransplant lymphoproliferative disorder, colon cancer, malabsorption).[39] Gastrointestinal panel and infectious tests came back negative, which suggests diarrhea is likely not due to infectious causes. CA is not on any antiarrhythmic, antidiabetic, laxative, proton pump inhibitor, or protease inhibitor. Since mycophenolate mofetil IR is a common cause of diarrhea, addressing this agent may be able to resolve CA's diarrhea, thereby improving his quality of life. CA is also experiencing a palatability problem with his nystatin oral suspension that so far has not impacted his adherence to this medication, but may cause adherence issues in the future.

Drug Therapy Problems:

- *Adverse drug reaction:* Intolerance to mycophenolate mofetil IR. The patient is continuing to take the medication with gastrointestinal discomfort (diarrhea).
- *Needs additional therapy:* Need for relief of mild-to-moderate diarrhea to reduce risk of diarrhea-induced dehydration or electrolyte imbalance and so the patient does not experience discomfort from his medication regimen to ensure there are no future adherence issues.
- *Adverse drug reaction:* Nystatin has a poor taste for the patient.

These conclusions drawn in the Assess step serve as the basis for the goal-setting and therapeutic decision-making that will occur in the Plan step.

Plan, Implement, and Monitor

PLAN: Goals (Posttransplant): Drug Therapy Problems—ADRs—Diarrhea, Medicine Palatability	
Conclusions	**Rationale: Information or Premise to Support the Conclusion**
Goals: 1. Decrease diarrhea incidence and improve quality of life by having no more loose stools within 1 to 2 weeks. 2. Achieve and maintain an acceptable improvement in nystatin palatability beginning with the next dose.	Current incidence of diarrhea: twice daily, Bristol Stool Scale 6.[44] Baseline: no diarrhea, stool once daily. Since the diarrhea is likely from the mycophenolate mofetil IR, 1 to 2 weeks would be a reasonable timeframe to ensure an appropriate washout period when medications are switched. This timeframe can also be extrapolated from pharmacokinetic data. A decreased incidence of gastrointestinal side effects such as diarrhea would result in improved quality of life by having the patient not use the bathroom as much. Achieving an acceptable improvement in nystatin palatability will help maintain the patient's adherence to his medication regimen.

Critical Thinking Checks for Developing This Patient's Goals for Resolving His Drug Therapy Problems

The SMART goals for CA's drug therapy problems were created and **clearly** communicated with **fair** consideration of the patient's wants and needs, and the patient's and caregiver's **clear** understanding of what can be achievable based on available options. They were **logically** developed with appropriate projected outcomes and timeframes, based on pathophysiology, patient assessment, relevant literature, potential therapies, and patient-specific parameters and with **deep** thinking about the complexity of his pharmacotherapy plan.

- SMART goals were developed for CA's drug therapy problems in consultation with him and his parents, as part of his transplant medication management and are focused on the acute stage where he is experiencing the side effects of diarrhea secondary to his mycophenolate mofetil IR and of poor palatability of nystatin suspension. Clearly, communicated SMART goals can be helpful for transplant patients who can be overwhelmed with the many medications and care plans to follow to prevent organ rejection, and achieving these goals should help CA improve his quality of life from the diarrhea resolution and improved nystatin palatability.

PLAN: Drug Therapy Problems—ADRs—Diarrhea, Medicine Palatability

Goals:
1. Decrease diarrhea incidence and improve quality of life by having no more loose stools within 1 to 2 weeks.
2. Achieve and maintain an acceptable improvement in nystatin palatability beginning with the next dose.

Conclusions	Rationale: Information or Premise to Support the Conclusion
Fluid replacement with a commercial oral rehydration solution to maintain hydration while patient is experiencing diarrhea (eg, Normalyte®—mix one packet with 500 mL of drinking water. May take 1 to 2 L within a 12- to 24-hour period)	The mainstay of therapy for transplant patients with mild-to-moderate diarrhea is fluid replacement, preferably with a commercial oral rehydration solution.[39] Cost of oral rehydration solutions can be an issue for some patients. If diarrhea does not resolve, diarrhea may be treated with over-the-counter loperamide after the transplant coordinator is notified and the diarrhea lasts longer than two days after the change in medication (see below), given that infectious causes of diarrhea have been ruled out by the medical team.[39]
Switch mycophenolate mofetil IR tablet to mycophenolic acid delayed-release tablet	Given that diarrhea is not infectious and likely related to the mycophenolate mofetil IR, it is a viable option to switch to mycophenolic acid delayed-release. It is very important to remember that switching mycophenolate mofetil IR to mycophenolic acid is not a 1:1 conversion, as 720 mg of mycophenolic sodium is equivalent to 1000 mg of mycophenolate mofetil IR.[45,46] Mycophenolic acid delayed-release tablets are enteric-coated tablets reported in the literature to have an improved gastrointestinal side effect profile compared to mycophenolate mofetil IR tablets.[46,47]
Split nystatin oral suspension 5 mL dose into two 2.5-mL volumes	Reducing the volume of nystatin suspension administered may improve its palatability (eg, splitting 5 mL into 2.5 mL each) based on previous clinical observations. One could also add 2 to 5 mL of cherry syrup to the nystatin to help with taste based on anecdotal evidence. Another consideration is to change to a clotrimazole troche formulation. Given the patient is not missing any doses and is willing to tolerate the nystatin, it would be suitable to have the patient continue taking nystatin.

KEY POINT

When creating pharmacotherapy plans for pediatric patients, palatability is an important consideration to ensure the patient is compliant with the medication regimen.

Critical Thinking Checks for This Patient's Plan for Resolving His Drug Therapy Problems

The complexity of the diarrhea has been **deeply** considered with different potential causes; the recommended options will likely help with quality of life by lowering diarrhea incidence.

I have considered all **significant** factors and therapeutic options to determine the best strategies for resolving the patient's drug therapy problems and thereby improve his quality of life and mitigate potential threats to his adherence to his medication regimen.

• I have considered alternative dosage forms of his medications and medication-use strategies.

I have collected and interpreted data and applied evidence-based practice to **objectively** make my best, **logically** sound pharmacological and nonpharmacological recommendations.

• I discussed concerns for dehydration with CA and his parents. They agreed the best course of action would be to start an oral rehydration solution for one to two days and switch the mycophenolate mofetil IR to mycophenolic acid delayed-release tablet. This discussion provided the family hope that quality of life would be increased, and I confirmed the cost associated with these changes would not be an issue for the family.

Chapter 1 describes therapeutic reasoning as the pharmacist empowers the patient in selecting goals of therapy and aids the patient in selecting from among the top offered plans. Based on the pharmacist's knowledge, experience, and evidence-based practice, potential strategies and supporting arguments are formed. Conclusions are typically formed in a patient-specific manner to help patients reach their specific goals. An argument map may be used to develop and show the premises for supporting an argument. An example of a map for supporting the argument for a recommendation of mycophenolic acid delayed-release is shown in **Figure 8-4** that depicts a hidden underlying structure of the argument, starting with inferences drawn to generate the Assessment, which supports inferences drawn for the SMART Goal, which underlies the premises—including one of the assumptions—that collectively help support the recommendation for mycophenolic acid delayed-release.

IMPLEMENT/MONITOR: Drug Therapy Problems—ADRs—Diarrhea, Medicine Palatability	
Conclusions	Rationale: Information or Premise to Support the Conclusion
Implement:	*Implement:*
• Recommend: Proper hydration with a commercial oral rehydration solution or water 2 to 4 L/day[39] (eg, Normalyte®—mix one packet with 500 mL of drinking water. May take 1 to 2 L within a 12- to 24-hour period).	Fluid replacement is a main replacement for patients with mild-to-moderate diarrhea, regardless of the cause.[39] This is to ensure proper hydration and to replenish electrolytes lost as needed.
Monitor:	*Monitor:*
• Continue hydration until diarrhea resolves.[39]	Diarrhea should be monitored to minimize fluid loss and ensure appropriate hydration.

Recommendation			
Discontinue mycophenolate mofetil IR 500 mg. Switch to mycophenolic acid delayed-release (DR) 360 mg PO every 12 hours.			
Mycophenolic sodium delayed-release tablets have been reported in the literature to have a reduced gastrointestinal side effect profile mycophenolate mofetil IR tablet.[46,47]	720 mg of mycophenolic sodium is equivalent to 1000 mg of mycophenolate mofetil IR.	There are no contraindications to mycophenolic acid for this patient.	Assumption to verify: Commercial insurance will cover mycophenolic acid.

SMART Goals
Decrease diarrhea incidence by having no more loose stools within 1 to 2 weeks. Within the next 1 to 2 weeks, improve quality of life by having no gastrointestinal side effects (eg, nausea, vomiting, diarrhea).

Assessment
Diarrhea is likely from mycophenolate mofetil IR 500 mg PO every 12 hours. Adverse drug reaction.

FIGURE 8-4. Argument map for mycophenolic acid delayed-release dosing recommendation.

Implement:

- Recommend: Discontinue mycophenolate mofetil IR 500 mg PO every 12 hours. Start mycophenolic acid DR 360 mg PO every 12 hours.

Education on proper use:

- Take as scheduled every 12 hours at the same time daily
- Take with or without food consistently
- Swallow tablet whole. Do not break, crush, or chew.
- Increased infection risk—wash hands often
- Monitor diarrhea frequency

Monitor:

- Patient and medical team monitor improvement in diarrhea
- Monitor CBC weekly
- Monitor for signs and symptoms of organ rejection

Implement:

The dosing conversion from mycophenolate mofetil IR 1000 mg to mycophenolic acid 720 mg should be used to advise safe dosing. Mycophenolic acid is available as a 360 mg DR tablet. Similar to mycophenolate mofetil IR, mycophenolic acid should be taken as scheduled every 12 hours at the same time daily and the patient should monitor diarrhea frequency.

Monitor:

The patient should be advised to monitor frequency of diarrhea and report any increased frequency or if diarrhea does not resolve.

The pediatric nephrology pharmacist and the medical team should continue to monitor CBCs to ensure no leukopenia. CBC should be monitored weekly for first month, twice monthly during the second and third months, and then monthly thereafter.[48]

Implement:	*Implement:*
• Continue with nystatin suspension 100,000 units/mL 500,000 units PO (swish for as long as possible and swallow) after meals and before bedtime • For each dose, draw up 2.5 mL twice • Education on proper use • Swish and swallow after meals and before bedtime • Place 5 mL in mouth and swish for as long as possible before swallowing • Expected duration of therapy is up to 1 year at our transplant center *Monitor:* • Adherence for missed doses of medication • Patient perception of palatability	Palatability of medications can influence adherence. It is important to give patients strategies to ensure medication is taken as prescribed. Drawing up 2.5 mL twice to have smaller doses, can help assure the taste is not as overwhelming for CA. *Monitor:* Encourage CA's parents to call the transplant coordinator if the palatability is unbearable or if there are missed doses. When that occurs, a new prescription may be called in to add 5 mL of cherry syrup to the nystatin or a switch to an alternative medication (eg, clotrimazole troches) can be recommended.

 KEY POINT

When managing diarrhea, it is crucial to remove the offending agent and ensure the patient is well hydrated.

 KEY POINT

When counseling on food intake with transplant medications, it is imperative to stress the importance of taking medications consistently with or without food to ensure consistent medication absorption.

 KEY POINT

When changing between different dosage forms and medications within a pediatric transplant medication regimen, it is important to double-check dosing conversions to avoid medication errors.

Critical Thinking Checks for This Patient's Implementation and Monitoring Plan

The medication therapy plan implemented was **clearly** communicated to the patient and caregiver. I ensured I incorporated the teach-back to ensure that I clearly understand the patient and caregiver, and they clearly understand me.

Given the complexity of this patient's transplant medication regimen, I chose to highlight the most **significant** changes and information needed to ensure success of the implementation of this plan.

I have evaluated the regimen to incorporate the patient's and caregiver's **relevant** needs and desires to ensure successful implementation of this plan.

I have developed this patient's transplant medication plan **fairly** by ensuring this patient would not be overwhelmed with changes and the patient's insurance covers the medication to avoid any additional barriers to the transplant regimen.

- After considering patient- and family-specific needs, I communicated the plan for the management of CA's diarrhea and used teach-back method to confirm CA and his parents understand the changes. The teach-back involved demonstration of drawing up a 5-mL syringe to the 2.5 mL mark to ensure the nystatin will be drawn to the correct syringe marking. It was also emphasized that this is done twice. I also specified the instructions for the Normalyte® solution and confirmed the family will have no issues affording this medication over the counter. I also communicated the change from mycophenolate mofetil IR to mycophenolic acid DR. The patient and parents confirmed that they understood the rationale for the medication and dose changes and will pick up the medication at the pharmacy on their way home from the clinic visit.

 KEY POINT

When utilizing liquid medications, it is crucial to educate using the teach-back method to ensure the caregiver and/or patient are able to demonstrate correct syringe technique.

 KEY POINT

When creating patient-specific pharmacotherapy plans, it is critical to evaluate the patient's financial status and insurance coverage to ensure there are no interruptions to plan implementation.

CONCLUSION

Pediatric nephrology is a complex service that requires the pharmacist to have knowledge of pediatric pharmacokinetics and pharmacokinetics of transplant medications. As a result, this requires patient-specific care plans that are developed in conjunction with the medical team and institutional patient care protocols. These patient-specific needs are also influenced by the phase of care the patient is in, such as pretransplant evaluation and posttransplant/ambulatory care settings.

 KEY POINT

The pediatric nephrology pharmacist uses the PPCP to create patient-specific care plans that are created in conjunction with the medical team, patient care protocols, and patient and caregiver needs.

The pediatric nephrology pharmacist in this setting effectively utilizes critical thinking and clinical reasoning skills to complete the necessary steps of the PPCP. Activities include collecting and evaluating pertinent data about medication adherence, side effect management, therapeutic drug monitoring, patient care plan development, and patient education. Being a pediatric nephrology pharmacist requires a lifelong learning process that involves the crafting of these critical thinking and clinical reasoning skills to better serve some of our most vulnerable patients.

Summary Points

- Pediatric pharmacy practice provides many opportunities for pharmacists to manage a wide range of age populations, from neonates to adulthood, and it includes not only general pediatric practice, but also several areas of specialization including critical care, neonatology, hematology/oncology, and nephrology.

- Pediatric nephrology pharmacists serve on the pediatric kidney transplant team during the three phases of transplant care (pretransplant, perioperative, posttransplant), applying their critical thinking and clinical reasoning skills and the PPCP to ensure patient-specific pharmacotherapy needs are identified and addressed, while ensuring side effects and complications are minimized.

- In their service on the pediatric kidney transplant team, pediatric nephrology pharmacists participate in multidisciplinary review board meetings, patient care rounds, and discharge planning meetings. In this role, it is imperative that the pharmacist engages with other medical professionals involved in the patient's care in a fair-minded and objective manner, free of any bias, to understand their perspectives and insights that can be important for pharmacotherapeutic decision-making.

- In the Collect step of the PPCP for pediatric kidney transplant patients, the pharmacist must complete a thorough patient history to understand the complexities of the many potential factors impacting kidney transplant medication management. It is best practice to collect information from the chart and the healthcare team and to verify the information with the caregiver and patient, as appropriate. Communication with the patient and caregiver must be clear and in a manner that best matches their health literacy. The pharmacist must obtain information with as much precision (detail) as possible, including information on the patient's history of adherence to medication regimens, to help uncover any adherence issues that may compromise the success of posttransplant medication therapy. The pharmacist must also be objective and fair when collecting a patient's social history as this may involve sensitive information and it is vital to obtain accurate and precise information on social factors that may affect the patient's medication usage.

- In the Plan step of the PPCP, the pediatric nephrology pharmacist thinks with precision, breadth, and depth to create patient-specific care plans in conjunction with the medical team, patient care protocols, and the needs of patient and caregiver. In developing the plan, it is important to be aware that the pediatric patient population has limited guidelines to guide therapy, and it is common to extrapolate recommendations from the adult primary literature while considering relevant pediatric-specific factors (eg, pharmacokinetics) to determine if the findings are clinically appropriate for a specific pediatric patient.

- In the Implement step, when discussing the posttransplant medication plan with the pediatric patient and caregiver, it is important for the pharmacist to be mindful of the lifestyle changes that they will experience, and to therefore be empathetic and receptive to open discussion and questions about the plan. Consistent education is recommended to empower the patient and caregiver to be successful with the transplant medication regimen.

Abbreviations

ABO	ABO Blood Group System: Type A, Type B, Type O, or Type AB Blood
ADR	Adverse Drug Reaction
AST	American Society of Transplantation
BP	Blood Pressure
CBC	Complete Blood Count
C. difficile	*Clostridioides difficile*
CKD	Chronic Kidney Disease
Clear ROAD for Logic	Clarity, Relevance, Significance, Objectivity, Fairness, Accuracy, Precision, Depth, Breadth, Logic
CMP	Complete Metabolic Panel
CMS	Centers for Medicare and Medicaid Services
CMV	Cytomegalovirus
CMV D+/R+	Cytomegalovirus: Donor Seropositive/Recipient Seropositive
DDKT	Deceased Donor Kidney Transplant
DR	Delayed Release
EBV	Epstein-Barr Virus
EBV: D+/R−	Epstein-Barr Virus Donor Seropositive/Recipient Seronegative
FDA	Food Drug Administration
g/dL	Grams Per Deciliter
GFR	Glomerular Filtration Rate
H&H	Hemoglobin and Hematocrit
HLA	Human Leukocyte Antigens
HR	Heart Rate
IR	Immediate Release
IU	International Units
IV	Intravenous
KDPI	Kidney Donor Profile Index
MRB	Medical Review Board
MWF	Monday, Wednesday, Friday
NKDA	No Known Drug Allergies
PCR	Polymerase Chain Reaction
PCV13	Pneumococcal Conjugate Vaccine 13
PGY1	Postgraduate Year 1
PGY 2	Postgraduate Year 2
PO	By Mouth
PPCP	Pharmacists' Patient Care Process
PPSV23	Pneumococcal Polysaccharide Vaccine 23
PRA	Panel of Reactive Antibody
QOL	Quality of Life
RR	Respiratory Rate
SMART Goals	Specific, Measurable, Attainable, Relevant, Time-Bound
TIBC	Total Iron Binding Capacity
UNOS	United Network for Organ Sharing
WNL	Within Normal Limits

References

1. Boucher EA, Burke MM, Klein KC, Miller JL. Update to the minimum requirements for core competency in pediatric hospital pharmacy practice. *J Pediatr Pharmacol Ther*. 2021;26(7):762-766.

2. Stucky ER; American Academy of Pediatrics Committee on Drugs; American Academy of Pediatrics Committee on Hospital Care. Prevention of medication errors in the pediatric inpatient setting. *Pediatrics*. 2003;112(2):431-436.

3. Pesaturo KA, Ramsey EZ, Johnson PN, Taylor LM. Introduction to pediatric pharmacy practice: reflections of pediatrics practitioners. *Am J Health Syst Pharm*. 2008;65(14):1314-1319.

4. Bhatt-Mehta V, Buck ML, Chung AM, et al. Recommendations for meeting the pediatric patient's need for a clinical pharmacist: a joint opinion of the Pediatrics Practice and Research Network of the American College of Clinical Pharmacy and the Pediatric Pharmacy Advocacy Group. *Pharmacotherapy*. 2013;33(2):243-251.

5. Eiland LS, Benner K, Gumpper KF, et al. ASHP-PPAG guidelines for providing pediatric pharmacy services in hospitals and health systems. *J Pediatr Pharmacol Ther*. 2018;23(3):177-191.

6. The Joint Commission Sentinel Event Alert 39. *Preventing Pediatric Medication Errors*. 2021. Available at https://www.jointcommission.org/resources/patient-safety-topics/sentinel-event/sentinel-event-alert-newsletters/sentinel-event-alert-issue-39-preventing-pediatric-medication-errors/; https://www.jointcommission.org/-/media/tjc/documents/resources/patient-safety-topics/sentinel-event/sea-39-ped-med-errors-rev-final-4-14-21.pdf. Accessed: January 16, 2022.

7. American Society of Health-System Pharmacists Required Competency Areas, Goals, and Objectives for Postgraduate Year Two (PGY2) Pediatric Pharmacy Residencies. Available at https://www.ashp.org/-/media/assets/professional-development/residencies/docs/pgy2-newly-approved-pediatric-pharmacy-2016.ashx. Accessed: January 16, 2022.

8. Joint Commission of Pharmacy Practitioners Pharmacists' Patient Care Process. 2014. Available at https://jcpp.net/wp-content/uploads/2016/03/PatientCareProcess-with-supporting-organizations.pdf. Accessed: January 16, 2022.

9. Maldonado AQ, Hall RC, Pilch NA, et al. ASHP guidelines on pharmacy services in solid organ transplantation. *Am J Health Syst Pharm*. 2020;77(3):222-232.

10. United Network for Organ Sharing (UNOS) Bylaws. 2015. Available at https://www.unos.org/wp-content/uploads/unos/UNOS_Bylaws.pdf. Accessed: January 16, 2022.

11. Department of Health and Human Services. *Organ Transplant Interpretive Guidelines Update*. 2008. Accessed: January 16, 2022.

12. Maldonado AQ, Tichy EM, Rogers CC, et al. Assessing pharmacologic and nonpharmacologic risks in candidates for kidney transplantation. *Am J Health Syst Pharm*. 2015;72(10):781-793.

13. Organ Procurement and Transplantation Network (OPTN) Policies. 2019. Available at https://optn.transplant.hrsa.gov/media/1200/optn_policies.pdf. Accessed: February 26, 2022.

14. Alloway RR, Dupuis R, Gabardi S, et al. Evolution of the role of the transplant pharmacist on the multidisciplinary transplant team. *Am J Transplant*. 2011;11(8):1576-1583.

15. Lee CH, Oh C, Lee S, Lee O, Lee KW, Park J-B. Kidney transplantation in children weighing 15 kg or less: technical challenges and outcome in a single center. *Adv Pediatr Surg*. 2021;27(2):67-72.

16. Sheldon CA, Churchill BM, Khoury AE, McLorie GA. Complications of surgical significance in pediatric renal transplantation. *J Pediatr Surg*. 1992;27(4):485-490.

17. Dharnidharka VR, Fiorina P, Harmon WE. Kidney transplantation in children. *N Engl J Med*. 2014;371(6):549-558.

18. Persky AM, Medina MS, Castleberry AN. Developing critical thinking skills in pharmacy students. *Am J Pharm Educ*. 2019;83(2):7033.

19. Sleath B, Bush PJ, Pradel FG. Communicating with children about medicines: a pharmacist's perspective. *Am J Health Syst Pharm*. 2003;60(6):604-607.

20. Deering CG, Cody DJ. Communicating with children and adolescents. *Am J Nurs*. 2002;102(3):34-42.

21. Spivey CA, Chisholm-Burns MA, Damadzadeh B, Billheimer D. Determining the effect of immunosuppressant adherence on graft failure risk among renal transplant recipients. *Clin Transplant*. 2014;28(1):96-104.

22. Martin JE, Zavala EY. The expanding role of the transplant pharmacist in the multidisciplinary practice of transplantation. *Clin Transplant.* 2004;18(Suppl 12):50-54.

23. Burckart GJ. Transplant pharmacy: 30 years of improving patient care. *Ann Pharmacother.* 2007;41(7):1261-1263.

24. Trofe-Clark J, Kaiser T, Pilch N, Taber D. Value of solid organ transplant-trained pharmacists in transplant infectious diseases. *Curr Infect Dis Rep.* 2015;17(4):475.

25. Andropoulos DB. Appendix B. Pediatric normal laboratory values. In: George A. Gregory DBA, eds. *Gregory's Pediatric Anesthesia.* 5th ed. Hoboken, NJ: Blackwell Publishing Ltd.; 2012.

26. Fleming S, Thompson M, Stevens R, et al. Normal ranges of heart rate and respiratory rate in children from birth to 18 years of age: a systematic review of observational studies. *Lancet.* 2011;377(9770):1011-1018.

27. Lampkin SJ, Gildon B, Benavides S, Walls K, Briars L. Considerations for providing ambulatory pharmacy services for pediatric patients. *J Pediatr Pharmacol Ther.* 2018;23(1):4-17.

28. Table 1. Recommended Child and Adolescent Immunization Schedule for Ages 18 Years or Younger, United States, 2021. Updated 2021. Available at https://www.cdc.gov/vaccines/schedules/hcp/imz/child-adolescent.html. Accessed: January 16, 2022.

29. Silverstein DM. Growth and nutrition in pediatric chronic kidney disease. *Front Pediatr.* 2018;6:205.

30. Aksoy N. Weight gain after kidney transplant. *Exp Clin Transplant.* 2016;14(Suppl 3):138-140.

31. Warner PR, Nester TA. ABO-incompatible solid-organ transplantation. *Am J Clin Pathol.* 2006;125 (Suppl):S87-S94.

32. Schinstock CA, Gandhi MJ, Stegall MD. Interpreting anti-HLA antibody testing data: a practical guide for physicians. *Transplantation.* 2016;100(8):1619-1628.

33. Hale DA. Basic transplantation immunology. *Surg Clin North Am.* 2006;86(5):1103-v. doi:10.1016/j.suc.2006.06.015.

34. Flynn JT, Kaelber DC, Baker-Smith CM, et al. Clinical practice guideline for screening and management of high blood pressure in children and adolescents [published correction appears in Pediatrics. 2017 Nov 30:] [published correction appears in Pediatrics. 2018 Sep;142(3):]. *Pediatrics.* 2017;140(3):e20171904.

35. KDOQI. KDOQI Clinical Practice Guideline and Clinical Practice Recommendations for anemia in chronic kidney disease: 2007 update of hemoglobin target. *Am J Kidney Dis.* 2007;50(3):471-530.

36. Kidney Disease: Improving Global Outcomes (KDIGO) CKD-MBD Update Work Group. KDIGO 2017 clinical practice guideline update for the diagnosis, evaluation, prevention, and treatment of chronic kidney disease-mineral and bone disorder (CKD-MBD) [published correction appears in Kidney Int Suppl (2011). 2017;7(3):e1]. *Kidney Int Suppl (2011).* 2017;7(1):1-59.

37. Joist H, Brennan DC, Coyne DW. Anemia in the kidney-transplant patient. *Adv Chronic Kidney Dis.* 2006;13(1):4-10.

38. Epogen (epoetin alfa) [prescribing information]. Thousand Oaks, CA: Amgen; 2018.

39. Angarone M, Snydman DR; AST ID Community of Practice. Diagnosis and management of diarrhea in solid-organ transplant recipients: Guidelines from the American Society of Transplantation Infectious Diseases Community of Practice. *Clin Transplant.* 2019;33(9):e13550.

40. Al-Absi AI, Cooke CR, Wall BM, Sylvestre P, Ismail MK, Mya M. Patterns of injury in mycophenolate mofetil-related colitis. *Transplant Proc.* 2010;42(9):3591-3593.

41. Helderman JH, Goral S. Gastrointestinal complications of transplant immunosuppression. *J Am Soc Nephrol.* 2002;13(1):277-287.

42. Asano T, Nishimoto K, Hayakawa M. Increased tacrolimus trough levels in association with severe diarrhea, a case report. *Transplant Proc.* 2004;36(7):2096-2097.

43. Nystatin oral suspension [prescribing information]. Greenville, SC: PAI Pharmaceutical Associates Inc; 2020.

44. Blake MR, Raker JM, Whelan K. Validity and reliability of the Bristol Stool Form Scale in healthy adults and patients with diarrhoea-predominant irritable bowel syndrome. *Aliment Pharmacol Ther.* 2016;44(7):693-703.

45. Gabardi S, Tran JL, Clarkson MR. Enteric-coated mycophenolate sodium. *Ann Pharmacother.* 2003;37(11):1685-1693.

46. Arns W, Breuer S, Choudhury S, et al. Enteric-coated mycophenolate sodium delivers bioequivalent MPA exposure compared with mycophenolate mofetil. *Clin Transplant.* 2005;19(2):199-206.

47. Cattaneo D, Cortinovis M, Baldelli S, et al. Pharmacokinetics of mycophenolate sodium and comparison with the mofetil formulation in stable kidney transplant recipients. *Clin J Am Soc Nephrol.* 2007;2(6):1147-1155.

48. CellCept (mycophenolate mofetil) [prescribing information]. South San Francisco, CA: Genentech USA Inc; 2021.

9

Inpatient and Outpatient Infectious Disease Care—Transitions of Care and Outpatient Parenteral Antimicrobial Therapy

Lindsey M. Childs-Kean and Barbara A. Santevecchi

CHAPTER AIMS

The aims of this chapter are to:

- Describe common medication-related problems encountered in Outpatient Parenteral Antimicrobial Therapy (OPAT) patients during the transition of care process.

- Discuss the roles of critical thinking, clinical reasoning and the Pharmacists' Patient Care Process (PPCP) in assessing and resolving medication-related problems as a part of collaborative care for patients receiving OPAT.

KEY WORDS

• OPAT • infectious diseases • transitions of care • clinical reasoning • clinical problem solving • medication-related problems • Pharmacists' Patient Care Process • critical thinking

INTRODUCTION

Infectious diseases (IDs) are encountered commonly across the healthcare system and affect all patient populations. These conditions range from nonsevere infections that may be treated in the self-care setting (eg, minor skin infections) and outpatient setting (eg, uncomplicated urinary tract infections) to critical illnesses requiring intensive hospital resources for management. In addition, patients with deep-seated infections may initiate therapy in the hospital and transition to the outpatient setting to complete a treatment course. Pharmacists fulfill vital roles in the prevention and management of IDs across various practice settings, including serving as members of antimicrobial stewardship teams, helping to manage transitions of care, and providing care in outpatient parenteral antimicrobial therapy (OPAT) programs.

Antimicrobial stewardship is defined as "coordinated interventions designed to improve and measure the appropriate use of antimicrobial agents by promoting the selection of the optimal drug regimen including dosing, duration of therapy, and route of administration."[1] One of the benefits of antimicrobial stewardship is a reduction in the incidence of antimicrobial-resistant microorganisms.[2] Antimicrobial resistance is recognized as a significant healthcare threat worldwide, and the Centers for Disease Control and Prevention report an annual incidence of 2.8 million antibiotic-resistant infections in the United States, with greater than 35,000 deaths as a result of these infections.[3] Additional goals of antimicrobial stewardship programs include improving patient outcomes and reducing the rate of secondary infections, such as *Clostridioides difficile* infection.[2] Several healthcare accreditation organizations require the presence of antimicrobial stewardship programs in the inpatient setting. Outpatient antimicrobial stewardship is an emerging area within the field of ID.

OPAT involves administration of intravenous antimicrobials outside of the hospital setting. As part of OPAT, patients may self-administer parenteral antimicrobials or receive these therapies with the assistance of a caregiver or healthcare provider at home. Patients may also receive treatment in an infusion center or institutional setting, such as a skilled nursing facility or long-term care facility. Benefits of OPAT include decreased hospital length of stay or avoidance of hospital admission, reduction in the risk of nosocomial-acquired infections, cost savings, and improved quality of life as compared to a prolonged inpatient stay.[4] It is important to ensure that patients receiving OPAT have a finalized treatment and monitoring plan in place prior to discharge from the hospital, including routine laboratory monitoring and plan for follow-up visits. The Infectious Diseases Society of America guidelines for the management of OPAT recommend that all patients undergo review by an ID expert or team of experts prior to initiation of this therapy.[4] In addition, ID-trained pharmacists are ideally suited as members of OPAT teams, and studies have demonstrated greater adherence to guideline-based therapies, increased interventions focused on safety and efficacy, reduction in costs, and decreased 30-day readmissions when pharmacists are involved in OPAT programs.[5]

 KEY POINT

OPAT refers to the administration of intravenous antimicrobials outside of the hospital setting and may be associated with several benefits including decreased hospital length of stay or avoidance of hospital admission, reduction in hospital-acquired infections, cost savings, and improved quality of life.

OUR PRACTICE—TRANSITIONS OF CARE INTERDISCIPLINARY ID CONSULT AND OPAT TEAM

Our practice consists of interdisciplinary teams working together to manage patients with an ID during hospital admission, through transitions of care, and in the outpatient setting. The practice manages adult patients who will be discharged from the hospital to receive intravenous antimicrobial therapy in the outpatient setting. A wide variety of IDs are encountered, including endocarditis and bone and joint infections. Within our practice, there are two primary ID pharmacists that serve different roles in providing care to patients with IDs: the inpatient ID pharmacist and the OPAT ID pharmacist (**Figure 9-1**). The inpatient ID pharmacist encounters the patient when they first enter into care. The main functions of the inpatient ID pharmacist include collecting, analyzing, and synthesizing information (such as diagnostic information that includes culture and susceptibility data) and developing a therapeutic plan in conjunction with the ID consult team. Inpatient ID consult teams typically consist of an attending physician, a fellow physician, an advanced practice provider (nurse practitioner and/or physician assistant), and an ID pharmacist. In addition, various health professions students may be part of the team (eg, medical, pharmacy). The OPAT ID pharmacist is engaged upon the patient's discharge from the hospital. Important responsibilities of the OPAT ID pharmacist include review of the therapeutic plan, monitoring of the patient following discharge (typically performed once weekly), and serving as a resource for any issues that arise over the course of the patient's outpatient antimicrobial therapy. In addition, this pharmacist may make interventions to alter therapeutic regimens based on patient-specific scenarios in the outpatient setting.

Hospital Admission
• Collect information (chart review, patient interview)

Discharge Planning
• Finalize therapeutic plan
• Assist in logistics of outpatient planning (e.g., access to antimicrobials, infusion strategy)

Outpatient Therapy
• Monitor patient weekly
• Serve as pharmacist resource through completion of therapy

Inpatient Course
• Participate in daily ID consult team rounds
• Develop therapeutic plan and monitor patient daily

Discharge from Hospital
• Receive notification of new OPAT patient
• Review therapeutic plan

Key
● **Inpatient ID Pharmacist**
○ **OPAT ID Pharmacist**

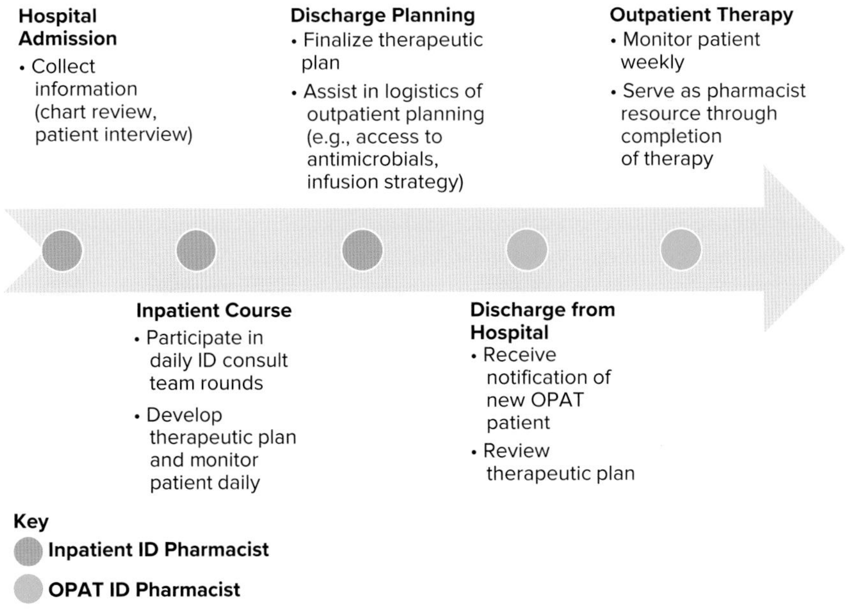

FIGURE 9-1. Timeline of pharmacist activities in our practice.

Patients admitted to the hospital with severe, deep-seated infections are often evaluated by the ID consult team that works closely with the primary medical team to assess patients and provide recommendations for diagnostic evaluation and treatment. If the inpatient ID consult team determines that a patient should receive a prolonged duration of intravenous antimicrobial therapy for optimal management of their infection (may be several weeks to months), the team works together to provide recommendations for OPAT. These recommendations include antimicrobial selection, dose (including infusion strategy: intermittent or continuous), frequency, monitoring, and duration of therapy. At this time, the inpatient ID consult team provides electronic notification and sign-off to the OPAT team who will be monitoring the patient in the outpatient setting. Once final recommendations have been made, the ID consult team signs off of the patient case, and the primary medical team, along with a case manager and/or social worker, secure home infusion services or admission to a facility, and transmit orders for outpatient intravenous antimicrobials and lab tests. The primary medical team and case manager work with the patient and/or caregivers to determine if OPAT may be safely administered at home or if this therapeutic approach requires admission to a facility. During this stage, the inpatient ID pharmacist is no longer actively following the patient, but is available to assist with issues that may arise during the transition if contacted by the primary medical team (such as inability to afford or access medications in the outpatient setting).

Following discharge from the hospital, patients are monitored by an OPAT team consisting of a physician assistant, an ID pharmacist, a nurse, a medical assistant, and an ID physician who is available if needed. To allow for continuity of care, the ID physician following the patient during OPAT is commonly the same physician who was part of the inpatient ID consult team. The OPAT team reviews routine laboratory monitoring (typically performed once weekly) and communicates with patients and outpatient healthcare providers (including home infusion companies and outpatient infusion pharmacies) to coordinate and manage the patient's antimicrobial regimen until completion. Some interventions that may be made in the outpatient setting by this team include adjustment of antimicrobial doses based on therapeutic drug monitoring or changes in renal or hepatic function, follow-up on pending culture and susceptibility data, and modification of antimicrobial regimens due to intolerance, laboratory abnormalities, or cost issues.

The interprofessional nature of our practice is vital to provide optimal care to patients with IDs. During the hospital course, the inpatient ID pharmacist works closely with the ID consult team by attending daily team rounds and serving as a resource to the team for pharmacotherapy-related questions. The typical format of daily team rounds involves a discussion on each patient (on average, the team may be following between 10 and 30 patients each day). This discussion includes a patient case presentation by a medical student, resident, or fellow; discussion of new or updated subjective or objective data (eg, laboratory results or surgical plans); and an open discussion on therapeutic plans and interventions. The physicians and advanced practice providers typically focus on diagnostic interventions and necessary procedures, while the pharmacist focuses on medications. However, there is overlap as all team members are focused on the patient's ID-related problem as a whole. During each patient discussion, the pharmacist may provide recommendations for interventions and/or answer questions posed by the team related to antimicrobials and pharmacotherapy. In the OPAT setting, the OPAT ID pharmacist typically performs self-directed, weekly reviews of patients, and contacts providers on the OPAT team if issues or interventions are identified (eg, dose modification required or adverse effect identified). In addition, the OPAT team may contact the OPAT ID pharmacist with questions related to the patient's antimicrobial regimen and therapeutic plan.

KEY POINT

A multidisciplinary healthcare team is vital for provision of safe and effective care to patients with complex infectious diseases across practice settings.

UTILIZING CRITICAL THINKING SKILLS IN OUR PRACTICE

Critical thinking is essential in all areas of our practice. When patients admitted to the hospital are being evaluated for OPAT, many factors must be considered to ensure this strategy is appropriate and safe for the patient. The ID pharmacist must work with the medical team to ensure OPAT is warranted (eg, oral antimicrobials are deemed not appropriate to treat the infection), feasible (including from cost and patient preference standpoints), evidence-based, and designed with a clear follow-up plan to promote patient safety. The team must continually reassess the plan as new information becomes available, such as updated culture and susceptibility results that may alter the treatment plan. In addition, the team must assess whether the plan for OPAT can be reasonably carried out based on the patient and/or caregiver's health literacy and ability to adhere to the antimicrobial regimen, and based on requirements for laboratory monitoring as an outpatient (especially when OPAT is administered in the home setting). Once patients are discharged on OPAT, the ID pharmacist must utilize critical thinking and communication skills to synthesize plans based on many sources of data, some of which may be incomplete. For example, a pharmacist may receive a laboratory result for a vancomycin concentration drawn in the outpatient setting without information readily available on the date or time of last vancomycin dose and whether this concentration is clinically evaluable as a trough concentration. **Table 9-1** provides several sample questions, based on critical thinking intellectual standards, that pharmacists in our practice can ask themselves to ensure that patients receive safe and effective therapy during transitions of care involving OPAT. The intellectual standards were described in Chapter 1. They are clarity, relevance, significance, objectivity, fairness, accuracy, precision, depth, breadth, and logic—embodied in the "Clear ROAD to Logic" mnemonic.

KEY POINT

The patient's health literacy, ability to adhere to the treatment regimen, and access to outpatient medical care must be critically assessed to determine if OPAT is a feasible consideration for an individual patient.

TABLE 9-1

Sample Standards-Based Questions That Can Be Applied to Assure That Intellectual Standards for Thinking Are Met as the Pharmacist Provides Patient Care as Part of ID Therapy and OPAT Transitions of Care

Clarity (explicit, unambiguous, intelligible, free from confusion or doubt)	• Is the antimicrobial plan clear and finalized with agreement between the primary medical team and ID consult team (eg, drug selection, dose, frequency, duration, and monitoring)? • Are the recommendations and plan for OPAT documented clearly in the electronic health record? • Is the patient able to clearly understand and adhere to OPAT (eg, based on his or her health literacy and understanding of the treatment plan?
Relevance (pertinent, applicable, germane)	• What collected information from patient assessment and laboratory data is pertinent to managing the infection? • Are appropriate resources and guidelines utilized to develop a plan that is optimal to the infection being treated?
Significance (important, nontrivial, necessary, critical, required, impactful)	• Have I identified the most important information from the primary medical team, ID team, and electronic health record to be able to design and monitor an OPAT regimen? • Am I missing information that could be significant for accurately evaluating this patient?
Objectivity (fact-based, unbiased)	• Is the plan free from bias related to the patient's socioeconomic status (such as unstable housing), past medical history (such as history of intravenous drug abuse leading to inability to receive intravenous antibiotics in an unmonitored setting) or healthcare literacy? • If available, did the team utilize the most current ID guidelines and/or peer-reviewed literature to objectively develop the treatment plan?
Fairness (unbiased, equitable, impartial)	• Is the patient involved in decision-making when determining whether OPAT is the best plan of action? • In fairness to the patient and other stakeholders, do I adequately understand the roles of other providers in this patient's care? • Are resources made available to all patients to facilitate appropriate use and monitoring of antimicrobials in the outpatient setting (eg, access to ID clinic staff for questions or issues that arise, or educating on home antimicrobial administration)?
Accuracy (verifiable, valid, true, credible, undistorted)	• Will the selected antimicrobial regimen treat the most common organisms causing the infection (empiric therapy) or the organism(s) identified as causing the infection (definitive therapy) if cultures are performed? • Was the narrowest antimicrobial regimen selected to appropriately treat the infection and minimize adverse effects (eg, acute kidney injury and *Clostridioides difficile* infection)? • Does the OPAT regimen documented in the electronic health record contain accurate information on the drug selection, dose, frequency, duration, and monitoring?

Precision (exact, specific, detailed)	• Have the most recent inpatient laboratory results been reviewed prior to discharge to assess for changes needed to the OPAT regimen (eg, dose adjustment due to therapeutic drug monitoring or changes in renal or hepatic function, or adjustment to antimicrobial regimen based on updated microbiology results)? • Has the patient been educated on and demonstrated understanding of the details of the OPAT plan, including monitoring and follow-up? • Does the selection of an antimicrobial regimen consider optimal outpatient infusion strategies (ie, once-daily dosing or continuous infusion)?
Depth (roots, fundamentals, complexities, interrelationships, cause/effect, implications)	• Has the source of infection been identified and addressed in order to provide the patient with the best chance for a successful outcome on OPAT? • How do patient social factors influence the treatment plan and its implementation? • What benefits may the patient experience as a result of OPAT compared to prolonged inpatient admission to receive intravenous antimicrobials?
Breadth (comprehensive, encompassing, alternative perspectives)	• Have alternatives to OPAT been considered and deemed not appropriate to treat the infection (eg, oral antimicrobial therapy)? • Have all stakeholders been identified and engaged prior to hospital discharge (eg, ID physician, primary care physician, outpatient pharmacist, home health nurse, and patient caregiver)? • Have all stakeholders been identified and engaged to put the OPAT plan into place (eg, case manager, social worker, home health agency, and outpatient infusion pharmacy)?
Logic (reasonable, rational, without contradiction, well-founded, sound)	• Is the antimicrobial plan evidence-based and supported by the most current guidelines and peer-reviewed literature? • Am I able to articulate the relevant evidence and rationale to support my conclusions? • Is OPAT feasible and able to be carried out following discharge (including from a cost perspective)? • Is there a sound plan in place for follow-up once OPAT is completed?

APPLICATION OF THE PPCP IN OUR PRACTICE

Application of the PPCP begins with collection of pertinent information, which is achieved through chart review, discussions with providers, and by patient interview. Examples of information collected include diagnostic data to support a specific infectious disease diagnosis, culture and susceptibility data, and allergy information. Once all relevant patient information is collected, the ID pharmacist uses this knowledge to assess the infection being treated, the goals of therapy, and the treatment plan (if already developed). The assessment serves as the basis to set appropriate goals and to determine interventions to develop and manage antimicrobial regimens as part of the Plan step. Both the inpatient and OPAT ID pharmacists work with providers to implement the therapeutic plan through coordination with the inpatient team, patients, home healthcare agencies, and outpatient infusion pharmacies. Lastly, the pharmacist is essential for both inpatient and outpatient monitoring for safety and efficacy of antimicrobial regimens through evaluation of laboratory results and communication with patients and caregivers. In all aspects of pharmacist-provided care, excellent critical thinking and clinical reasoning are paramount.

 KEY POINT

Multiple sources of data should be utilized to ensure the most current and pertinent patient information is collected, such as chart review, discussions with providers, and patient interview.

COLLECTION OF PATIENT INFORMATION IN OUR PRACTICE

Typically, data collection begins with a review of the information to date in the medical record and additional medication information from outside sources. This can then be followed by a patient interview, which will include a medication history and an assessment of the ability to continue IV antibiotics outside of the hospital. Additional sources of data can include other members of the healthcare team, including but not limited to physicians and case managers. Examples of the type of information that is collected during a chart review in preparation for a patient interview are provided in **Table 9-2**.

TABLE 9-2

Examples of Data That Can Be Collected During Chart Review in Preparation for the Patient Interview

Data to Collect During Chart Review	Rationale for Collecting Specific Data
Patient diagnosis, including any relevant imaging (eg, MRI, CT, X-ray)	This information will allow the pharmacist to verify the need for antimicrobial treatment. The pharmacist would review the imaging reports to verify the infection-related diagnosis. It will also aid the pharmacist in antimicrobial selection, ensuring the antimicrobial is active at the site of infection. For example, daptomycin is inactivated by lung surfactant and would not be a good choice for pneumonia. The pharmacist will also use this information to guide antimicrobial dosing and duration recommendations.
Microbiology (cultures and susceptibilities) and other lab results (including any relevant therapeutic drug monitoring)	This information will allow the pharmacist to recommend an active antimicrobial regimen for the given infection based on culture and susceptibility results. The pharmacist may also use this information to guide antimicrobial dosing and duration recommendations. This includes any dose modifications necessary due to renal and/or hepatic dysfunction.
Recent antimicrobial use	This information will help the pharmacist determine the patient's risk for multidrug-resistant organisms and guide empiric antimicrobial selection recommendations or antimicrobial selection if no pathogens are grown in cultures. If organisms are grown in culture(s), then the antimicrobial selection recommendations are tailored to those results.

Patient allergies/ intolerances	This information will help the pharmacist to recommend an antimicrobial regimen that limits the risk of allergic and adverse reactions.
Medication list	The pharmacist should review the patient's complete inpatient medication list and any medications that will be continued after discharge to help screen for potential drug–drug interactions.
Insurance coverage	The pharmacist should be aware of the patient's insurance coverage in order to limit cost to the patient.

With a thorough chart review completed, the Collect step continues with a patient interview. **Table 9-3** describes examples of data that can be collected during the interview.

The Case of Daniel D.: Overview

Daniel D. (DD) is a 45-year-old male who was admitted to the hospital with fevers. He was previously admitted one month ago with gangrene of both second toes. X-rays at that time showed soft tissue gas and osteomyelitis in the right second digit and erosion of the distal phalanx of the left second digit concerning for osteomyelitis. During that admission, he was taken to the operating room for bilateral second toe amputation and right first toe amputation through the proximal phalanx. Cultures were not sent; however, per vascular physicians, source control was achieved. The ID consult team saw the patient and recommended IV vancomycin, cefepime, and metronidazole on admission, with transition to oral doxycycline, ciprofloxacin, and amoxicillin/clavulanate on discharge to complete a 2-week course. When questioned on medication adherence, the patient reports that he misses several doses of his insulin regimen each week; however, he confirms that he took all of his antibiotic doses. He was seen in the vascular clinic one week ago and was told the wounds looked good. After that appointment, the patient states he did a lot of walking around at home and noted soreness in his right foot and fevers up to

TABLE 9-3

Patient Interview: Examples of Data That Can Be Collected During the Patient Interview

- Patient's baseline understanding of the need for antimicrobial treatment and the proposed treatment plan
- Patient's/caregiver's desire for treatment at home with home health nursing or in a more monitored setting (eg, skilled nursing facility)
- Patient's/caregiver's comfort level with administering medication and caring for IV-line access at home
- Patient's/caregiver's desired antimicrobial administration frequency and duration
- Patient's goal(s) for treatment
- Any potential transportation issues for patient to attend follow-up appointments
- Complete medication review, including indication, dosing, side effects, allergies, insurance coverage, etc.
- Any anticipated issues with medication costs after discharge

101 degrees Fahrenheit at home. He had purulent drainage from the right foot. He did not note any streaky erythema on his feet. He had nasal congestion but denied coughing or shortness of breath. The patient reported no nausea, vomiting, diarrhea, dysuria, or flank pain. On admission, DD had slightly elevated temperatures, WBC was 6.2, procalcitonin 0.19, CRP 53.95. He had open wounds on his right foot near the remaining toes and left great toe. Wound culture is showing MRSA. MRI results indicated the patient had either postsurgical changes or early osteomyelitis. He is currently receiving vancomycin 1250 mg IV q8h.

The patient is being set up to receive OPAT at home to complete 6 weeks of treatment, so the OPAT team (including the OPAT pharmacist) is paged to review antimicrobial therapy.

Past Medical History:
Diabetes Mellitus Type 2
Peripheral Vascular Disease
Hypertension
Past Surgical History:
Bilateral second toe amputation and right first toe amputation through the proximal phalanx (1 month ago)
Tonsillectomy (20 years ago)
Insurance coverage: State Medicaid

CLINICAL REASONING, CRITICAL THINKING, AND THE PPCP FOR THE CARE OF DANIEL D.

The following series of tables delineates the PPCP as it is applied for the provision of pharmacy care to DD. For each step, from Collect to Monitor, there is a description of the pharmacist's clinical reasoning along with examples of how the critical thinking standards can be applied to optimize the pharmacist's clinical reasoning. Clinical reasoning is described in terms of the conclusions drawn along with their rationale: the case information or premises on which the conclusions are based. Critical thinking intellectual standards are expressed in the form of past-tense statements, instead of the question format introduced in Chapter 1. This is because the case analysis was performed in *reflection* upon the clinical encounter. An exception to this past-tense format of critical thinking statements is with the Collect step, where the future-tense is used to illustrate how the standards can be applied in *preparation* for the clinical encounter. As a reminder, the critical thinking standards are embodied in the mnemonic "Clear ROAD for Logic". They are clarity, relevance, significance, objectivity, fairness, accuracy, precision, depth, breadth, and logic.

Collect

In this step, the pharmacist collects the subjective and objective information about the patient in order to understand the relevant medical and medication history and clinical status of the patient. This will include information from the chart review conducted by the pharmacist in preparation for the counseling session and verified with the patient during the session.

COLLECT: Current Medications and Immunizations

Conclusions	Rationale: Information or Premise to Support the Conclusion
Complete a comprehensive medication review during discussion with the patient. *(To be collected through chart review and patient interview.)* For each medication, identify the indication. During patient discussion, review the indication, dosing, administration, and possible adverse effects of each medication.	• While the focus will be on antimicrobial management, the pharmacist should have a thorough understanding of the full medication regimen. • Identifying any potential drug–drug interactions that would limit antimicrobial choice or require additional monitoring is vital. • Matching each medication to an indication will allow the pharmacist to recognize any unnecessary therapeutic duplications and/or recognize any untreated indications. • A thorough medication review can reveal any drug therapy problems (adverse events, adherence concerns, etc.) • Reviewing indication, dosing, administration, and adverse effects of each medication will aid in optimizing the patient's understanding of and adherence to the medication regimen.
Determine if immunizations are up-to-date. *(To be collected during chart review.)*	• Ensuring the patient's immunizations are up-to-date is vital to helping protect the patient from other IDs.

Critical Thinking Checks for the Collect Plan for This Patient's Current Medications and Immunizations

In the medication review for this patient, it will be important to collect information with sufficient **accuracy** and **precision** that will enable me to draw sound conclusions on medication effectiveness, safety, and adherence, and any barriers negatively impacting the patient's medication use experience.

• During the discussion with the patient, he confirms he has no issues with adherence, either to his current medications or to the prior course of oral antibiotics he was prescribed. He confirms no adverse reactions from any of his chronic medications.

As optimizing medication use is an essential part of my practice, it will be critical in our discussion of medications that I **clearly** understand the patient and that he clearly understands me.

Given that the patient has several medical conditions and takes several medications, it will be important for me to think **deeply** as we discuss his medication usage so that I can gather the information needed for me to grasp the complexity of his medication experience.

• Because the patient's case and medication regimen are complex, it is important that I listen to his explanation of how he takes his medications at home and ask clarifying questions when needed. Once I have collected this information, I need to think deeply about how the conditions interrelate and can impact therapy goals. For example, uncontrolled diabetes likely led to the osteomyelitis requiring toe amputations and IV antibiotics, and continued lack of diabetes control could impair wound healing.

Collected Current Medication and Immunization Information Entered into Health Record

Current inpatient medication regimen:

• Aspirin 81 mg PO daily. Indication: heart attack prevention. No ADRs.
• Atorvastatin 20 mg PO qhs. Indication: heart attack prevention. No ADRs.
• Enoxaparin 40 mg subq daily. Indication: clot prevention. No ADRs.

- Insulin 70/30 NPH/regular 18 units subq bid before meals. Indication: diabetes. No ADRs.
- Insulin aspart 0 to 15 units (sliding scale) subq qid before meals and bedtime. Indication: diabetes. No ADRs.
- Lisinopril 5 mg PO daily. Indication: hypertension. No ADRs.
- Pioglitazone HCl 30 mg PO daily. Indication: diabetes. No ADRs.
- Vancomycin HCl 1250 mg IV q8h. Indication: bone infection. No ADRs.

Proposed outpatient medication regimen by ID and primary surgery teams:
- Aspirin 81 mg PO daily. Indication: heart attack prevention.
- Atorvastatin 20 mg PO qhs. Indication: heart attack prevention.
- Insulin 70/30 NPH/regular 18 units subq bid before meals. Indication: diabetes.
- Lisinopril 5 mg PO daily. Indication: hypertension.
- Pioglitazone HCl 30 mg PO daily. Indication: diabetes.
- Vancomycin HCl 1500 mg IV q8h. Indication: bone infection.

Current immunizations:
- Influenza vaccine: up-to-date
- Pneumococcal vaccine: up-to-date
- COVID-19: up-to-date
- Tetanus/diphtheria: up-to-date
- Hepatitis A: up-to-date
- Hepatitis B: up-to-date

Allergies: NKDA

COLLECT: Vital Signs, Labs, and Imaging	
Conclusions	Rationale: Information or Premise to Support the Conclusion
Complete a review of the patient's vital signs during chart review.	• Reviewing the patient's vital signs will allow the pharmacist to determine appropriate antimicrobial dosing and confirm that the patient is stable enough to be discharged. For example, a patient's weight would be used to dose antibiotics that are generally dosed on a mg/kg basis.
Complete a comprehensive review of patient's labs and lab trends during chart review. Complete a comprehensive review of patient's microbiology (culture/susceptibility) results during chart review.	• Reviewing labs and lab trends will allow the pharmacist to recommend appropriate antimicrobial choice and dosing, and establish a baseline for lab comparison after discharge. For example, knowing the patient's renal function while inpatient will allow both the ID pharmacist to recommend an antimicrobial dose for discharge and allow the OPAT ID pharmacist to monitor for any changes after discharge and adjust the antimicrobial dose if needed. • Reviewing the microbiology results will allow the ID pharmacist to recommend appropriate antimicrobial therapy, including an agent that will be active given the susceptibility results. The minimum inhibitory concentration (MIC) reported in the susceptibility results will allow the ID pharmacist to ensure adequate antimicrobial dosing is recommended.

| Complete a review of patient's imaging results during chart review | • Reviewing imaging results will allow the pharmacist to verify the diagnosis made by the physician(s), which can impact antimicrobial choice, dosing, and duration. For example, confirming a diagnosis of osteomyelitis is important because treatment of osteomyelitis requires a longer treatment duration (~6 weeks) compared to other infections. |

Critical Thinking Checks for the Collect Plan for This Patient's Vital Signs, Labs, and Imaging

In the chart review and medication review for this patient, it will be important to collect a **breadth** of information with sufficient **accuracy** and **precision** that will enable me to draw **sound conclusions** on anticipated medication effectiveness, safety, and adherence, and identify any barriers negatively impacting the patient's medication use experience.

• The information in the patient's chart is substantial, but focusing on collecting the **relevant** objective data that support the need for long-term IV antibiotics will be critical. Examples of this type of data include patient's weight, WBC, serum creatinine, inflammatory markers (ESR, CRP), therapeutic drug monitoring (eg, vancomycin concentrations), and cultures/susceptibilities. Of this data, it will also be critical to determine what is most **significant** for a complete and accurate assessment that will form the basis for therapeutic planning.

Relevant Vital Signs, Lab, and Imaging Information Present in the Health Record

Current vital signs:

4/9/2022: Temp 36.9°C, Pulse: 82 beats/minute, Resp: 16 breaths/minute, BP: 119/74 mm Hg, Height: 74 in, Weight: 90 kg

Labs:

Lab	04/07/2022	04/08/2022	04/09/2022
WBC	6.2	7.0	7.1
Hgb	12.0	11.9	11.3
Hct	34.7	34.3	33.2
Plt	189	195	210
Neutrophil (%)	45.5	50.4	48.8
Lymphocyte (%)	34.7	35.3	36.2
Monocyte (%)	16.6	10.7	10.7
Eosinophil (%)	2.3	2.8	3.4
Basophil (%)	0.9	0.8	0.9

Lab	04/06/2022	04/07/2022	04/08/2022	04/09/2022
Na	-	136	136	137
K	-	3.9	3.8	3.7
CO_2	-	29	27	29
BUN	-	13	19	13

Creatinine	-	0.68	0.63	0.56
Glucose	-	271	258	243
Albumin	3.6	-	-	-
T Bili	0.5	-	-	-
AST	14	-	-	-
ALT	9	-	-	-
EGFR	-	117	120	124
A1C	-	8.1	-	-

Lab	03/08/2022	03/10/2022	04/06/2022
HS-CRP	56.45	49.33	53.95
ESR	38	38	-

Vancomycin concentrations:
Concentration 1 collected 04/09/2022 at 1100: 18.5 mcg/mL
Concentration 2 collected 04/09/2022 at 1530: 9 mcg/mL
Pharmacist vancomycin pharmacokinetic monitoring note:
Calculated AUC is subtherapeutic at 358 mg*h/L on 1250 mg IV q8h dosing (goal AUC range 400 to 600 mg*h/L). Recommend increasing dose to 1500 mg IV q8h (calculated AUC 429 mg*h/L on this regimen). Recommend targeting goal trough concentration range of 10.5 to 17 mcg/mL (corresponds to AUC range of 401 to 601 mg*h/L). Based on the evaluation of patient's vancomycin clearance, it will not be possible to achieve therapeutic AUC utilizing every 12-h dosing frequency without exceeding 2000 mg IV q12h dosing.
Culture results:

Date	Culture Type	Result
04/06/2022	Blood Culture Set 1	No growth
04/06/2022	Blood Culture Set 2	No growth
04/06/2022	Respiratory Virus Panel	No pathogens detected
04/06/2022	SARS-CoV-2 PCR	Not detected
04/07/2022	Wound Culture, Right Foot	4+ Staphylococcus aureus

04/07/2022 Wound Culture: *Staphylococcus aureus*		
Drug	**MIC (mcg/mL)**	**Interpretation**
Penicillin	≥0.5	Resistant
Ciprofloxacin	≤0.5	Susceptible
Clindamycin	0.25	Susceptible
Daptomycin	0.25	Susceptible
Erythromycin	≥8	Resistant

Gentamicin	≤0.5	Susceptible
Levofloxacin	≤0.12	Susceptible
Linezolid	2	Susceptible
Minocycline	≤0.5	Susceptible
Moxifloxacin	≤0.25	Susceptible
Oxacillin	≥4	Resistant
Ceftaroline	0.5	Susceptible
Rifampin	≤0.5	Susceptible
Tetracycline	≤1	Susceptible
Vancomycin	≤0.5	Susceptible
Trimethoprim/ Sulfamethoxazole	≤10	Susceptible

Imaging on current hospitalization:
Ultrasound Leg Venous Duplex Bilateral, 04/06/2022
No evidence of an acute DVT in the lower extremities to the level of the popliteal vein.
Right Foot X-ray, 04/06/2022
No evidence of acute fracture. Amputation of the first and second phalanges with soft tissue swelling. No frank cortical destruction to suggest osteomyelitis radiographically. Osseous mineralization within normal limits.
Left Foot X-ray, 04/06/2022
No evidence of acute fracture. Amputation of the second phalange with soft tissue swelling. No frank cortical destruction to suggest osteomyelitis radiographically. Osseous mineralization within normal limits.
Chest X-Ray Portable 1-View, 04/06/2022
No acute cardiopulmonary abnormalities. No focal consolidation.
Left Forefoot MRI, 04/09/2022
Postsurgical changes of second toe amputation, with an open wound along the dorsum of the foot at the second toe metatarsal head. Mild edema and enhancement within the metatarsal head, which likely reflects evolving postsurgical changes, although early osteomyelitis could also have this appearance.
Right Forefoot MRI, 04/09/2022
Given proximity to recent surgery, findings involving the second metatarsal head are indeterminate for postoperative edema versus early osteomyelitis. Findings involving the dorsal surface of the first metatarsal head, medial sesamoid, and proximal phalangeal stump are favored to be reactive given involvement of multiple osseous structures but also could represent early osteomyelitis.
Imaging on last hospitalization (prior to amputation surgery):
Right Toes X-ray, 03/10/2022
Soft tissue swelling with subcutaneous gas at the great toe and second toe. No frank cortical destruction to suggest osteomyelitis radiographically. Mild great toe MTP osteoarthritis. Osseous mineralization within normal limits. No other abnormalities of the bones, alignment, or soft tissues identified.

Right Toes X-ray, 03/08/2022

Soft tissue swelling at the level of the second digit without osseous erosion indicates osteomyelitis at this level. However, there is subcutaneous gas seen around the second digit, and also at the medial aspect of the second digit at the level of the distal phalanx. These findings support soft tissue infection. Necrotizing infection could be present. Vascular calcifications are present.

Left Toes X-ray, 03/10/2022

Soft tissue wound, with subcutaneous air, at the distal tip of the second toe with underlying bone destruction of the tuft of the second toe distal phalanx, concerning for osteomyelitis. Osseous mineralization is otherwise within normal limits. No other abnormalities of the bones, alignment, or soft tissues identified.

Left Toes X-ray, 03/08/2022

Full-thickness skin defect seen at the level of the distal second digit with underlying associated osseous erosion of the phalangeal tuft. This is concerning for osteomyelitis.

COLLECT: IV Access and Discharge Planning Needs	
Conclusions	Rationale: Information or Premise to Support the Conclusion
Complete a review with the team regarding IV access options.	Discussing the options for the patient's IV access with the team will allow the pharmacist to determine if any antimicrobials are not feasible due to a need for central line access for infusion.
Complete a review with the team and patient regarding the patient's destination after discharge and other needs after discharge.	Discussing with the team and patient about the setting following discharge will allow the pharmacist to assess if any antimicrobial agents are not feasible or not preferred, and assess for any issues with transportation to follow-up appointments.

Critical Thinking Checks for the Collect Plan for This Patient's IV Access and Discharge Planning Needs

In the review of this patient's IV access and discharge planning needs, it will be important to collect information with sufficient **accuracy** and **precision** that will enable me to draw sound conclusions about the optimal type of IV access and the place patient could receive their OPAT, and any barriers that may negatively impact the patient's medication use experience.

• It is critical that there is a discussion with the patient regarding his (and/or his partner's) comfort level with administering IV antibiotics at home. This, in addition to overall health status, will help determine if the patient can safely receive OPAT at home or if the patient needs to be placed in a higher level of care (eg, skilled nursing facility).

As IV access and discharge planning are critical to optimizing OPAT medication use, it will be critical in our patient and team discussions that the team and I **clearly** understand the patient and his partner and that they clearly understand us. To accomplish this, I need to be certain to communicate with a vocabulary that they understand, is free of jargon that they may not understand, and is communicated with an empathetic understanding of each of their perspectives and in a manner that assures they are empowered to confidently assume their roles in implementing the OPAT plan.

Collected IV Access and Discharge Planning Needs Based on Current Patient Status and Patient Interview

IV Access Options due to need for more than two weeks of antimicrobial treatment:

- Peripherally Inserted Central Catheter (PICC)
- Tunneled Central Line
- Anticipated currently to have a PICC line placed since patient has no other IV infusion needs and is anticipated to go home with home health and infusion pharmacy services.

Discharge planning needs:

No need for skilled nursing placement, so anticipate discharge to home with home health and infusion pharmacy services.

Partner is able and willing to help with any infusion and line care needs.

No anticipated issues with transportation (patient and partner have their own vehicles) or paying for outpatient medications.

 KEY POINT

A thorough assessment of discharge planning needs is required to ensure a smooth transition between inpatient and outpatient settings with minimal risk to the patient.

Example Collect Statement for DD

DD is a 45-year-old male who was admitted for fevers and right foot soreness. Patient has a recent history of gangrene of both second toes and resulting osteomyelitis. He underwent amputation of his bilateral second toes and right first toe. The patient completed two weeks of oral antibiotics (doxycycline, ciprofloxacin, and amoxicillin/clavulanate) after discharge. However, he developed fevers and soreness in his right foot, bringing him to the hospital. On admission, he had slightly elevated temperatures and an elevated CRP. Imaging during this admission shows possible osteomyelitis of left second metatarsal and right forefoot. Wound culture from the right foot grew MRSA, which is susceptible to multiple antibiotics, including vancomycin and daptomycin. He is currently receiving vancomycin 1250 mg IV q8h. AUC-guided dosing of vancomycin suggests a dose of 1500 mg IV q8h. The patient prefers to receive the remainder of his antibiotic therapy at home with the help of his partner and home health nursing, and there is no medical need for skilled nursing placement. DD prefers as simple of a regimen as possible since he and his partner will be responsible for the majority of the infusions. A PICC line is anticipated to be placed prior to discharge to facilitate long-term IV antibiotic therapy. The patient confirms no medication allergies, insurance through state Medicaid, and up-to-date vaccinations. The patient does not anticipate any issues paying for outpatient medications or issues with transportation to follow-up appointments. He has a past medical history of hypertension, type 2 diabetes mellitus, peripheral vascular disease, and a past surgical history of tonsillectomy and multiple toe amputations. Recent labs are WNL or stable. Notably, the patient's serum creatinine is WNL and his glucose is elevated but stable compared with prior inpatient results. The patient denies any history of illicit drug use.

Assessment of Collected Information

The Assess step involves applying critical thinking and clinical reasoning in the evaluation of information gathered during the Collect phase to identify, characterize, and prioritize the patient's main problems that may benefit from pharmacist intervention. Critical thinking must be utilized during all PPCP steps, and standards-based questions such as those delineated in Table 9-1 may be employed to help assure high-quality critical thinking. In order to develop optimal plans, it is vital for the pharmacist to work together with the OPAT team to appropriately identify and assess the patient's main issues requiring intervention. In addition, it is important to recognize that issues may overlap and there may be several contributing factors identified for any one problem. When evaluating patients with IDs, it is important to assess the source of infection and the medications that will be used for treatment of the infection in order to develop an optimal treatment plan with the goals being infection cure and prevention of progression and relapse. The pharmacist should consider the feasibility of the treatment approach and identify any potential issues during the Assess step, such as inability to adhere to the antimicrobial regimen or selection of a regimen that does not treat the causative organism(s) or is associated with adverse effects. Previous treatments and interventions performed for the infection should also be evaluated in order to develop a complete and appropriate therapeutic regimen. In addition, the prevention of IDs should be assessed through review of the patient's vaccination history, for example.

KEY POINT

It is important to consider both appropriate antimicrobial treatment and management of the source of infection when treating patients with infectious diseases.

KEY POINT

Prior treatments and interventions utilized for the infection should be considered in order to develop a complete and appropriate therapeutic regimen.

ASSESS: Osteomyelitis of Right and Left Feet	
Conclusions	Rationale: Information or Premise to Support the Conclusion
Osteomyelitis of both feet caused by MRSA, due to a failure of oral antibiotics and surgical procedures to eradicate a diabetic foot MRSA infection. Potential additional contributing factors: • Uncontrolled type 2 diabetes mellitus	The patient presents with fevers, soreness, and drainage from right foot in the setting of recent right and left lower extremity infections. Physical examination reveals open wounds on the right foot near the remaining toes with purulent drainage and on the left great toe. Objective findings include elevated CRP and fever. MRI of right and left forefeet is concerning for early osteomyelitis, which fits with the patient's current clinical presentation and history. Although X-rays of both right and left feet did not show findings consistent with osteomyelitis, MRI has higher sensitivity to identify bony changes consistent with osteomyelitis and is the recommended imaging study when evaluating for osteomyelitis in the setting of diabetic foot infection.[6] The location of osteomyelitis

• Peripheral vascular disease • Frequent walking on affected lower extremities	appears similar to prior imaging from about 1 month ago, indicating surgical intervention may not have removed all infected bone, leading to ongoing infection. Given the history of uncontrolled diabetes mellitus, it is likely that the patient's lower extremity infections began as diabetic foot infections and progressed to osteomyelitis. A wound culture is obtained and growing MRSA. The isolate is determined to be MRSA based on reported resistance to oxacillin. Surgical cultures were not sent from amputations about 1 month ago. Although intraoperative cultures are preferred to wound cultures to determine the causative pathogen(s), MRSA will be treated as the likely causative organism as it is a known pathogen in osteomyelitis, including in the setting of moderate-to-severe diabetic foot infection as is the case for this patient.[6] The patient previously received a two-week course of oral antibiotics to treat osteomyelitis following surgical intervention. The regimen included doxycycline, which provides appropriate coverage of MRSA based on wound culture results indicating susceptibility to tetracycline. Of note, the patient was also receiving ciprofloxacin, which the culture report indicates as susceptible; however, fluoroquinolones are not considered reliable options for treatment of MRSA due to potential for rapid development of resistance while on therapy. He confirmed adherence to this regimen during patient interview. Despite treatment with doxycycline, the patient's infection progressed, which may have been due to incomplete surgical source control if all infected bone was not removed, potential for decreased penetration at site of infection with oral antibiotics, and/or a duration of therapy that was too short. In addition, the patient's type 2 diabetes mellitus is documented as uncontrolled, as evidenced by elevated hemoglobin A1C. Uncontrolled diabetes mellitus is a known causative factor for both development of infection and delay in healing and resolution of infection.[7] Peripheral vascular disease may also predispose the patient to develop foot infections and impair wound healing. Lastly, frequent walking on lower extremities may increase the risk of trauma, such as development of blisters or pressure sores, which may progress into wounds and increase risk of infection.
Needs additional therapy: Requirement for outpatient intravenous antibiotic therapy	As the patient's infection was not eradicated and progressed following a course of oral antibiotics, the team has decided to treat with a prolonged course of intravenous antibiotics. Consultation with vascular surgeons should be considered to determine if further surgical intervention (eg, removal of infected bone via amputation) is warranted. Initiation of OPAT requires several logistical considerations, including selection of an appropriate antimicrobial regimen, establishment of IV access to receive medications, and determination of the location in which patient will receive IV antibiotics (eg, home, skilled nursing facility, etc.).

Critical Thinking Checks for Assessing This Patient's Osteomyelitis of Right and Left Feet

In order to evaluate the patient's osteomyelitis, it was necessary to collect and analyze all **relevant** subjective and objective information, including clinical presentation, vital signs and laboratory data, imaging results, and culture and susceptibility results. In addition, information about prior interventions employed for the infection that were deemed **significant** and important for proper assessment were also considered (including previous surgical intervention and oral antibiotic treatment). The **accuracy** of information was confirmed prior to developing clinical assessments.

- It is important to both understand and consider prior interventions that did or did not work when developing the current therapeutic plan. For example, without knowledge that the patient had previously completed a course of oral antibiotics followed by progression of infection, the pharmacist may have considered an oral antibiotic regimen for ease of treatment as compared to an IV regimen. Proper analysis of previous therapeutic interventions is vital to completing an appropriate assessment that leads to development of optimal, patient-centered plans.

In order to perform a **fair** and **precise** assessment, it was vital to assess the information in an **objective** manner, including awareness and avoidance of unnecessary biases or false conclusions that were not supported by the available information. One potential bias includes fundamental attribution error, which may have occurred if the clinician assumed that the patient's infection progressed due to lack of adherence to the previous oral antibiotic regimen without evidence to support this conclusion.

In addition, an appropriate **depth and breadth** were utilized to evaluate for etiologies of ongoing infection (such as potential for nonadherence to previous antimicrobial therapy, incomplete surgical source control, or uncontrolled diabetes mellitus), assess for alternative treatment options, and identify key components necessary to pursue a transition to OPAT for the patient.

ASSESS: Type 2 Diabetes Mellitus and Peripheral Vascular Disease

Conclusions	Rationale: Information or Premise to Support the Conclusion
Uncontrolled type 2 diabetes mellitus	The patient is documented as having uncontrolled type 2 diabetes mellitus in the case. This is confirmed by an elevated hemoglobin A1C of 8.1%. Inpatient blood glucose values ranging from 243 to 271 mg/dL are higher than the estimated average glucose associated with an A1C of 8.1%. Contributing factors could include stress of hospitalization and ongoing infection. Outpatient medications used by DD for treatment of his type 2 diabetes mellitus include insulin 70/30 NPH/regular and pioglitazone. Uncontrolled type 2 diabetes mellitus is a known risk factor for both development of infection and impaired healing and resolution of infection once present.[7] One reason for uncontrolled diabetes mellitus includes suboptimal adherence with the insulin regimen as reported by the patient.
Peripheral vascular disease that is being monitored	Peripheral vascular disease is documented in the patient's past medical history and the patient is followed in the vascular clinic for this condition. The case indicates the patient was recently evaluated in the vascular clinic and told the wounds "looked good," suggesting good perfusion to the wound area. Current medications related to peripheral vascular disease include aspirin and atorvastatin as secondary prevention measures to reduce the risk of heart attack.

Critical Thinking Checks for Assessing This Patient's Type 2 Diabetes Mellitus and Peripheral Vascular Disease

To evaluate and assess the patient's past medical history, including type 2 diabetes mellitus and peripheral vascular disease, it was important to collect **relevant** and **accurate** information from the patient's chart. It was necessary to identify the most **significant** information to assess the disease states, such as hemoglobin A1C value to assess whether type 2 diabetes mellitus is under control.

In addition, an appropriate **depth** of analysis was utilized to form connections between disease states and the infection being treated, such as determination that uncontrolled type 2 diabetes mellitus is likely contributing to ongoing infection.

- When performing an assessment, the pharmacist must use caution not to focus solely on the therapeutic issue at hand, but rather utilize a more global approach to identify other factors that may be contributing to the condition. For example, in this patient's case, the pharmacist identified that the patient has uncontrolled type 2 diabetes mellitus, which is likely contributing to development of infections, delayed healing, and progression of current infection.

ASSESS: Drug Therapy Problems	
Conclusions	Rationale: Information or Premise to Support the Conclusion
Needs additional therapy—OPAT	Vancomycin has been selected for OPAT based on wound cultures growing MRSA. The patient is currently receiving vancomycin in the hospital at a dosing frequency of every 8 hours, which is supported by therapeutic drug monitoring and stable renal function. Vancomycin AUC dosing calculations were performed and indicate that a q12h dosing frequency is not possible without utilizing unconventional dosing above 2000 mg IV q12h that is not preferable in the outpatient setting where close monitoring is not possible. Vancomycin q8h dosing frequency is required to achieve a therapeutic AUC and optimize efficacy of vancomycin for treatment of the infection. Given the requirement for q8h dosing frequency, additional therapy is required for the patient's OPAT plan.
Inappropriate adherence—Insulin therapy	The patient is documented as having uncontrolled type 2 diabetes mellitus. Upon patient interview, the patient reports that he is not always adherent to his insulin regimen at home and misses several doses per week. Consultation with the patient's primary care physician or endocrinologist who manages diabetes care may be beneficial in developing a plan to optimize the patient's diabetes control and reduce risk of infection.

Critical Thinking Checks for Assessing This Patient's Drug Therapy Problems

Review of the patient's vancomycin dosing required both **precision** and **accuracy** to confirm that a regimen dosed less frequently than every 8 hours is not an option and may compromise efficacy of vancomycin based on therapeutic drug monitoring results.

In addition, attention was paid to **clarity** of the OPAT plan as it relates to the antimicrobial regimen selected (drug and dosing frequency).

Assessment of information collected during patient interview on medication adherence was important to **accurately and objectively** identify the patient's adherence issues to outpatient insulin therapy for treatment of diabetes mellitus, rather than assuming an alternative reason for uncontrolled diabetes mellitus.

Given the complexity of this patient, who has several co-current conditions and is taking several medications, it can be useful to create a concept map to help grasp some of the interrelationships that contribute to the complexity (**Figure 9-2**). Understanding these interrelationships can be useful to create a comprehensive assessment of this patient, which is expressed in the Assess statement below.

Example Assess Statement for DD

DD is a 45-year-old male presenting with fever and purulent drainage from right foot and diagnosed with osteomyelitis involving both right and left lower extremities.

(1) Osteomyelitis of right and left feet caused by MRSA

The patient's clinical presentation (soreness and purulent drainage from right foot, fevers), laboratory results (elevated CRP), and imaging findings are consistent with a diagnosis of osteomyelitis involving bilateral lower extremities. Based on the history of uncontrolled type 2 diabetes mellitus and the location of infection, it is likely that the patient's infection began as diabetic foot infection that progressed to osteomyelitis. Although results of X-rays of left and right feet do not indicate changes consistent with osteomyelitis, MRI findings are consistent with the diagnosis, which is supported by this study's increased sensitivity for detection of osteomyelitis, making MRI the recommended imaging strategy to evaluate for osteomyelitis in the setting of diabetic foot infection.[6] A wound culture is obtained and is growing MRSA, which is deemed to be the causative pathogen of infection. MRSA is a common pathogen associated with osteomyelitis, including in the setting of moderate-to-severe diabetic foot infection as is the case for DD.[6] Several contributory factors are identified that may explain the patient's ongoing infection, including potential for lack of complete surgical source control with prior amputations, possible decreased or impaired penetration at site of infection with oral antibiotics, and a duration of therapy that was too short. IDSA guidelines on treatment of diabetic foot infection with osteomyelitis recommend a prolonged antibiotic duration of at least 4 weeks when there is persistent infected or necrotic bone following surgical intervention.[6] Persistent infected bone may not have been a concern at the time of prior amputations due to documentation indicating the surgical team felt adequate source control was achieved. It is recommended to send intraoperative specimens of bone at the margin of debridement for histopathologic evaluation, which may be useful in determining presence of remaining infected bone.[8]

(2) Uncontrolled type 2 diabetes mellitus

The patient is documented as having uncontrolled type 2 diabetes mellitus as evidenced by an elevated hemoglobin A1C. In addition, inpatient blood glucose values are elevated, though this may be caused in part by ongoing infection and stress related to hospitalization. DD is receiving outpatient therapy for diabetes management including insulin and pioglitazone. The patient reports suboptimal adherence with his insulin therapy. The current infection may be worsened by uncontrolled diabetes mellitus due to impairment of the immune system as a result of hyperglycemia.[7]

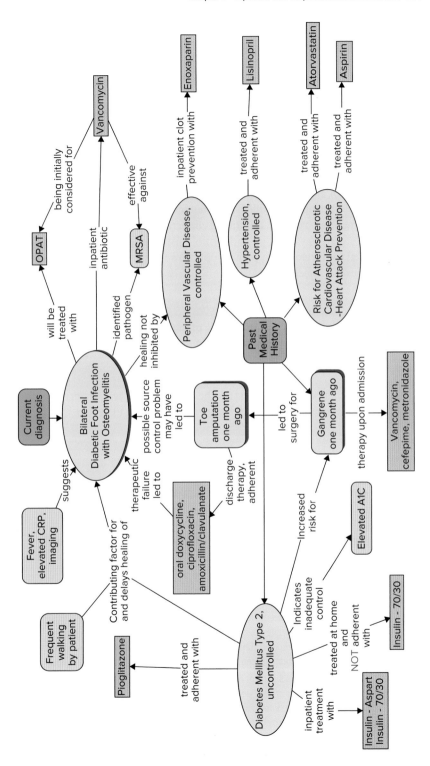

FIGURE 9-2. Concept map depicting interrelationships between this patient's disease states, medications, and related factors.

(3) Drug therapy problems

Needs additional therapy—OPAT: The team is considering discharge with OPAT to receive vancomycin. Although inpatient therapeutic drug monitoring indicates a requirement to receive vancomycin at every 8-hour dosing frequency to achieve pharmacokinetic targets for efficacy, an alteration to the vancomycin regimen is required for OPAT due to the risk for suboptimal adherence with vancomycin q8h dosing in the outpatient setting. It is typically not possible for patients to adhere to dosing frequency more often than every 12 hours in the outpatient setting due to negative impacts on quality of life and activities of daily living.[9]

Inappropriate adherence—Insulin therapy: Upon patient interview, the patient reports that he is not always adherent to his insulin regimen at home and misses several doses per week. Uncontrolled diabetes may be contributing to ongoing infection and increase risk of additional infections. Consultation with the patient's primary care physician or endocrinologist who manages diabetes care may be beneficial in developing a plan to optimize the patient's diabetes control and reduce the risk of infection.

 KEY POINT

Attention should be taken to ensure that goals of therapy are focused on both direct and indirect contributors to the patient's main infectious disease-related issues.

The conclusions that are developed in the Assess step will determine the subsequent steps to be taken for clinical decision-making in the Plan step.

Plan, Implement, and Monitor

PLAN: Goals	
Conclusions	Rationale: Information or Premise to Support the Conclusion
Goals include: 1. Resolution of signs/symptoms of infection associated with osteomyelitis of bilateral feet after 6-week course of IV antibiotics.	Current signs/symptoms of infection include soreness and purulent drainage from right foot, fevers, laboratory results (elevated CRP), and imaging findings consistent with a diagnosis of osteomyelitis involving bilateral feet.
	Goal is for resolution of signs/symptoms of infection through completion of IV antibiotic course. A 6-week IV antibiotic course is sufficient for goal of eradication of infection.[6]
2. Improve blood glucose control through achievement of A1C <7% within 3 months from diabetes treatment plan modifications.	Requirements for OPAT regimens include an antibiotic that provides appropriate coverage for causative pathogen (MRSA), dosing frequency of q12h to q24h if possible, ability to monitor regimen in outpatient setting, and ability for patient to afford OPAT regimen.
	Patient's current A1C is above goal at 8.1%. Goal A1C is likely <7% for this patient per American Diabetes Association guidelines, though determination of patient's specific goal will be performed by the provider managing his diabetes care.[10] The A1C represents a 3-month average of blood glucose levels. 2022 American Diabetes Association guidelines recommend assessment of glycemic status at least quarterly in patients who are not achieving glycemic goals.[10]

Critical Thinking Checks for Developing This Patient's Goals

The patient's SMART goals were developed with specific goals and targets **clearly** defined so that a **logical** and **precise** plan may be developed to achieve these goals.

The SMART goals were developed with **logic** and **objectivity** through appropriate assessment of the disease state pathophysiology and treatment, and utilization of the most up-to-date clinical guidelines for the respective disease states.

- For example, the time frames of 6 weeks for osteomyelitis resolution and 3 months for improved blood glucose control were logically based on evidence, the patient assessment, and what is known about these conditions.

The SMART goals were created in a **fair-minded** manner with an empathetic consideration of the patient's ability to afford and monitor the OPAT regimen.

The SMART goals were created with considerations of their **relevance** to the patient's main drug therapy-related problems identified.

PLAN: Osteomyelitis of Bilateral Lower Feet and Development of OPAT Regimen

Goal: Resolution of signs/symptoms of infection associated with osteomyelitis of bilateral feet after 6-week course of IV antibiotics

Conclusions	Rationale: Information or Premise to Support the Conclusion
Initiate daptomycin 550 mg (6 mg/kg) IV q24h for 6 weeks of therapy.	An alternative antibiotic to vancomycin is needed for treatment of the patient's MRSA osteomyelitis, as vancomycin therapeutic drug monitoring utilizing AUC dosing indicates a required dosing frequency of q8h. It is difficult for patients to administer antibiotics more frequently than q12h to q24h in the outpatient setting; therefore, an antibiotic that can be administered less frequently is preferable.[9] The patient confirmed this. In addition, the patient reported suboptimal adherence with insulin therapy outpatient, which heightens concern for adherence issues with q8h antibiotic dosing outpatient. Alternative options that provide coverage for MRSA include daptomycin (generally well-tolerated and q24h dosing), linezolid (also available as an oral agent and dosed q12h), ceftaroline (typically dosed q8h for off-label treatment of MRSA infections), and long-acting lipoglycopeptides (ie, oritavancin or dalbavancin). Since the patient has developed a progressive infection following a course of oral antibiotics, it may be preferable to treat with IV antibiotics in this case. A prolonged duration of linezolid (>2 to 4 weeks) may be associated with emergence of toxicities, such as thrombocytopenia and peripheral and optic neuropathy; therefore, this agent was not selected for treatment.[11] Ceftaroline also requires consideration for q8h dosing when used off-label for MRSA infections; therefore, this antibiotic was not selected as an alternative to vancomycin.[12] Based on the drug half-lives, dalbavancin and oritavancin provide approximately 8.5 to 10 days of antibiotic coverage following a dose, respectively, and therefore patients may require repeated dosing in the outpatient setting for prolonged antibiotic courses, which may be associated with logistical issues.[13,14] This leaves daptomycin as a potential option for the patient given coverage of MRSA within its spectrum of activity, q24h dosing, and as this agent is generally well tolerated.

	It is recommended to monitor creatine phosphokinase (CPK) at baseline and at least once weekly in patients receiving daptomycin to monitor for development of myopathy or rhabdomyolysis.[15]
	Since the patient takes atorvastatin for heart attack prevention due to peripheral vascular disease, the medical team will need to carefully evaluate the risks and benefits of continuing atorvastatin while the patient is receiving daptomycin. If the patient is deemed to be at low risk for a cardiovascular event by the primary medical team, the decision may be made to hold atorvastatin during daptomycin therapy. The literature is mixed regarding whether statins should be held during treatment with daptomycin to reduce risk of myopathy and rhabdomyolysis, and this is often a patient-specific decision.[16,17]
Educate patient on appropriate wound care.	Appropriate wound care is important for healing of the current infection. This includes moist wound care through use of wound dressings (selection of dressing is based on the size and depth of wound and characteristics of the ulcer) and off-loading of pressure from the affected area of the foot.[6] Education on wound care is often initiated in the inpatient setting through consultation with a wound care specialist.
Limit excessive walking on lower extremities, educate and assess availability of appropriate footwear.	It is important to address factors that may be related to poor wound healing including frequent walking on lower extremities that prevents off-loading of pressure and potential for improper footwear. This will promote healing of current wounds and the infection.

 KEY POINT

It is difficult for patients to administer antimicrobials more frequently than once or twice daily in the outpatient setting; therefore, selection of a medication that can be administered less frequently is preferable.

Critical Thinking Checks for This Patient's Treatment Plan for Osteomyelitis and Development of OPAT Regimen

Assessment of the feasibility and appropriateness of several alternative antibiotic regimens was evaluated in order to provide a **logical** and **relevant** antimicrobial plan with appropriate **breadth**.

- The pharmacist must identify several therapeutic options, as alternative plans are often necessary if the first plan is not desirable or feasible. In this situation, the pharmacist carefully assessed and analyzed several therapeutic alternatives to appropriately treat the infection, including vancomycin, linezolid, ceftaroline, long-acting lipoglycopeptides (eg, oritavancin, dalbavancin), and oral antibiotics. Incorporation of information pertinent to the patient's specific scenario (such as inability to administer an antibiotic every 8 hours at home) and prior interventions utilized helped the pharmacist decide on daptomycin in this case.

An appropriate **depth** of thinking was applied to integrate nonpharmacological measures with the pharmacological strategy and patient education to maximize the chances of achieving the SMART goals.

PLAN: Uncontrolled Type 2 Diabetes Mellitus	
Goal: Improve blood glucose control through achievement of A1C <7% within 3 months from diabetes treatment plan modifications	
Conclusions	Rationale: Information or Premise to Support the Conclusion
Refer to primary care provider (PCP) or endocrinologist who is managing diabetes care for adjustment to therapeutic regimen as needed.	As the patient's A1C is not at goal, and uncontrolled diabetes mellitus may delay resolution of infection and increase risk of developing further infection, it is important to refer the patient to the medical team currently managing diabetes care for adjustments. Since management of diabetes is not typically performed by the ID consulting team, referral and discussion with the physician(s) currently treating this disease state is appropriate and important to ensure continuity of care.
Educate patient on lifestyle modifications that may aid in improved glycemic control.	Aside from modification of medication regimens, lifestyle changes may be associated with significant benefits and an increase in achievement of therapeutic goals in patients with diabetes. Examples of lifestyle modifications include reducing intake of foods high in sugar and carbohydrates and increasing exercise and physical activity as tolerated.
Educate patient on prevention of diabetic foot infections.	Frequent walking and use of improper footwear (such as shoes that are ill-fitting or too tight) may predispose patients with diabetes to development of blisters or ulcers and subsequently increase risk of diabetic foot infection. Guidelines recommend providing education on foot self-care to all patients with diabetes, such as performing regular foot self-exams.[18]

Critical Thinking Checks for This Patient's Uncontrolled Type 2 Diabetes Mellitus

In order to develop a comprehensive plan for treatment of current infection and prevention of future infections, evaluation of the patient's current diabetes management was deemed **relevant** and **significant**.

Discussion of lifestyle modifications should be approached with the patient with an **objective** and **fair** mindset, free of bias or judgment, and with a goal of **clarity** of understanding that will encourage and empower the patient to self-manage his health and health behaviors.

In order to ensure that strategies for this patient's diabetes care are **logical** and complete, it is important to refer the patient to the current provider(s) managing his diabetes who will have the **depth** and **breadth** of understanding of his disease state and therapy needed to optimize his diabetes care.

To develop an appropriate therapeutic plan for the patient, the pharmacist must utilize knowledge and understanding of the issue at hand, and the best available evidence to construct a feasible and appropriate plan. One way in which this may be achieved is through argument mapping, which involves the synthesis and development of several conclusions that come together to support a final recommendation. **Figure 9-3** provides an example of an argument map supporting the recommendation to initiate daptomycin for the patient.

Recommendation				
Daptomycin 6 mg/kg IV infusion q24h × 6 weeks				
Daptomycin provides appropriate coverage for MRSA and is not an inferior option to vancomycin therapy.	Daptomycin may be administered as a once-daily medication via IV infusion.	If daptomycin is effective, an end result would be eradication of osteomyelitis, including resolution of signs and symptoms of infection.	There are no contraindications to daptomycin for this patient.	Assumption to verify: Patient is able to afford outpatient daptomycin (requires case management assistance to investigate cost to patient on current insurance).

SMART Goal

Following 6-week course of IV antibiotics, resolution of signs/symptoms of infection associated with osteomyelitis of bilateral lower extremities.

Assessment

Uncontrolled osteomyelitis of bilateral lower feet with contributing factors, including failure of oral antibiotics and surgical procedures to eradicate infection, uncontrolled type 2 diabetes mellitus, peripheral vascular disease, and frequent walking on affected lower extremities

FIGURE 9-3. Argument map for daptomycin selection.

IMPLEMENT/MONITOR: Foot Wounds: Postsurgical Changes Versus Early Osteomyelitis	
Conclusions	Rationale: Information or Premise to Support the Conclusion
Implement: Educate patient on the importance of wound care Confirm follow-up appointments with surgical team.	*Implement:* Wound care and follow-up with the surgical team is important for continued healing and progress.
Monitor: OPAT team to monitor attendance to follow-up appointments and progress via surgical team notes.	*Monitor:* Longitudinal education on the importance of attending surgical team appointments and adequate wound care.

Implement:	*Implement:*
Recommend: Daptomycin 550 mg (6 mg/kg) IV infusion q24h to complete 6 weeks of treatment.	Educating the patient and partner on proper at-home daptomycin administration, measures of infection improvement, and signs of adverse infusion site problems and adverse drug effects will be vital to optimizing treatment outcomes and minimizing adverse events, such as infections around the IV insertion site.
Educate patient and partner on proper administration.	
• A clinic nurse or home health nurse will train the patient and his partner on how to administer the infusion.	
Educate patient and partner on wound improvement and possible adverse events.	
• Anticipate less redness and inflammation at wound sites in coming weeks.	*Monitor:*
• Pain in toes may continue, but should improve in coming weeks.	Wound signs and symptoms may take at least a week to start to improve. Labs should remain stable during OPAT and improvement may be seen in the inflammatory markers as treatment proceeds. Daptomycin is generally well-tolerated, but the most common adverse effect is muscle pain and weakness.
• Redness/inflammation around IV insertion site is a possible adverse event and should be reported to the home health nurse and OPAT team.	
• Muscle pain/weakness is a possible adverse event with daptomycin and should be reported to the OPAT team.	
Monitor:	
• Patient and interdisciplinary team to monitor for improvement in wound signs and symptoms. Patient will monitor daily. Interdisciplinary team will evaluate at follow-up appointments.	
• OPAT ID pharmacist to monitor for stability in weekly labs (CBC, CPK, Serum Creatinine, AST/ALT) and improvement in the inflammatory markers (ESR and CRP).	
• Patient and OPAT team to monitor for any potential adverse effects, including muscle pain and weakness. Patient will monitor daily. OPAT team will monitor at follow-up appointment.	

IMPLEMENT/MONITOR: Diabetes and Peripheral Vascular Disease	
Conclusions	**Rationale: Information or Premise to Support the Conclusion**
Implement:	*Implement:*
Direct patient to schedule an appointment with PCP for further evaluation of diabetes and peripheral vascular disease.	While the antimicrobial regimen will likely improve the wound infection, it is important that the patient be evaluated and monitored for diabetes and peripheral vascular disease, the conditions that put the patient at risk of foot wounds.
Monitor:	*Monitor:*
During OPAT follow-up period, check to ensure patient is scheduled with PCP and review any PCP notes.	It is important to verify that the patient has at least one PCP appointment scheduled after hospital discharge to provide continuity of care and disease state management.

Critical Thinking Checks for This Patient's Implementation and Monitoring Plan

In **fairness** to the patient, the implementation plan has been developed and communicated with an empathetic understanding of his preferences for long-term IV antibiotic therapy. This will allow him to be empowered to self-manage his health and health behaviors.

The implementation plan was developed **fairly**, considering the fact that the patient can be overwhelmed with the required care that he will need to take on in order for his infection to be successfully treated.

In developing and providing **clear** education to the patient, I carefully considered potential ambiguities, jargon, poor grammar, or other potential causes of unclear understanding by the patient.

The steps for implementing the treatment plan were **clearly** outlined and provided both verbally and in writing with enough **clarity**, **accuracy**, and **details** to facilitate their implementation by the patient.

To facilitate successful implementation of strategies that may be complicated to the patient, I have outlined and conveyed the most **significant** actions for strategy implementation.

In thinking **broadly** about this patient's care, I have determined that wound care and the surgical team will play a significant role in this patient's wound healing and infection management.

CONCLUSION

Evaluation and management of infectious diseases spans the healthcare continuum. Pharmacists fulfill a vital role in the design and monitoring of therapeutic regimens for infections in both inpatient and outpatient settings through collaboration with other healthcare providers. In their efforts to provide optimal care for their patients, pharmacists utilize excellent critical thinking and clinical reasoning as they effectively employ the PPCP in clinical problem-solving. As discussed in the case provided in this chapter, it is important to involve patients in decision-making and ensure therapeutic plans are feasible prior to implementation to promote achievement of optimal outcomes. As utilization of OPAT becomes more frequent, ID-trained pharmacists are well-suited to serve an important role in optimizing outcomes for patients receiving this treatment modality.[5]

 KEY POINT

Pharmacists serve a vital role in the design and monitoring of therapeutic regimens for treatment of infectious diseases across healthcare settings through interprofessional collaboration.

Summary Points

- The provision of safe and effective care to patients with complex infectious diseases requires a multidisciplinary team approach to care that includes pharmacists in the design and monitoring of therapeutic regimens in both inpatient and outpatient settings, which may include Outpatient Parenteral Antimicrobial Therapy (OPAT). OPAT has the benefits of decreased hospital length of stay or avoidance of hospital admission, reduction in hospital-acquired infections, cost savings, and improved quality of life. The provision of optimal PPCP-guided care by ID pharmacists can be achieved through the use of strong critical thinking and clinical reasoning skills in each PPCP step.

- In the Collect step, to ensure a comprehensive collection of the most current and pertinent patient information during PPCP-guided care of the infectious disease patient, the pharmacist utilizes multiple sources of information, including the chart review, discussions with providers, and the patient interview.
- For the Assess step, in order to fully evaluate the patient's infection and to identify and explain drug therapy problems, it is necessary to collect and analyze all relevant subjective and objective information, including the clinical presentation, vital signs and laboratory data, imaging results (when warranted), and culture and susceptibility results.
- For the Plan step, in developing the therapeutic plan for the OPAT patient, specific goals and targets are clearly defined so that a logical and precise plan may be developed to achieve these goals. The feasibility and appropriateness of several alternative antibiotic regimens are evaluated, as alternative plans are often necessary if the first plan is not desirable or feasible. Additionally, an appropriate depth of thinking is required to factor in the patient's other conditions and medications in therapeutic planning, and for developing nonpharmacological measures that can be integrated with the pharmacological strategy and patient education to maximize the chances of achieving therapeutic goals.
- In the Implement and Monitoring steps, for OPAT to be successful, it is important for the pharmacist to engage and educate the patient and caregiver(s) with an empathetic, fair-minded attitude knowing the critical role they play in OPAT care. The pharmacist must communicate to the patient with a vocabulary and level of detail that will ensure a clear understanding of the implementation and monitoring steps required to ensure the success of the OPAT plan.

References

1. Fishman N, Patterson J, Saiman L, et al. Policy statement on antimicrobial stewardship by the Society for Healthcare Epidemiology of America (SHEA), the Infectious Diseases Society of America (IDSA), and the Pediatric Infectious Diseases Society (PIDS). *Infect Control Hosp Epidemiol*. 2012;33(4):322-327.

2. Barlam TF, Cosgrove SA, Abbo LM, et al. Implementing an antibiotic stewardship program: guidelines by the Infectious Diseases Society of America and the Society for Healthcare Epidemiology of America. *Clin Infect Dis*. 2016;62(10):e51-e77.

3. CDC. *Antibiotic Resistance Threats in the United States, 2019*. Atlanta, GA: U.S. Department of Health and Human Services, CDC; 2019. doi:10.15620/cdc:82532.

4. Norris AH, Shrestha NK, Allison GM, et al. 2018 Infectious Diseases Society of America clinical practice guideline for the management of outpatient parenteral antimicrobial therapy. *Clin Infect Dis*. 2019;68(1):e1-e35.

5. Rivera CG, Mehta M, Ryan KL, et al. Role of infectious diseases pharmacists in outpatient intravenous and complex oral antimicrobial therapy: Society of Infectious Diseases Pharmacists insights. *J Am Coll Clin Pharm*. 2021;4:1161-1169.

6. Lipsky BA, Berendt AR, Cornia PB, et al. 2012 Infectious Diseases Society of America clinical practice guideline for the diagnosis and treatment of diabetic foot infections. *Clin Infect Dis*. 2021;54(12):132-173.

7. Chávez-Reyes J, Escárcega-González CE, Chavira-Suárez E, et al. Susceptibility for some infectious diseases in patients with diabetes: the key role of glycemia. *Front Public Health*. 2021;9:559595.

8. Allahabadi S, Haroun KB, Musher DM, et al. Consensus on surgical aspects of managing osteomyelitis in the diabetic foot. *Diabet Foot Ankle*. 2016;7:30079.

9. Hamad Y, Dodda S, Frank A, et al. Perspectives of patients on outpatient parenteral antimicrobial therapy: experiences and adherence. *Open Forum Infectious Diseases*. 2020;7(6):ofaa205.

10. American Diabetes Association Professional Practice Committee. 6. Glycemic targets: standards of medical care in diabetes-2022. *Diabet Care*. 2022;45(Suppl. 1):S83–S96.

11. Zyvox (linezolid) [package insert]. New York, NY: Pfizer Inc.; 2021.

12. Cosimi RA, Beik N, Kubiak DW, et al. Ceftaroline for severe methicillin-resistant staphylococcus aureus infections: a systematic review. *Open Forum Infect Dis*. 2017;4(2):ofx084.

13. Orbactiv (oritavancin) [package insert]. Lincolnshire, IL: Melinta Therapeutics, LLC.;2021.

14. Dalvance (dalbavancin) [package insert]. Madison, NJ: Allergan USA, Inc.; 2021.

15. Cubicin (daptomycin) [package insert]. Whitehouse Station, NJ; Merck & Co. Inc.; 2022.

16. Kido K, Oyen AA, Beckman MA, et al. Musculoskeletal toxicities in patients receiving concomitant statin and daptomycin therapy. *Am J Health Syst Pharm*. 2019;76;206-210.

17. Dare RK, Tewell C, Harris B, et al. Effect of statin coadministration on the risk of daptomycin-associated myopathy. *Clin Infect Dis*. 2018;67(9):1356-63.

18. American Diabetes Association Professional Practice Committee. 11. Microvascular complications and foot care: standards of medical care in diabetes-2021. *Diabetes Care*. 2021;44(Suppl. 1):S151-S167.

Appendix

A. Worksheet for Determining Standards-Based Questions That Can Be Applied to Assure That Intellectual Standards of Thinking Are Met as the Pharmacist Provides Care

This worksheet can be used to create important critical-thinking standards-based questions that can be asked to help assure that intellectual standards of thinking are met as pharmacists provide patient care in their specific practice.

Note:

- Please refer to the following tables in Chapter 1 as needed to stimulate ideas for completing the worksheet:
  - Table 1-4: Critical Thinking Intellectual Standards
  - Table 1-6: Examples of Questions Pharmacists Can Ask Themselves to Help Them Meet Intellectual Standards in Each Step of the PPCP
- In addition, each clinical chapter has examples of standards-based questions specific to the clinical focus of the chapter. These questions are usually in Table 1 in these chapters.

Sample standards-based questions that can be applied to assure that intellectual standards for thinking are met as the pharmacist provides care for patients with:	
Clarity (explicit, unambiguous, intelligible, free from confusion or doubt)	
Relevance (pertinent, applicable, germane)	
Significance (important, nontrivial, necessary, critical, required, impactful)	
Objectivity (fact-based, unbiased)	
Fairness (unbiased, equitable, impartial)	
Accuracy (verifiable, valid, true, credible, undistorted)	
Precision (exact, specific, detailed)	

Depth (roots, fundamentals, complexities, interrelationships, cause/effect, implications)	
Breadth (comprehensive, encompassing, alternative perspectives)	
Logic (reasonable, rational, without contradiction, well-founded, sound)	

B. Worksheet for Integrating Clinical Reasoning and Critical Thinking in Patient Cases Using the PPCP

Using the same format used by the authors of clinical chapters, this worksheet can be used to integrate clinical reasoning and critical thinking through the application of your reasoning and the critical thinking standards as you work through cases using the PPCP. Please note that you can be selective as to which standards you believe are most important for you to apply in each PPCP step.

Please refer to the following tables in Chapter 1 as needed to stimulate ideas for completing the worksheet:

- Table 1-2: Common Inferences and Conclusions for Each Step of the PPCP
- Table 1-4: Critical Thinking Intellectual Standards
- Table 1-6: Examples of Questions Pharmacists Can Ask Themselves to Help Them Meet Intellectual Standards in Each Step of the PPCP

Please see the table below for a review of the standards and some examples of their application.

Critical Thinking Standards: Clear ROAD to Logic	
Standard	**Examples of the Application of the Standard**
Clarity (explicit, unambiguous, intelligible, free from confusion or doubt)	• Unclear words used by the patient or you • Something you don't clearly understand that you might need to research
Relevance (pertinent, applicable, germane) *Significance* (important, nontrivial, necessary, critical, required, impactful)	• The relevant data to collect or questions to ask • The critical information to gather • The significance of particular data • The relevant strategies to consider
Objectivity (fact-based, unbiased) *Fairness* (unbiased, equitable, impartial)	• Threats to objectivity such as your emotions, stress, or something visceral about the patient • Fairly considering other perspectives or impacts on others
Accuracy (verifiable, valid, true, credible, undistorted) *Precision* (exact, specific, detailed)	• Accuracy of information obtained from the patient • Details of symptoms • Medication reconciliation accuracy • Appropriate detail in patient education or professional communication

Depth (roots, fundamentals, complexities, interrelationships, cause/effect, implications) **Breadth** (comprehensive, encompassing, alternative perspectives)	• Drug-condition or condition–condition relationships • Potential consequences or implications of a recommendation • Considering a broad array of data to form a strong conclusion • Considering multiple perspectives and psychosocial factors • Considering multiple strategies to meet goals
Logic (reasonable, rational, without contradiction, well-founded, sound)	• Why this explanation of the data is better than competing explanations of the data • How the argument for a particular recommendation follows logically from the assessment, the patient's goals, and evidence

Information to Collect for this Patient's...

Conclusions	Rationale: Information or Premise to Support the Conclusion	Application of Critical Thinking Standards (Clear ROAD to Logic)

Assessment of This Patient's...

Conclusions	Rationale: Information or Premise to Support the Conclusion	Application of Critical Thinking Standards (Clear ROAD to Logic)

Plan: SMART Goals for This Patient's...

Conclusions	Rationale: Information or Premise to Support the Conclusion	Application of Critical Thinking Standards (Clear ROAD to Logic)

Plan: Nonpharmacological Plan for This Patient's...		
Conclusions	**Rationale:** Information or Premise to Support the Conclusion	**Application of Critical Thinking Standards** (Clear ROAD to Logic)

Plan: Pharmacological Plan for This Patient's...		
Conclusions	**Rationale:** Information or Premise to Support the Conclusion	**Application of Critical Thinking Standards** (Clear ROAD to Logic)

Implementation and Monitoring Plan for This Patient's...		
Conclusions	**Rationale:** Information or Premise to Support the Conclusion	**Application of Critical Thinking Standards** (Clear ROAD to Logic)

C. Worksheet for Identifying Potential Biases and Approaches to Avoid or Mitigate Them

This worksheet can be used to identify potential biases that might affect your reasoning and for determining debiasing strategies that can help you prevent these biases from adversely impacting your reasoning.

Bias	Examples of How Bias Can Manifest in My Practice or with This Patient	Examples of How I Can Prevent These Biases from Adversely Impacting My Reasoning
Anchoring		
Relying too heavily on the first piece of information offered. *For example, creating an initial impression based on salient features in the patient's initial presentation, and failure to adjust this initial impression when warranted by later information.*		
Availability		
Being biased towards more recent information or information that most readily comes to mind when making judgments. *For example, failing to persevere and look at other information can prevent the clinician from considering alternative plausible therapeutic strategies.*		
Bandwagon Effect		
Believing and doing certain things because many others are doing so. *Groupthink* is an example that can have a detrimental impact on team decision-making and patient care.		
Blind Spot Bias		
Believing yourself to be less susceptible to bias than others. *For example, this can cause clinicians to fail to adequately recognize and consider their own biases when working with patients, or fail to effectively implement de-biasing strategies.*		

Confirmation Bias		
The tendency to favor or look for information that confirms what we think, without being adequately alert to or open to refuting information, even if it is more persuasive. *For example, this can cause the pharmacist to favor looking for information to confirm a hypothesis that a medication is the cause of a particular sign or symptom, at the expense of adequately considering other plausible explanations.*		
Diagnosis Momentum		
Failure to consider other plausible diagnostic conclusions when interacting with patients, due to an earlier conclusion that was accepted by others without sufficient independent scrutiny, and therefore gathered increasing momentum as the accurate diagnostic conclusion in subsequent interactions with the patient. *For example, this can affect future patient workups and how handoffs are "framed" if practitioners do not properly evaluate patient information independently.*		
Framing Effect		
The tendency to allow our thinking and judgment about issues or information to be influenced by how it is presented to us (e.g., how it is framed by the patient, other clinicians, or other stakeholders). As with other biases, this can cause the clinician to think without sufficient depth, breadth, or objectivity.		

Fundamental Attribution Error		
The tendency to be inappropriately judgmental and explain illnesses or behavior on internal factors of a patient, such as personality or disposition, without adequately considering external factors or circumstances. *For example, there may be socioeconomic factors or certain stressors impacting a patient's health that may be significant and therefore should be considered.*		
Information Bias		
The tendency to believe that the more evidence one can accumulate to support a conclusion, the better. While gathering *sufficient* information to make a decision is important, it is also important to know the relevance and significance of information for making the decision, and not assume that the more information the better, regardless of its significance.		
Overconfidence Bias		
The tendency to have more confidence in our knowledge or abilities than is objectively reasonable. Overconfidence reflects a tendency to act on incomplete information, intuitions, or hunches. *For example, not being self-aware of the limits of our knowledge or skills in particular situations may cause failure to adequately recognize and consider important features, complexities, or consequences in diagnostic or therapeutic decision-making.*		

Premature Closure		
The tendency to stop an inquiry or reasoning process once a decision or conclusion has been made, before it has been adequately validated.		
Search Satisficing		
The tendency to search through the available alternatives until an acceptability threshold is met and then call off the search once something plausible is found. Although this can be valuable in formulating initial hypotheses, it can be detrimental if it stops the consideration of other plausible hypotheses.		
Visceral Bias		
The influence of the clinician's affective response (e.g., emotions or state of mind) about a patient on decision-making. This can cause a visceral arousal that may be positive or negative and can undermine objectivity and lead to poor decisions. *For example, feeling friendly, humored, unsafe, untrusting, irritated, or sad about a patient can have a negative impact on a clinician's objectivity during patient interactions.*		
Implicit Bias		
Attitudes and stereotypes that unconsciously affect one's understanding, actions, and decisions.		(The following strategies are from Chapter 1, but there can be other strategies as well: perspective-taking, emotional regulation, partnership creation, cultural understanding, bias understanding, individuating, and performing teach-back).

Index

Page numbers followed by *f* and *t* denote figures and tables, respectively.